BIOMEDICAL COMPUTING

The Johns Hopkins University
Studies in Historical and Political Science

130th Series (2012)

BIOMEDICAL COMPUTING

Digitizing Life in the United States

Joseph November

The Johns Hopkins University Press

Baltimore

The Johns Hopkins University Press
2715 North Charles Street
Baltimore, Maryland 21218-4363
www.press.jhu.edu

Library of Congress Cataloging-in-Publication Data

November, Joseph Adam, 1975–
Biomedical computing : digitizing life in the United States / Joseph November.
p. ; cm. — (Johns Hopkins University studies in historical and political science ;
130th ser., 2)
Includes bibliographical references and index.
ISBN-13: 978-1-4214-0468-4 (hdbk. : alk. paper)
ISBN-10: 1-4214-0468-0 (hdbk. : alk. paper)
I. Title. II. Series: Johns Hopkins University studies in historical and political science ;
130th ser., 2.
[DNLM: 1. National Institutes of Health (U.S.) 2. Biomedical Research—history—United
States. 3. Medical Informatics Computing—history—United States. 4. History, 20th
Century—United States. 5. United States Government Agencies—history—United States.
W 20.5]
610.72′40285—dc23   2011029753

A catalog record for this book is available from the British Library.

*Special discounts are available for bulk purchases of this book. For more information,
please contact Special Sales at 410-516-6936 or specialsales@press.jhu.edu.*

The Johns Hopkins University Press uses environmentally friendly book materials, including
recycled text paper that is composed of at least 30 percent post-consumer waste,
whenever possible.

For Sultana

CONTENTS

ACKNOWLEDGMENTS

I have become indebted to many people in the course of researching and writing this book. What follows is by no means a comprehensive account of that debt. Foremost, I wish to extend my gratitude to my wife, Sultana Banulescu. Her unwavering faith in my ability to write a good book was the main force propelling my work. Sultana's expertise in biology, medicine, and creative writing helped me make this book much more accurate and internationally accessible. My parents, Robert and Hannah November, and my sister and brother-in-law, Elizabeth November and Tavian Cardwell, provided a steady stream of encouragement, support, and good humor.

This book evolved from my dissertation for the History of Science Program at Princeton University. Many of the questions I ask here and the approaches I take to answering them were shaped by my teachers and fellow graduate students at Princeton. Most influential were the dissertation's four readers: Michael Mahoney, Angela Creager, Michael Gordin, and Soraya de Chadarevian. Many of the book's better qualities have roots in their recommendations. Although my dissertation began as an exploration of how biomedicine was changed by computing, Mike Mahoney's guidance (grounded in his unique knowledge of both the history of science and the history of computers) made it possible for me to also explore how computing was transformed by biomedicine. In short, he gave me the tools to tell a much more interesting and much more important story than what I had originally envisioned. Sadly, Mike did not live to see my dissertation take form as a book. His sudden death in 2008, besides being a great personal loss to me, deprived the history of science and the history of technology of an irreplaceably insightful and rational voice.

The graduate students who trained alongside me at Princeton will, I hope, be pleased to see how their feedback on class papers, conference talks, and my presentations to the weekly Program Seminar all helped to improve what finally became a book manuscript. My cohort-mates, Tania Munz, Carla Nappi, and Matt Wisnioski, saw my project from the very beginning and deserve special recognition for their input over the years. Others at Princeton who shared their time and knowledge in relation to what appears in this book included Eric Ash, Sultana Banulescu, Daniel Bouk, Emily Brock, Jamie Cohen-Cole, Manfred Laubichler, Ole Molvig, Aaron Moore, Jane Murphy, Nicholas Popper, Gail Schmitt, Suman Seth, Alistair Sponsel, Laura Stark, and Doogab Yi.

Without good sources, I would not have had much of a story to tell, and my access to those sources was made possible by the hard work and generosity of many people. These include Janice Goldblum (National Academy of Sciences Archive), Henry Lowood and Margaret Kimball (Stanford University Archives), Michelle Lyons (National Institutes of Health), and Dag Spicer (Computer History Museum). Access to personal or private institutional collections was graciously provided by Wesley Clark and Maxine Rockoff, Nelson Kiang, Robert Ledley, Fred Ledley, Elenora Serotek (National Biomedical Research Foundation), and Donna Molnar. Access to artifacts was provided by Deborah Douglas (LINC, LINC-8, ARC), Robert Ledley (FIDAC and several other early computers), Scott Robinson (LINC), and Gio Wiederhold (ACME).

Two of the book's main subjects, Wesley Clark and Robert Ledley, have my gratitude for patiently sharing their unique knowledge with me as well as for reviewing parts of the manuscript. Other subjects whose conversations with me form an integral part of this work are Jerome Cox, Edward Feigenbaum, Nelson Kiang, Joshua Lederberg, Terry Ledley, Severo Ornstein, and Gio Wiederhold. I also gained much valuable information from discussions with Edwin Becker, Robert Berger, Judy Dayhoff, Ruth Dayhoff and Vincent Brannigan, Fred Ledley, James Lynch, Maxine Rockoff, and William Talbot.

From professional historians I have received a tremendous amount of useful feedback. The reviewer of the manuscript, Nathan Ensmenger, proved both erudite and capable of cutting to the heart of some tricky conceptual and historiographic issues. My efforts to follow his recommendations have, I hope, brought the book closer to the potential he saw in the early versions of the manuscript. Careful reading of portions of the manuscript by Richard Burian, Veronika Hofer, Ann Johnson, Johannes Lenhard, and Bruno Strasser yielded suggestions that greatly helped me to craft a more cohesive and more useful narrative. Jeffrey Yost, by pointing me to his *Bibliographic Guide to Resources in Scientific Computing*, made me aware of the existence of several of the sources I cite heavily here. Though not a historian by training or profession, biomedical computing expert R. P. Channing Rodgers offered dozens of corrections to the manuscript—his fixes and encouragement made a big difference.

While writing this book I received a wide range of support from my colleagues at the University of South Carolina (USC). At USC, my fellow historians of science and technology, Emily Brock, Ann Johnson, Allison Marsh, and Thomas Lekan provided excellent feedback and advice. My discussions with Christine Ames and Kathryn Edwards about the process of writing a book helped me to work much more efficiently. I thank department chairs Patrick Maney, Lacy Ford, and Lawrence Glickman for providing me the resources I needed to get this book done. USC-based philosophers Davis Baird, Kevin Elliott, George Khushf, and Michael Stoeltzner all provided insights and material that helped me to better see the epistemological and ethical implications of the story I am telling.

My year at the NIH as a Stetten fellow, made possible by the research-friendly policies of USC Deans Mary Anne Fitzpatrick and Timothy Mousseau, provided me with the raw material and knowledge I needed to attempt to elucidate the agency's role in introducing computers to biology and medicine. My sponsor at the NIH, the Center for Information Technology, gave me both a pleasant work environment and access to many of the people who first worked with computers in biomedical research. Robert Martensen, director of the Office of NIH History, helped me to frame my ideas in such a way that they would make sense in a book. Two former directors of the ONH, Alan Schechter and Victoria Harden, also provided me with valuable information and personal contacts. For their insights and for showing me the ropes at the NIH, I am grateful to David Cantor, Caroline Hannaway, Deborah Kraut, Michele Lyons, and Buhm Soon Park.

The production of a scholarly book was a new process to me. I therefore owe much to my editor at the Johns Hopkins University Press, Robert J. Brugger, for his patience and careful guidance. His suggestions went a long way toward making this book more coherent and easier to read. David Coen, through his careful copyediting, has saved readers from having to endure many of my typographical, grammatical, structural, and factual errors. Any shortcomings found in the following pages are purely my own.

ABBREVIATIONS, ACRONYMS, AND INITIALISMS

650	IBM 650 Magnetic Drum Data Processing Machine
1410	IBM 1410 Data Processing System
7090	IBM 7090 Data Processing System (variants include the 7094)
ACCR	Advisory Committee on Computers in Research (NIH)
ACM	Association for Computing Machinery
ACME	Advanced Computer for Medical Research (Stanford University)
ACTA	Automatic Computerized Transverse Axial (NBRF)
A-D	analog-to-digital (often spelled A/D)
ADAD	Automatic Device for Antibiotic Determination
AIL	Airborne Instruments Laboratory
AMA	American Medical Association
ARC	Average Response Computer (MIT)
ARDC	Air Research and Development Command (US Air Force)
ARPA	Advanced Research Projects Agency (known as DARPA 1972–93)
ASWORG	Anti-Submarine Warfare Operations Research Group (USA)
BBN	Bolt Beranek and Newman
BCL	Biomedical Computer Laboratory (Washington University)
BRI	Brain Research Institute
CBL	Communications Biophysics Group (MIT; widely called the Communications Biophysics Lab)

CDC	Control Data Corporation
CPC	Computer Policy Committee (Stanford University)
CRSS	Computer Research Study Section (NIH; successor to ACCR)
CRT	cathode ray tube
CSL	Computer Systems Laboratory (Washington University)
DARPA	Defense Advanced Research Projects Agency (also known as ARPA 1960–72, 1993–present)
DCRT	Division of Computer Research and Technology (NIH)
DEC	Digital Equipment Corporation
DENDRAL	Dendritic Algorithm (Stanford University)
DRFR	Division of Research Facilities and Resources (NIH; now National Center for Research Resources)
DRG	Division of Research Grants (NIH; now Center for Scientific Review)
EDSAC	Electronic Delay Storage Automatic Calculator (Cambridge University)
EDVAC	Electronic Discrete Variable Automatic Computer
ENIAC	Electronic Numerical Integrator And Computer (University of Pennsylvania)
EPAM	Elementary Perceiver and Memorizer
FIDAC	Film Input to Digital Automatic Computer (NBRF)
FORTRAN	The IBM Mathematical Formula Translating System (often spelled Fortran)
HSCF	Health Sciences Computing Facility
IBM	International Business Machines
IEEE	Institute of Electrical and Electronic Engineers
IRE	Institute of Radio Engineers (now part of IEEE)
IRL	Instrumentation Research Lab (Stanford University)
KP	Kaiser Permanente
LAP	Linc Assembly Program (MIT)

LCS   Laboratory of Computer Science (MGH)

LINC   Laboratory Instrument Computer (MIT/Lincoln Laboratory;
               previously known as Linc)

MGH   Massachusetts General Hospital

MIT   Massachusetts Institute of Technology

MRB   Mathematical Research Branch (NIH)

MTC   Memory Test Computer (MIT/Lincoln Laboratory)

MULTICS   Multiplexed Information and Computing Service

MUMPS   Massachusetts General Hospital Utility Multi-Programming System
               (now known as M)

NASA   National Aeronautics and Space Administration

NAS   National Academy of Sciences

NBRF   National Biomedical Research Foundation

NBS   National Bureau of Standards (now known as National Institute of
               Standards and Technology)

NCBI   National Center for Biotechnology Information (NIH)

NIH   National Institutes of Health

NRC   National Research Council (NAS; often abbreviated as NAS-NRC)

NSF   National Science Foundation

OD   Office of the Director

OR   Operations Research

ORS   Operational Research Section (UK)

ORSA   Operations Research Society of America

PARC   Xerox Palo Alto Research Center (also known as Xerox PARC)

PDP   Programmed Data Processor (e.g., PDP 1, PDP 11; built by DEC)

PHS   US Public Health Service

RAND   Research and Development Corporation (aka RAND Corporation)

SCC   Stanford Computation Center

SEAC	Standards East Coast Automatic Computer (NBS)
SMC	Stanford Medical Center
SUMEX-AIM	Stanford University Medical Experimental Computer–Artificial Intelligence in Medicine
SWAC	Standards Western Automatic Computer (NBS)
TX	Transistorized Experimental Computer (e.g., TX-0, TX-2; built at MIT's Lincoln Lab)
UCLA	University of California, Los Angeles
WESTEX	West coast group of the Panel on Extraterrestrial Life

Introduction

One does not need to be a scientist, a physician, or a computer expert to have felt the effects of the introduction of computers to biology and medicine. For most recipients of healthcare services in a Western society chances are good that much of the research as well as the diagnostic and treatment protocols used by their care providers involved the use of computers. Yet, the machines that are now nearly ubiquitous in biomedicine were barely being imagined, let alone built, seventy years ago. This transformation has cut the other way too—for through its presence at the laboratory's bench and the clinic's bed the computer itself has also changed, with consequences reaching far beyond biomedicine. The many millions of people who daily use electronic digital computers at work and at home have often come to depend on machines and software—and ways of using them—that have roots in early efforts to computerize biology and medicine.

Among those involved in—or those who closely watch—biomedical research or computing, the convergence of information technology and the study of life has been the source of tremendous excitement. Over the last two decades, that excitement has proven infectious, as became acutely evident during the heady dot-com bubble years between 1995 and 2000. One of the major forces propelling the tech-laden NASDAQ stock index to dizzying heights unseen before or since was the notion that computer technology was profoundly changing the way people looked at and worked with life. The buzz surrounding one computer-dependent biomedical research endeavor, the Human Genome Project, was particularly intense. It reached a crescendo on June 26, 2000, when US president Bill Clinton and UK prime minister Tony Blair jointly announced that the "working draft" of the human genome was complete. In Washington, DC, Clinton, flanked by Francis Collins, the head of the International Human Genome Project, and J. Craig Venter, president of the Celera Genomics Group, hailed the genome as "the most important, most wondrous map ever produced by humankind." To rapturous applause, President Clinton predicted that knowledge of the genome "will revolutionize the diagnosis, prevention and treatment of most, if not all, human diseases." Blair, speaking from London via satellite, called the project "the first great technological triumph of the 21st century," classifying it as the kind of "breakthrough that takes humankind across a frontier and into a new era."[1]

For many observers circa 2000, the success of the Human Genome Project (HGP) indicated that they were living in exceptional times. In the new millennium, with its promise of new technologies and new knowledge, they felt society would leave behind the traditional economic constraints on creative human activities. The HGP was a case in point. When the project to sequence the 3 billion base pairs of DNA in a human cell was formally launched in 1990 by the Department of Energy and the National Institutes of Health (NIH), its sponsors predicted it would be complete by 2005 and cost more than $3 billion.[2] Typically, both budgets and timeframes are lowballed at the outset and tend to expand dramatically as large projects progress. However, thanks mostly to leaps in microprocessor technology, the HGP harnessed ever-faster and ever-cheaper computers to finish years ahead of schedule and within its budget.[3] From a computational standpoint, the project was immense. Celera's contribution alone, for instance, required 500 million trillion (5×10^{20}) sequence comparisons. What would have taken about a decade to process on the fastest machine available in 1990 could be completed in 2000 using Celera's supercomputer in a mere matter of months.[4] Hence, when the HGP "working draft" was announced in 2000 rather than 2005, the enthusiasm surrounding the genome's potential in biomedical research was compounded by an exhilarating sense that with enough computing power one could overcome many of the traditional bounds of human endeavors.[5]

A decade and a major downturn later, we are far less sanguine about the prospects of using technology to escape old economic and institutional forces, but enthusiasm surrounding the union of computing and the study of life has, if anything, only grown more intense. Not only has the use of electronic digital computers emerged as the sine qua non in many areas of biological and medical research, but their presence has also shaped the way life itself is regarded. In 2003, renowned evolutionary biologist Richard Dawkins articulated this new relationship when he proclaimed, "Genetics has become a branch of information technology. The genetic code is truly digital, in exactly the same sense as computer codes. This is not some vague analogy, it is the literal truth. Moreover, unlike computer codes, the genetic code is universal."[6] Indeed, the bond between computing and the study of life had become so intimate that nobody publicly challenged Leroy Hood, prominent California Institute of Technology (Caltech) lab chief and founder of the Institute for Systems Biology and developer of the automatic nucleotide sequencer, when he declared that "the reason for the convergence between biotechnology and information technology is that at its heart, biology is the only science that is digital in nature. DNA is the digital source code of life. Other sciences—physics, chemistry, geology, and so on—are basically derived from analog measurements." As Hood saw it, "The deepest question in biology is how the digital source code is converted into a four-dimensional living creature."[7]

Computer developers, meanwhile, were returning that embrace with equal warmth. In 2004, Microsoft's Bill Gates informed an audience of college students that he had come to regard biology as a "sister science" to computer science. By way of career advice, Gates encouraged the students to double-major in biology and computer science, telling them, "I think a lot of the breakthroughs will be made by people who were trained in biology and computer science."[8] On the more speculative side, the Singularity University, funded in large part by the founders of Google, envisions a near future in which biotechnology, nanotechnology, and information technology will converge. During this convergence, according to Raymond Kurzweil, who made his fortune pioneering optical character recognition (OCR) and who now is the éminence grise behind the Singularity University, humans and machines will merge to form hyper-intelligent and immortal "transcendent" beings, thereby radically and irrevocably altering human existence.[9]

In more immediate, pragmatic terms, computerized biomedicine has already, through its expected contribution to the American economy, shaped the political and social landscapes along with the scientific and technological ones. In the depths of the 2008–9 recession, when so many budgets were slashed in the name of austerity, biomedical research projects—and disproportionately those that made heavy use of computers—enjoyed increased funding. Under the 2009 American Recovery and Reinvestment Act (a.k.a. "the Stimulus"), over $10 billion was added to the NIH's annual $30 billion budget and directed toward research. The rationale was that NIH-funded projects "have exceptional potential to create new jobs and improve the economy while leading the way toward important medical discoveries that can benefit the health of Americans nationwide."[10] In awarding the stimulus grants, the agency placed special emphasis on supporting researchers who wanted to acquire new technology: a quick look at the NIH's RePORT database shows that hundreds of grants went toward computer-dependent projects.[11]

The NIH continues to pursue computing even as doubts have surfaced about the usefulness of the previous decade's great triumph of computerized biomedicine, the HGP. The agency's general response to the HGP's inability (so far) to produce the expected medical breakthroughs has not been to seek alternatives to computation-oriented research but rather to invest in approaches that can apply still more computational force to biomedical problems. Ten years after the completion of the human genome's "rough draft," it has become apparent that a general map of human genes does not suffice to show the genetic roots of diseases such as Alzheimer's or cancer. The consensus now holds that to make significant progress in combating such dread diseases, each individual patient's genome must be sequenced, and the complex interactions between proteins and DNA must be much better understood. Computationally, these two problems pose an enormous challenge. Sequencing an individual's genome requires as many calculations as did the initial HGP, while modeling proteins—dynamic molecules often composed of thousands of atoms—in a reasonable amount of time would require computer systems that are orders of magnitude more powerful than those available today. In the face of this challenge, the NIH has effectively doubled down on its investment in computing, as is illustrated by the agency's present emphasis on developing "high-throughput technologies," which typically rely on cutting-edge computer systems to quickly process enormous volumes of nucleotide and protein-related data collected from organisms. Francis Collins, who has risen from head of the HGP to become director of the

NIH, has made promoting such technologies a key part of the research agenda he is setting for the agency.[12] While post-genomic fields like proteomics are pursued on the molecular level, neuroscientists are using NIH funds to put similarly powerful computers to use to build the *connectome*, a map of the 100 billion connections in the human brain.

Meanwhile, years after the "genomics bubble" had burst, the major pharmaceutical companies, which had invested billions in genomics research, now report to their more wary shareholders that the genome was but the first step toward using quantitative means to achieve rational drug design. That is, they intend to craft drugs to specifically target particular molecular processes as opposed to today's norm of using relatively crude trial-and-error methods to determine the effect of a new substance on potential patients. Given the sheer volume of data involved in the process of determining which genes interact with which proteins and which drugs, the companies have identified "information overload" as one of their core future challenges, and have enlisted computer experts in their efforts to manage that information.[13] The total investment in research computing resources by established companies like Johnson & Johnson and Merck measures in the billions.[14] At the same time, many biotech firms— the largest of these, such as Amgen and Genzyme, could also be viewed as major pharmaceutical companies—continue to have as their core businesses projects that depend almost entirely on computing.

On the clinical side, computers are now commonplace in healthcare settings and there is rising pressure from the American public to make still greater use of information technology. Amid national efforts to reform healthcare, computers have been championed as tools that would give Americans access to inexpensive yet high-quality care. For instance, the increased use of computers in clinics is a key part of the Obama administration's plan to cover most of the costs of healthcare reform by reducing waste in Medicare and Medicaid. Indeed, Obama held up Utah's Intermountain Healthcare system, which aggressively employs computers in many aspects of diagnosis and treatment, as an example for other hospital systems to follow, praising its ability to "offer high-quality care at costs below average."[15] Concurring was John Wennberg, founder of the Center for Evaluative Clinical Services at Dartmouth Medical School, who described Intermountain as "the best model in the country of how you can actually change health care."[16] The ambitious goal of Intermountain's next-generation Enterprise Clinical Information System (ECIS), expected to be complete in 2015, is to provide hospital staff the capability to diagnose and treat patients based on protocols automatically developed from information—gathered via the Internet—produced by scientific publications and by compatible databases in other hospital systems.

In contrast to biologists, among physicians there remains significant resistance to the heavy use of computers in diagnosis and treatment. Fears abound among physicians that reliance on computers would lead to an overstandardized "cookbook medicine" or "McDonald's medicine" that would, in turn, threaten doctors' professional authority and autonomy as well as dangerously minimize the circumstances and needs of individual patients.[17] Already, critics have loudly decried the increasing amount of time physicians spend using computers as time taken away from their visits with their patients.[18] Nevertheless, in an environment where patients are themselves regular computer users and where physicians are publically castigated as "luddites" for their sluggishness in adopting information technology, it is likely that heavily computerized systems like Intermountain will soon become the norm.[19]

The Unexpected Computerization of the Study of Life

From today's perspective, it seems that biomedicine and computing will be crucially important to each others' futures. Yet, just fifty years ago the study of life was by far the least computerized area of science. The opportunities that came for the physical sciences during World War II to collaborate in large numbers and use new technologies—including information technology—seemed to have passed biology and medicine by. When Vannevar Bush, who had been broadly in charge of US research and development efforts during the war and who would become a major patron of computing, surveyed the war's consequences for American science, he asked, "What are the scientists to do next?" Bush found that "for the biologists, and particularly for the medical scientists, there can be little indecision, for their war has hardly required them to leave the old paths. Many indeed have been able to carry on their war research in their familiar peacetime laboratories. Their objectives remain much the same."[20]

From the 1940s to the early 1960s, most biologists and physicians regarded their subject matter as inherently incompatible with the newfangled electronic digital computers so many others were rushing to adopt. Living systems, they argued, were too complex and too dynamic to be reduced to the level where they could be meaningfully studied using machines that, while speedy, were strictly limited to simple, purely logical operations. Furthermore, small laboratories and care-oriented hospitals could hardly afford or even accommodate computers, which typically cost hundreds of thousands or millions of dollars and whose operation required specially prepared rooms and trained staff.

In 1959, in the wake of Sputnik and in the face of rising public demand for better healthcare, the US Congress became so alarmed by the hesitancy among biologists and physicians to adopt computers that it provided the NIH with over $50 million in emergency funding for the express purpose of introducing computers to biomedical research.

Between the late 1950s and the present, electronic digital computers became a critical component of almost all research in biology and medicine. However, for all the billions of dollars and thousands of careers invested in the computerization of the study of life and its diseases, the origins of and motives for this process are only vaguely understood. Therefore, the broad aim of this book is to explore the crucial early years of the introduction of computers to biology and medicine some if of the phenomenon's far-reaching consequences, both in biomedicine and in computing. To that end, it examines the conditions that made possible the computerization of biology and medicine, and it clarifies how these fields' objects of study—from the structure and function of molecules to cognitive and physiological processes—evolved from exemplars of systems that computers could not describe into exemplars of systems that computers could indeed describe. Where information technology and the life sciences intersected, computer scientists also came away deeply changed, leading to important developments in computer architecture and software design.

Through its exploration of early biomedical computing, this book shows that there was nothing inevitable about the way in which biology and medicine became computerized, or the enormous degree to which the process continues. A familiarity with the early struggles to promote and make productive use of computers in biomedicine will help readers move beyond the triumphal narratives of the rising importance of computers to research and healthcare that pervade so many discussions of the matter. Most educated readers already know a few variants of the popular account of computerizing the life sciences. It is essentially a tale of technological contingency, one that diminishes the importance of the hard-fought campaigns, intellectual priorities, and unique institutional circumstances that together created enormous demand for computers in biology and medicine. The conventional narrative holds that in the 1950s it was inconceivable that computers could process the enormous amounts of information found in living systems. Over the decades, it goes, computers improved so dramatically that it became feasible to model life's processes, and therefore researchers began to use the machines in large numbers. Moore's law is frequently invoked.

Ever-speedier and ever-cheaper computers have indeed opened many important paths of inquiry, but such explanations obscure the fact that in the life sciences—including the supposed bellwether, molecular biology—the groundwork for computerization was laid decades before computers became small, fast, and inexpensive. Today's life scientists are only able to take advantage of computers because they have access to tools and methods developed during a costly, ambitious, and largely forgotten attempt to computerize biology and medicine undertaken by the NIH in the late 1950s and early 1960s. The NIH campaign, inspired by the polymath and digital electronic computing pioneer Robert S. Ledley (a dentist–turned–operations researcher–turned–computer specialist) and led by his cohort Lee B. Lusted (a radiologist with a background in radar engineering), sought to restructure biology and medicine by computerizing them. Decades later, its effects are still being felt.

This book also shows that from the time of their introduction to the life sciences, computers served not only as tools but also as overt agents of intellectual, institutional, and social change. In trying to harness what Nobelist Joshua Lederberg (1925–2008) wryly called the "phylum Automata," many biomedical researchers structured their experiments to include quantitative methods and to exclude the nondigital or nonquantitative types of data computers could not process.[21] To gain access to large, centralized computers, they also integrated— or were pushed to integrate—their centers of research into the infrastructures of both government and corporate power. Once computers came into a scientist's or physician's life the changes their presence wrought proved both profound and irreversible. In the following pages, case studies in molecular biology, physiology, psychology, and medicine will show that computer technology both opened new realms for exploration and created an environment in which everyday work became dependent on access to computers.

Just as important as the story of how computers changed biology and medicine is the story, explored in the following chapters, of how those fields changed computing. Rather than treat computers as "black boxes," this account strives to consider what historian Michael S. Mahoney calls the "many agendas of computing." The electronic digital computer, Mahoney explains, "became what various groups of people made of it. The computer thus has little or no history of its own. Rather, it has histories derived from the histories of the groups of practitioners who saw in it, or in some yet to be envisioned form of it, the potential to realize their agendas and aspirations."[22] The various types of computers adopted by—and some cases explicitly developed for—life scientists were built to realize a wide variety of intellectual, institutional, and personal agendas. The room-sized IBM 7090 met one set of agendas, while the refrigerator-sized LINC (Laboratory Instrument Computer) met another. Examining these agendas illuminates many of the reasons computers were used in particular ways and settings. In the case of the LINC, where the unique needs of biologists played a significant role in shaping the computer architect's agenda, the influence of the life sciences on computer design becomes clear as well. Software, the programs and procedures that run and run on computers, also was influenced heavily by the life sciences. DENDRAL (Dendritic Algorithm), an exemplary expert system (that is, a program that solves problems by drawing from a knowledge base generated by human experts), and M (originally MUMPS or Massachusetts General Hospital Utility Multi-Programming System), a programming language used in and far beyond the hospitals for which it was developed, were both built to satisfy the agenda of biologists or physicians. Although these projects are well known in computing, their origins in the life sciences have not been examined thoroughly until now.

Biology, Medicine, and Computers amid the "American High"

Before delving into the story of early biomedical computing, it is worth becoming familiar with some basic aspects of the life sciences and computing in the years leading up to the period most intensely covered by this book, 1955 to 1965. Like today, the late 1940s and early 1950s were a time of tremendous change and optimism in biology and medicine. In the years following World War II, particularly intense excitement surrounded new explorations of life on the molecular level, such as those undertaken by the Phage Group at Caltech and the protein crystallographers of Cambridge University. In both cases, physicists and chemists drawn to biology applied their training to try to make sense of the structure and function of genes and proteins. The most celebrated outgrowth of this work was James Watson and Francis Crick's 1953 double-helix model of DNA.

Many imaginations were captured by the notion that important aspects of the workings of living things could be reduced to DNA's long sequence of As, Ts, Gs, and Cs, each letter representing one nucleotide base—or (more figuratively) one rung on the spiraling double-helical ladder. However, Crick's oft-recalled pronouncement that he and Watson had "discovered the secret of life" has retrospectively masked the enormous chasm between conceiving how DNA worked and actually being able to read the sequence of bases in the molecule. To those who hoped to bring about a more quantitative approach to biology, DNA's four-digit code indeed beckoned as early as the mid-1950s, but the raw data needed to sustain such an approach was for many years sorely lacking. The 1965 *Atlas of Protein Sequence and Structure*, which printed most of the sequences that had been discovered to date, fit into a small book. It was not until the early 1970s, when rapid sequencing of nucleotide bases was developed, that it became possible to determine the order of bases for portions of DNA larger than those that generated individual proteins. The first fully sequenced genome (completed in 1977), that of the virus *phi X 174*, contained just 5,386 base pairs, a paltry number compared to the 3 billion base pairs in humans. Furthermore, many obstacles related to procuring data, namely isolating DNA from the rest of the cell and then obtaining enough of it to actually sequence, were not overcome until the development of polymerase chain reaction (PCR) amplification techniques in the 1980s.

While the potential of DNA was the topic of much optimistic discussion, X-ray crystallography also seemed to hold great—and arguably more immediate—promise. Beginning in the 1930s, the technique had been employed to help create three-dimensional models of the structure of molecules important to biology and medicine. Dorothy Crowfoot Hodgkin, working in England, had used crystallographic methods to determine the structures of cholesterol in 1937 and penicillin in the late 1940s; by the early 1950s, she was building knowledge of the structures of vitamin B-12 and insulin. Crystallographers and their admirers shared a growing confidence that even large proteins, which consisted of many thousands of atoms, could be modeled if one could somehow manage the millions of simple calculations involved in extrapolating structural information from crystallographic data. By the late 1940s, Cambridge crystallographers had put dozens of young women to full-time work as "computers," in order to carry out the arithmetic component of their research into the structure of proteins.

The feeling during the 1940s and 1950s that world-changing breakthroughs loomed on the horizon was not limited to the areas of investigation that would eventually become known under the name molecular biology. In physiology, where many of the early adopters of computer technology would be found, a host of new projects, especially those related to the brain, drew inspiration from cybernetics, a way of examining complex mechanical systems in terms of regulation and feedback developed by mathematician Norbert Wiener during the war. The parallels between organisms and self-regulating machines that cybernetics posited proved difficult to investigate in reality, and very few explicitly cybernetics projects were pursued.[23] However, many young scientists and engineers were motivated to use information technology to investigate physiology upon hearing the excited discussion about cybernetics at the Macy Conferences, a series of interdisciplinary conferences on the workings of living systems held by the Josiah Macy Jr. Foundation between 1946 and 1953, and by reading Wiener's books *Cybernetics or Control and Communication in the Animal and the Machine* (1948) and *The Human Use of Human Beings* (1950).[24]

Although early explorations of life's molecules and ruminations about the mechanics of living processes tended to be fairly abstract, they were also grounded in the belief that a new understanding of the living world would yield enormous medical benefits. Decoding DNA appeared to hold great promise for combating disease, while the discussions that surrounded cybernetics, which were often strikingly close to some of today's speculative talk, portrayed humanity as entering a new kind of relationship with machines and thereby being on the precipice of transcending its purely organic form and behavior.[25] In many countries during the postwar years, enthusiasm and expectations for medical research ran high, but only in the prosperous, relatively unscathed United States was that research the target of significantly increased funding. In addition to support from philanthropic trusts like the Rockefeller Foundation, American medical researchers drew funding from the military and from rapidly growing civilian agencies like the NSF and especially the NIH. For-profit healthcare systems, medical instrument manufacturers, and drug companies, meanwhile, also generously devoted resources to the pursuit of medical research. Among these diverse patrons of research was a general consensus that new technology would be a boon for science and medicine and that breakthroughs were, if not imminent, inevitable.[26]

Behind the belief that new technologies would transform biomedicine were the stunning advances in electronics during the early twentieth century. From the perspective of the mid-1950s, the view was breathtaking. Just in the course of their own lives many of the decision makers in biology and medicine had watched the electric grid spread across the United States and other Western societies, and had then seen electronic devices like radios and televisions become commonplace. In the sciences, the use of instruments with embedded electronics had opened vast new realms of inquiry within just years of their introduction. Electron microscopes, ultracentrifuges (with electronic speed control), and a wide array of electronic biotechnical recording devices were all by the mid-1950s being used to pursue agendas that had not even been conceivable just decades before.

Starting in the early 1940s a new type of electronic device emerged, one capable of performing programmed logical operations. The first stored-program electronic digital computer, the Electronic Numerical Integrator And Computer (ENIAC), was built in secrecy during the war by J. Presper Eckert and John Mauchly at the University of Pennsylvania's Moore School of Electrical Engineering, in Philadelphia. Eckert and Mauchly designed ENIAC to quickly and accurately carry out the millions of simple calculations involved in constructing artillery firing tables, which were used to predict the path of a shell given the angle at which it was fired and local atmospheric conditions. These tables, which generally held data for three thousand trajectories, would take about twenty thousand hours of labor to complete using a mechanical desk calculator. Thus it would take a team of one hundred human computers a month to complete one table. On ENIAC, the process of carrying out these computations could be replicated by routing an electrical signal through a carefully arranged series of switches and relays, while the instructions for the calculation could be stored in vacuum tubes.

To handle the task of making firing tables by integrating seven-variable differential equations, ENIAC had many times more components than any other electronic machine of its day. ENIAC's circuit elements consisted of 17,468 vacuum tubes, seventy-two hundred crystal diodes, forty-one hundred magnetic elements, and tens of thousands of resistors and capacitors. Once constructed, the machine occupied eighteen hundred square feet and when running it consumed 174 kilowatts of power, enough to power about fifty modern homes.[27] When wired up to run a program, ENIAC appeared at first glance to resemble a busy telephone exchange, with hundreds of patch cords plugged into various components of the machine, carrying electrical signals from one part to another. To change a program on ENIAC meant spending days rearranging the cords.[28] Once up and running, though, ENIAC was inhumanly fast and accurate—it could accomplish in mere hours what a large team of human calculators could do in a month.

In the late 1940s, owing to ENIAC's complexity, expense, and difficulty of operation, there seemed to be little demand for general-purpose electronic digital computers. Howard Aiken, architect of the electromechanical Harvard Mark I calculator, has been quoted often (and erroneously) as predicting that no more than five or six such machines would be needed in the entire United States.[29] However, by this time ENIAC had already drawn much attention from beyond the worlds of mathematics or artillery. When it was unveiled to the public in 1946, ENIAC quickly captured the imagination of business and scientific leaders as well as of the general public.

Popularly hailed as a "giant brain," ENIAC spawned the UNIVAC, designed by Eckert and Mauchly and sold by Remington Rand starting in 1951.[30] By the mid-1950s, two dozen or so UNIVACs were sold to customers so hungry for its ability to crunch numbers that they tolerated its high cost and cumbersomeness. Besides the military and the US Census Bureau, early UNIVAC customers included insurance companies, utilities, and large technologically oriented firms such as General Electric, US Steel, and Westinghouse. On election night in 1952, UNIVAC became an American household name when, as a publicity stunt, Remington Rand teamed up with CBS television to use the computer to predict the outcome of the presidential race between Dwight Eisenhower and Adlai Stevenson. Contradicting the polling firms, which had predicted a very close race, programmers using UNIVAC to project the results based purely on data from early election returns calculated a landslide victory for Eisenhower and were dramatically proven correct.[31]

Seeing such high demand for the UNIVAC, Remington Rand's much larger rival, IBM, which had been developing computers almost exclusively for the military, decided to enter the civilian market, hoping that by bringing its immense technological resources to bear on the problem of building effective electronic digital computers, it would be able to seize a share of a rapidly growing market. IBM's 700-series computers, publicly marketed beginning in late 1952 and intended to compete with UNIVAC, used new magnetic drum memory and were assembled from modules that could be easily transported to the customer. By 1956, the somewhat more convenient and reliable IBM 700 was dominating the market, with orders for almost two hundred compared to around fifty for UNIVAC. Meanwhile, the much smaller (and substantially less powerful) IBM 650, first announced in 1953, and dubbed by IBM's head, Thomas Watson Jr., as the "Model T of computing," was quietly racking up hundreds of orders from smaller companies and universities.[32] Whether the computer was from Remington Rand, IBM, GE, RCA, or Honeywell, once it arrived there was generally no going back to the way things were before. Once an organization computerized, it generally remained that way. Thus, even before the transistor made electronic computing so much more feasible, the information age was arriving.[33]

In the 1950s and early 1960s, when digital computing took off, Americans were generally more forward-looking and broadly optimistic than they had been in the decades before or since. Though the debate over racial segregation divided the nation, and though the issue of gender discrimination smoldered largely unacknowledged, it was a time when dissent was unusual. "In that era of general good will and expanding affluence," David Halberstam wrote, "few Americans doubted the essential goodness of their society."[34] For the millions of men and women who had as children endured the Great Depression and whose early adulthood was consumed by war, the peaceful prosperity of postwar America presented an opportunity to build their lives, and they enthusiastically seized it. Even the Cold War, and the prospect of nuclear annihilation that came with it, did little to dampen their spirits. Driving the boom was what William L. O'Neill pithily characterized as an "American High," that is, "the faith, that given enough effort, anything could be accomplished."[35] This trust in America's possibilities fed upon itself. It propelled—and, in turn, was propelled by—unprecedented socioeconomic mobility, a generally expanding economy, thriving industry, and stunning new scientific, medical, and technological developments.

For 1950s Americans, biomedical research was a particularly potent source of confidence in the future of their society. Millions participated in the tests of Jonas Salk's polio vaccine, which were often the top story in the news. A Gallup poll showed in 1954 that more Americans could correctly identify the Francis Field Trial as a test of the Salk vaccine than could give the full name of President Eisenhower. When the vaccine was deemed safe and effective on April 12, 1955, euphoria erupted on a national scale.[36] The excitement surrounded biomedical work led to exceptional mobility—even by 1950s standards—for many of those directly involved in it. Robert Ledley and Lee Lusted, two American subjects of this book, had between them a dozen different full-time positions during the decade. For the most part, these jobs were secure, high-paying, and prestigious. When they left one job—or one region—for another it was most often by choice. Though in some senses both men were marginal in biomedical establishments, being at the institutional margins did not for them translate into economic insecurity or uncertainty.

That Ledley and Lusted each enjoyed such mobility was largely a consequence of the expanding science and technology research budgets throughout the 1950s and early 1960s. Between 1950 and 1959, the NIH's budget grew from $52 million to almost $292 million. By the mid-1960s, the agency's budget had mushroomed to more than $1 billion.[37] The growth was only slowed in the late 1960s by the escalating expense of the conflict in Vietnam. Thus, during the years examined in this book, biologists and computer developers worked in an environment where they could usually expect to receive not only continued support for their projects but increased support in the future. Though competition for grants was intense, the rapidly growing allocations of funding bodies like the NIH and the Department of Defense provided many back channels—some with very little oversight—through which projects could receive support. Many of this account's subjects learned to become expert navigators of those channels.

The Past in the Biomedical Future

This book makes the case that the computerization of biology and medicine was an irreversible process shaped by intellectual, institutional, political, and technological forces. Broadly, it shows why and how computer technology was first adopted in biology and medicine, and it explores the changes using those machines brought to each area. It also reveals that computing itself was profoundly altered by early efforts to introduce computers to the study of life. Although this work's narrative spans a decade and examines many of the people, institutions, and machines involved in the introduction of computers to the study of life, it is by no means comprehensive. Relatively greater coverage is given to endeavors that left behind the most extensive records and whose participants were able to take part in interviews in recent years. For further historiographic discussion, see the Essay on Sources.

To read this book, you do not need to be an expert in biology, medicine, or computing. Readers primarily interested in the history of biology or medicine will find here a story that demystifies the capabilities of computers in research from the 1940s to the 1960s. A better appreciation of the early use of computers in biology and medicine will provide a firmer grounding for the still-unfolding histories of computer-dependent endeavors like the Human Genome Project and indeed of whole disciplines such as bioinformatics, computational biology, and medical informatics. Meanwhile, readers seeking to learn more about the history of computing will find case studies of how the demands of biological and medical research shaped computer design. Finally, readers examining the consequences of government and philanthropic support for emerging technologies will find that early decisions to sponsor the proliferation of information technology in the life sciences were heavily contested, and even those now hailed as great successes did not appear as such until quite recently.

To bring to light the major causes and effects of the use of computers in the life sciences, this book takes several approaches—each roughly encompassed by one chapter—to the story of how biomedicine became computerized. The first chapter examines the earliest efforts, beginning in the late 1940s, to use computers in biology and medicine. It focuses on how operations research (OR), a collection of mathematical methods initially used to optimize British radar systems during World War II, served as the main waypoint through which computers entered biology and medicine. Though OR had military origins, its methods and priorities deeply influenced the early biomedical computing activities of biochemist and crystallographer John Kendrew in the United Kingdom and Robert Ledley and Lee Lusted in the United States.

The second chapter views early computerization from a more institutional perspective by examining the first major effort, undertaken in the late 1950s and early 1960s by a deeply divided National Institutes of Health, to promote computer use among American biomedical researchers. By closely investigating the challenges faced by the NIH's outspoken and often-outmaneuvered supporters of computing, namely the Advisory Committee on Computers in Research (ACCR), guided and led (respectively) by Ledley and Lusted, the chapter reveals the massive potential seen in computers but also the many reasons behind the life sciences' initial inability to realize that potential.

The third chapter shows the influence of biology on early computing by closely following the 1961–65 development of the LINC, an important but often overlooked precursor to the modern personal computer. Conceived and built by an MIT Lincoln Laboratory team led by Wesley Clark and supported by the NIH, the LINC was both an outgrowth of Clark's iconoclastic design philosophy and of his solutions to problems related to the unique practical and institutional requirements of biomedical research.

The fourth chapter investigates the use and development of NIH-sponsored computers—especially the LINC—in laboratories, hospitals, and Robert Ledley's National Biomedical Research Foundation (NBRF) during the 1960s. By combining evidence drawn from broad surveys and technical reports from individual researchers or institutions, it makes explicit the effects of computers on research and patient care as well as the challenges associated with early—but also contemporary—efforts to use computers in these areas. In its survey of the NBRF's key work in the 1960s and 1970s, this chapter explores: the origins of bioinformatics in Margaret Dayhoff's *Atlas of Protein Sequence and Structure*; the roots of the recently exploding field of pattern recognition in Ledley's Film Input to Digital Automatic Computer (FIDAC); and Ledley and the NBRF's role in promoting digital computing technologies in clinical settings via its best-known instrument, the 1974 Automatic Computerized Transverse Axial (ACTA) scanner, the first full-body CT/CAT scanner.

Building on but also further elucidating the themes of the previous chapters, the fifth and final chapter examines Stanford University's emergence as a leading nexus for the exchange of ideas between life scientists and computer scientists during the 1960s. In this study of a single institution, the chapter makes the case that computer science and life science shaped each other through several convergences—of the research agendas of ambitious young scientists who wanted to transform their fields, grand institutional aspirations of deans and provosts attempting to restructure their ailing university, nation-spanning visions of federal administrators eager to use information technology to advance biology and medicine, and dreams of wealth among computer manufacturers seeking a lucrative new market. The chapter shows that often these interests did not align well and that Stanford's rise as a center of biomedical computing, therefore, while a tale of success, is not a story of cascading triumphs but rather one also marked by multimillion-dollar cancelations and abandoned careers. Extraordinary ambition and deep frustration alike would be found in the stories of the university's aborted first attempt to acquire a large computer from the NIH, led by renowned computer scientist George E. Forsythe in 1962 and 1963, and of the influential mid-1960s DENDRAL and ACME projects, led by geneticist Joshua Lederberg, as part of his quest of "finding another branch of evolution." Finally, the chapter shows how projects initially localized to Stanford, such as the Stanford University Medical Experimental Computer–Artificial Intelligence in Medicine (SUMEX-AIM), grew into national resources.

Readers who are already familiar with today's biomedical computing should be prepared to set aside the modern conception that computing in biology and computing in medicine are separate entities. Presently, the fields of bioinformatics and medical informatics are indeed distinct, the former pertaining mostly to computer use in molecular biology (especially DNA sequencing) while the latter broadly covers the use of computers in medicine. Relative to the period covered in this book, however, both terms are new; "bioinformatics" was coined by Paulien Hogeweg and Ben Hesper in 1978, and "medical informatics" was introduced by John Anderson, Jean-Claude Pages, and François Gremy in 1974.[38] Prior to the 1970s, both fields fell under the rubric of "biomedical computing," and extensively shared personnel and patronage networks. Consequently, this book treats computing in biology and medicine as they were generally viewed in the United States in the 1950s and 1960s, as a single entity. Though it may be clear in retrospect that biology and medicine each presented its own set of challenges to computing, this did not become generally apparent until the mid-1960s, when the NIH computerization effort was well under way.

Taken together, the contents of this book show how computers came to and began to become central to biology and medicine, and how the life sciences, in turn, changed computing. Today, if we are to believe many of the leading figures in the study of life as well as in computing, it is clear that these areas are not only mutually important but will increasingly shape each other in the years to come. The future consequences of our society's multibillion-dollar investment in biomedical computing remain unclear, though high expectations and institutional momentum have committed us to a path that can only be navigated by harnessing the forces of biomedicine and computing. Knowing why and how that journey began should help us prepare for the road ahead.

Putting Molecular Biology and Medical Diagnosis into Metal Brains

Operations Research and the Origins of Biomedical Computing

On any given Monday morning," wrote Arnold "Scotty" Pratt of his early years as director of the National Institutes of Health's computing facility, "it was often necessary for the staff to make a new commitment to self and country." The IBM 650 that Pratt's team operated in the late 1950s, due mostly to its deep unpopularity among NIH researchers, was housed in the basement of Building 12, a space deemed "unsatisfactory for human occupancy." Immediately above the 650 were hundreds of cages for mice and monkeys, the source of animal odors that permeated the building. Meanwhile, the ventilation system, which drew air from just downwind of the agency's fuel depot and incinerator, filled the data processing center with fumes and grit. "Lighting a match on gasoline delivery day, with our exchange system frequently belching finely charred particulate matter, challenged even the most intrepid souls."[1]

Why were Pratt and his staff subjected to such miserable conditions? The official explanation by NIH administrators was that the agency lacked any other space on its Bethesda, Maryland, campus to accommodate the bulky 650. It was indeed difficult to place. Weighing in at three tons, the "moderate-sized" IBM 650 Magnetic Drum Data Processing Machine—before 1960 the term *computer* generally referred to humans who performed calculations—required a two-hundred-square-foot air-conditioned room equipped with high-voltage electrical outlets and reinforced floors. A much larger space was needed near the 650 to accommodate its dozen operators (who worked in three eight-hour shifts) and the many thousands of punch cards on which programs and data were stored. Although there were several suitable locations on the campus for the 650, only the space in Building 12 went uncontested.

That none of the NIH's score of research institutes welcomed the 650 was also a consequence of the broader problem. Of IBM's first generation of general-purpose electronic digital computers, the 650 was by far the most popular, with some two thousand units sold. At the NIH, however, the 650 was received very poorly by the community of researchers it was intended to serve. As one group of early computing advocates noted, "The biomedical researcher, who for fifty years was reaping success after phenomenal success using only experimental means and qualitative notions, looked on the computer with suspicion and apprehension." The question in most life scientists' minds, it seemed, was, "How could a computer that only handles numbers be of fundamental importance to a subject that is qualitative in nature and deals in descriptive rather than analytic terms?"[2]

Particularly troubling to the biomedical researchers was the way in which early computers like the 650 handled numbers. Strictly limited to performing simple logical operations (albeit very quickly), the 650 and other first-generation computers were unable to process data that had not been carefully prepared beforehand. For instance, finding the statistical mean of a sample of ten thousand cases took several steps. First, one had to prepare one punch card for each case, being sure to punch the correct spot every time. Then the computer had to be instructed to add up all the values of all the cards, and then finally to divide the sum by the number of cases. This was accomplished by preparing another set of punch cards containing routines, written in the FORTRAN programming language or machine code, which the 650 would follow. If the data and the program were prepared correctly, the 650 could flawlessly perform the task of finding the mean of a large sample in a small fraction of the time it would have taken a team of trained human beings.

For users with little or no quantitative data to crunch, the days spent preparing data and programs for the 650—not to mention the months of training required beforehand—were hardly worthwhile. The major obstacle preventing NIH researchers from using computers was that they did not readily have quantitative data or equations that computers could manipulate. This circumstance set life scientists apart from those who had used computers effectively during the 1950s. In areas like physics, where many important problems involved equations that were straightforward to develop, it was also fairly straightforward to develop computer programs to help solve those problems. In the study of life, however, most problems seemed far too complex to describe as simple equations or otherwise reduce to a form that a computer could process. In short, the vast majority of biologists and physicians deemed computers to be useless.

While the 650's impracticality merely alienated most NIH researchers, its high cost generated outright resentment across campus. The initial $300,000 spent in 1958 to purchase and install the 650 had come from the discretionary fund of NIH director James Shannon, who had been persuaded of computers' value to research by a small group of colleagues and by a weeklong course offered by IBM. But it was unclear how the agency would pay the projected $700,000 to operate and maintain the 650 over the next five years. Pointing out that "digital computers—like all other computers—are justified by being kept busy," one opponent to acquiring the 650 noted that there were nowhere near enough research tasks to occupy the machine's run time.[3] With a shortage of research projects, much of the 650's time was to be dedicated to processing payroll data, which NIH's outspoken computer enthusiasts conceded was "sort of a backlog of food for these monsters that can keep them somewhat alive and healthy while more research people are coming to appreciate their capabilities."[4]

For help overcoming hostility to computing among NIH researchers, Shannon turned to an outsider, a young computer expert named Robert Ledley. During the previous decade Ledley had pioneered the application of digital computers to a wide variety of problems in biology and medicine, including simulating jaw movements during chewing, modeling DNA-to-protein translation, and creating a logical basis for automating many aspects of medical diagnosis. Beyond using computers in his own work, Ledley firmly believed they would be a boon to biology and medicine, and by the late 1950s he had become a vocal public promoter of biomedical computing. He found, however, that few who studied life shared his enthusiasm for computers, a point driven home after his 1957 survey of computer use among American biomedical researchers revealed that few envisioned ever using the machines in their work. Only a tiny minority of researchers reported having data that could be processed by computers, and fewer still believed they could learn to use computers.

In 1959, encouraged by Shannon as well as the National Academy of Sciences, Ledley published two widely read articles in the journal *Science* setting forth his vision of how biology and medicine would benefit from the use of computers and how workers in those fields should prepare to use the machines. To better enable life scientists to harness the power of computers in the service of their research, Ledley proposed that they follow the route that had enabled him to productively apply computers to problems in biology and medicine. To that end, he called on biologists and physicians to learn the methods of operations research, the heavily quantitative approach to studying and optimizing complex systems developed during World War II—and then, as he had done in the early 1950s, apply those methods to biomedical problems. In essence, Ledley hoped to train biomedical researchers to emulate skilled computer programmers, who are able to accurately describe complex real-world phenomena in purely logical and arithmetical terms so that they can be simulated and meaningfully explored using a computer capable of performing only simple logical operations.

Ledley's plans did little to win over opponents of the 650, but the proposals captured the imaginations of NIH administrators and the agency's patrons on Capitol Hill. Consequently, Ledley's particular approach to computing inspired the NIH's early 1960s effort, funded directly by Congress, to computerize biology and medicine. While computing languished on the NIH campus itself, the agency was directing tens of millions of dollars toward establishing dozens of major biomedical computing centers across the country. Led by Ledley's collaborator, Lee Lusted, the NIH computerization effort gave rise to many of the technologies and institutions that would shape computer use in biology and medicine for decades to come. It also shaped perceptions, within science and medicine and among the general public, of how using computers could change the study of life.

By drawing heavily from OR, the NIH computing effort brought many of OR's methods, priorities, and assumptions to biology and medicine. It may seem odd that OR, which was developed to optimize weapons systems and logistical planning, would have applications so far removed from its military origins. However, the strong influence of OR on biomedical computing becomes clear when we examine how Ledley and an even earlier pioneer of biomedical computing, the UK's John Kendrew, independently applied the techniques they learned during their careers as military operations researchers to major problems in biology and medicine. In both cases, the experience of developing methods for the military to manage and improve complex systems enabled these men to imagine that electronic digital computers—then a brand new and not altogether promising technology—could be a crucial tool for learning about the natural world.

Operations Research in War and Early Computing

Beginning as they do with OR, most paths to computerized biology and medicine began with a way of thinking we do not readily associate with either area. Brought about by the exigencies of war, OR and closely related fields were crucibles for the two men who arguably did the most to introduce computers to the study of life, the Englishman John Cowderey Kendrew (1917–1997) and American Robert Steven Ledley (b. 1926). At first inspection, Kendrew and Ledley would appear to have little in common. Kendrew is best known for his work in protein crystallography, for which he was awarded the Nobel Prize in 1962. Ledley, meanwhile, is remembered primarily for developing and patenting the full-body CT scanner in the mid-1970s. However, by looking beyond their best-known accomplishments, one can see that the two men shared an approach to scientific problems. Namely, they both translated their knowledge of OR into computerized solutions to problems in biology and medicine. Furthermore, they worked for some time in the same milieu—the areas of inquiry that later would become known as molecular biology—though after Ledley teamed up with Lee Lusted his work would also extend deep into the early development of medical computing.

So important to early biomedical computing, OR was "born of radar."[5] In the years leading up to World War II, Britain invested heavily in radar in the hope that the new technology would, if war came about, stave off attacks from German aircraft. For the engineers and scientists responsible for developing radar, the burden was heavy. Not only did the integrity of Britain's air defense seem to depend on their work, but they were building an enormously complex system on a very small budget. Their objective was to build a series of radar stations along the coast, called Chain Home, to detect incoming aircraft in time for British planes to take off and intercept them. In that way, the smaller British force would be able to prevent the larger German force from reaching its targets. Getting this system to work, however, was difficult. First, Radio Direction Finding was a new technology that required extensive refinement before it could reliably detect airplane-sized targets. Second, there was the problem of collecting information from the radar stations and then transmitting it to the interceptor bases closest to the projected path of the incoming planes.

The engineers responsible for troubleshooting the Chain Home stations called their work "operational research."[6] In essence, OR was developed to model the behavior of complex systems using a wide variety of statistical and probabilistic methods with the goal of making those systems more efficient and reliable. Initially, OR was not a formal discipline or even a way of thinking but rather a collection of quantitative methods used by a politically active (and generally left-leaning) segment of the British scientific community—notably including Patrick Blackett, J. D. Bernal, and Robert Watson-Watt—to influence military policy makers. Specifically, operations researchers used statistics-based efficiency reports and probabilistic simulations—war games, in essence—to guide government resources to their projects in a time of scarcity.

During the war, the methods used to craft reports that persuaded politicians to support radar transformed into a set of tools used by scientists participating directly in military work.[7] Starting in 1939, the focus of OR activity was the Royal Air Force's Coastal Command Operational Research Section (ORS), which had two major responsibilities: to determine how to most effectively operate and deploy personnel and equipment to detect and neutralize the enemy, and to optimize radar and weapons for ease-of-use and durability in battlefield conditions. Following the Battle of Britain (1940), the ORS's mission was expanded to the North Atlantic Theater of Operations, where it was charged with defending convoys from U-boat attacks.

What distinguished the ORS from other forms of military research and development was not only its mix of civilian and military researchers but also its aim to provide a "total system" to defend Britain. The ORS technologists—or boffins, in the British descriptor for such experts—were encouraged to examine the military's mission in the abstract in order to make assessments, often based on aggregate statistical data rather than individual combat reports, on the efficiency of weapons and tactics and of the organizations that employed them in battle.[8] Granted extraordinary leeway by a government desperate to find means to counter attacking aircraft and submarines, early OR workers not only influenced decisions of designers and manufacturers of crucial equipment but also developed training regimens and guidelines to be followed by the military when it came to deploying that equipment.[9]

Based on this new approach to military data, the ORS offered advice concerning, in the words of one former section member, the "prediction of the outcome of future operations either in the tactical or strategic field with the object of influencing policy."[10] Consequently, the ORS placed heavy emphasis on the speedy collection and analysis of large amounts of operational data, which, in turn, required that its officers be familiar with how the apparatus they were trying to improve worked and with the means to organize the data their studies produced. Collecting such data during wartime was an unenviable task. ORS analysts not only were "called upon to face physical danger" to gather combat data firsthand, but their quantitative work "was frequently dull and boring, highly repetitive, and under extreme pressure for results."[11] By treating in the abstract the data they painstakingly gathered from early phases of Germany's aerial campaign against Britain in 1940, the ORS were able to spot trends that otherwise would have gone unnoticed in the heat of battle. Piecing together their knowledge of German air strategy with observations of which British strategies for stopping the bombers were most effective, the ORS gave advice that allowed the Royal Air Force to push the Luftwaffe's losses to the point where Germany was forced to cease its bombing campaign.

Following the war, OR was applied to problems related to a wide variety of complex systems in military planning, corporate and government organization, healthcare, and science. OR reduction and optimization methods also became central to a new type of work, describing problems in such a way that they could be solved using a machine capable of only logical and arithmetic operations, the electronic digital computer. Herbert Simon, a Nobel Prize–winning economist and a pioneer in the field of artificial intelligence, described OR as an "applied science" that would bring about the "procedural rationality" needed to create effective and efficient computer programs. "Linear programming, integer programming, queuing theory, and linear decision rules"—all used in creating "algorithms for handling difficult multivariate decision problems"—were in Simon's words, "examples of widely used OR procedures" in early computer programming.[12]

Many early computer workers had extensive backgrounds in OR, which was reflected in the way they went about formulating problems for computers to solve. The techniques used by OR workers during the war to break down a complex system so that it could be examined using mathematical models could also be used to reduce complex problems to a form that could processed by a computer. "To permit computers to find optimal solutions with reasonable expenditures of effort when there are hundreds or thousands of variables," Simon noted, "the powerful algorithms associated with OR impose a strong mathematical structure on the decision problem." However, in both the war effort and in early computing there was a price associated with using OR methods, namely that "their power is bought at the cost of shaping and squeezing the real-world problem to fit their computational requirements: for example, replacing real-world criterion function and constraints with linear approximations so that linear programming can be used." Simon found on the one hand that "the decision that is optimal for the simplified approximation will rarely be optimal in the real world." Yet he also found through experience that many simplified models, while not perfectly accurate, were "satisfactory" in terms of providing useful information.[13] A skilled operations researcher, therefore, could balance the requirements of describing a real-world phenomenon with the requirements of reductive models to produce a piece of analysis or perhaps a computer program that would be viewed as reliable and accurate.

Molecular Biology at the Dawn of Electronic Computing

The dawn of the age of computers was an exciting time to be studying life. The 1930s through the 1950s, the same turbulent decades that gave rise to OR, were also a period of extraordinary developments in biology, especially in the areas that would become known as molecular biology. In the span of about twenty years, researchers found in life's atoms and molecules many of the mechanisms that control important vital processes like heredity, development, metabolism, and respiration. In their attempts to make sense of these processes on the molecular level, biologists set up problems that later would be approached using computers. In the United States, early computers were brought to bear on molecular studies of heredity—how traits pass from one generation to the next—and regulation—how an organism maintains its form in a chaotic environment. In the UK, meanwhile, computers would become an indispensible part of an effort to understand the molecular structure of important proteins such as hemoglobin, which transports oxygen in the blood.

In the mid-1930s, a decade before the first electronic digital computers were built, the notion of looking at how proteins functioned on the molecular level began to generate major attention as well as raise problematic questions. By that time, biologists had obtained much of the knowledge we currently possess about cell function, but they could only explain how cell heredity and regulation worked in the broadest physical and chemical terms. Physical and chemical evidence, such as Wendell Stanley's 1935 work with tobacco mosaic virus (TMV) crystallization, pointed to proteins as the key for unlocking the secrets of genetics and development.[14] However, the precise way the molecules comprising proteins acted to determine heredity, govern growth, or carry out functions like metabolism and respiration eluded study.

The mystery of how life worked on the molecular level attracted attention far beyond biology. Among those drawn in was theoretical physicist Max Delbrück, who quickly came to believe that that genetics "was, in fact, a domain of biological inquiry in which physical and chemical explanations might turn out to be insufficient."[15] As Delbrück began to explore the physical structure of organic molecules, he found that physiological functions and life's complexity defied scientific or even logical explanation. "Listening to the story of modern biochemistry," he wrote, "[the physicist] might become persuaded that the cell is a sack full of enzymes acting on the substrates converting them through various intermediate stages into cell substance or waste products . . . it looks sane until paradoxes crop up."[16]

The paradox causing Delbrück the most trouble was that genetic molecules—again, then thought to be proteins—remained stable in the face of the second law of thermodynamics, which states that elements in a closed system tend to seek their most probable distribution; that is, in a closed system entropy always increases. Given that organizations of molecules eventually degrade into disorder and that genes/proteins are organizations of molecules, the molecules that comprise genes should therefore be subject to this law. But, as we know, genes remain stable for millions of years, seemingly in defiance of a law that applies to all other molecular organizations. "How," asked physicists like Delbrück, "does the tiny gene of the Hapsburg lip manage to preserve its specific structure for centuries while being maintained at 310 degrees Kelvin?"[17] The resolution of this paradox, Delbrück believed, could yield not only an understanding of how proteins carried genetic information but also "other laws of physics."[18]

The early attempts to resolve Delbrück's paradox were generally straightforward: physicists would simply try to learn more about the gene's three-dimensional (3-D) structure and hope to find something compatible with both the second law of thermodynamics and the observations of geneticists. Physicist-turned-biologist Gunther Stent recalled that in 1940 the study of molecular structure in biology by physicists was "entirely rational," by which he meant that physicists interested in molecular biology tried to understand organisms purely in terms of structure—what was 3-D on the visible scale was also 3-D on the molecular scale.[19] For instance, British X-ray crystallographers W. H. and

W. L. Bragg "had acceded to the idea that the physiological function of the cell can be understood only in terms of the three-dimensional configuration of its elements."[20]

Delbrück's own approach to the paradox focused not on building a better 3-D model of the organism but on how proteins carried information. His first formal attempt to study genes was laid out in a 1935 collaborative paper, "The Nature of Genetic Mutations and the Structure of the Gene," which was based on observations of *Drosophila melanogaster* (fruit flies) bombarded with radiation.[21] Known more widely as the "Three Man Paper," this study speculated that "genes were very small, relatively stable, physical structures, molecules whose configurations could be rearranged when targeted by X-rays."[22] The paper also introduced the notion that the stability of genetic molecules stems from their staying put in "energy wells."[23] In his search for the physical basis of heredity, however, Delbrück soon abandoned *Drosophila* for bacteriophages, viruses that infect bacteria (and arguably the simplest form of life), collaborating first with biochemist Emory Ellis and then with microbiologist Salvador Luria and bacteriologist Alfred Hershey in an early 1940s study of reproductive mechanisms of bacteriophages.[24] As Delbrück's enthusiasm for bacteriophage research grew, he attracted considerable funding, especially from the Rockefeller Foundation, to himself and the scientists who gathered around him at Caltech to be part of his Phage Group.

Among those inspired by the "Three Man Paper" was the quantum physicist Erwin Schrödinger, who popularized Delbrück's work in his 1945 book *What Is Life?* "Life," posited Schrödinger, "seems to be orderly and lawful behavior of matter, not based exclusively on its tendency to go over from order to disorder, but based partly on existing order that is kept up."[25] The question, then, was how did life maintain order in an entropic universe? By way of an answer, Schrödinger conjectured that the gene was an aperiodic crystal: an irregular array of units in which there was a very limited number of types of individual units.[26] He explained, "The gene is most certainly not just a homogenous drop of liquid. It is probably a large protein molecule, in which every atom, every radical, every heterocyclic ring plays an individual role, more or less different from that played by any of the other similar atoms, radicals, or rings."[27] Schrödinger's gene preserved information and maintained order through simplicity. His gene was a "long linear molecule in which units are not identical but consist of a small number of moieties that can serve as the symbols in the code script."[28] This "codescript," according to him, was responsible for the design and control of all life: "The term code-script is, of course, too narrow. The chromosome structures are at the same time instrumental in bringing about the development they foreshadow. They are law-code and executive power—or to use another simile, they are the architect's plan and the builder's craft—in one."[29]

Following the war, two distinct but nevertheless tightly intertwined groups formed to study life on the molecular level. In California, Delbrück's Phage Group focused on the questions he and Schrödinger had raised, while in Cambridge, England, a motley collection of crystallographers set out to determine the structure of crucial molecules in living systems. Each group, in its groundbreaking work, would draw from the methods of OR in order to harness the power of electronic digital computers. Among the British group was John Kendrew, a young chemist who became, after his wartime service as a Radio Operational Research officer in the Royal Air Force, the leader of the earliest major effort to employ computers in life sciences research.

EDSAC and the Crystallographers

It was in the OR-steeped laboratories of the British crystallographers that computers and the life sciences initially came together. Starting in the late 1940s, Kendrew and Max Perutz, both of the unit for the Study of Molecular Structure of Biological Systems at Cambridge University's Cavendish Laboratory, each led teams that were employing crystallographic methods to determine the structures of the oxygen-transport proteins hemoglobin and myoglobin. Each team faced an enormous amount of calculation work, but only Kendrew's employed an electronic digital computer, the Electronic Delay Storage Automatic Calculator (EDSAC), to overcome the task. Perutz's group, on the other hand, relied extensively on human computers and the services of commercial firms that automated simple calculations via Hollerith punched card tabulating machines.

Hemoglobin and myoglobin are large, complex molecules, and to create maps (in the form of electron density projections) of their structure on the basis on crystallographic data required an enormous amount of arithmetic.[30] For each density point found via crystallography, roughly seven thousand Fourier terms would be summed to determine which part of the molecule's structure that density point represented. For hemoglobin, Kendrew and Perutz found 58,621 density points, thus necessitating more than 400 million arithmetic operations to map the points. As Perutz later quipped to historian Soraya de Chadarevian, calculation by hand of this amount of data was "beyond the patience of even a crystallographer!"[31]

Most crystallographers had neither the time nor the resources to perform the massive amount of arithmetic required to model the large molecules found in living systems. In a retrospective for *Crystallography News*, Robert O. Gould recalled the immensity of the task the crystallographers faced circa 1950, noting, "It is difficult for the modern crystallographer, whose Fourier syntheses are calculated so quickly that they don't even give time for a good swig of coffee, to realise the appalling task of actually carrying out even a two dimensional synthesis." He explained that "A modest grid of 30 × 30 and 400 data meant that for a centrosymmetric structure, cos [2π (hx + ky)] had to be evaluated 36,000 times. This seriously limited the possibility of using Fourier methods at all, and made three-dimensional summations almost unthinkable."[32]

Nevertheless, for those determined to create models of complex molecules from crystallographic data, there was a shortcut, the Beevers-Lipson strip, that allowed them to skip the time-consuming step of consulting sine-cosine tables, thus making the task possible, though still extremely demanding.[33] The Beevers-Lipson strips, which were printed on cardboard and came in sets of a few thousand, served two purposes. First, "to simplify the calculations greatly by factorising the trigonometric expressions to reduce the two-dimensional calculations to many fewer one dimensional ones." And second, "to provide a convenient technique for carrying out the summations—the strips themselves. The factorisation technique is still at the heart of many computer programs."[34]

Using the strips was simple, though onerous. No flipping through catalogs of tables was involved; all one had to do was select the right strips and line them up. Gould provides an example of a Beevers-Lipson summation: "For a one dimensional sum, the appropriate strips were arranged one under the other and the columns summed: The following shows the start of an array of cosine strips, here for [lattice points] h = 0, 1, 2, and 3 and [reflection values generated by Fourier transform] F = 46, –35, 28 and –19" (fig. 1.1).[35] Some crystallographers tried to ease their mathematical burden by employing calculating machines to perform the Beevers-Lipson summations, but such machines were so slow and difficult to operate that most chose to do the figuring in their heads. Thus, to use the strips, a knack for arithmetic was indispensable; as Gould notes: "It should be admitted that their efficient use depended on a standard of mental arithmetic not so common today as then!"[36]

By the late 1940s, Beevers-Lipson strips could be found in most major crys-

F	h	Degrees (0–90)															
2πx(*)>		0	6	12	18	24	30	36	42	48	54	60	66	72	78	84	90
46 C	0	46	46	46	46	46	46	46	46	46	46	46	46	46	46	46	46
−35 C	1	−35	−35	−34	−33	−32	−30	−28	−26	−23	−21	−18	−14	−11	8	−4	0
28 C	2	28	27	26	23	19	14	9	3	−3	−9	−14	−19	−23	−26	−27	−28
−19 C	3	−19	−18	−15	−13	−6	0	6	13	15	18	19	18	15	13	6	0
Sum			20	20	23	23	27	30	33	36	35	34	33	31	27	25	21	18

Fig. 1.1. Beevers-Lipson summation. Robert O. Gould, "The Mechanism of Beevers-Lipson Strips," *Crystallography News* (Dec. 1998)

tallographic laboratories, including Kendrew and Perutz's operation at the Cavendish.[37] For Kendrew and Perutz, the strips had made possible the projection of a two-dimensional (2-D) model of hemoglobin from X-ray crystallographic data, but using them entailed days and even weeks of arithmetic drudgery that dampened many a scientist's enthusiasm, especially considering that the 2-D structure they ended up producing was, "because the molecule is so complex . . . too confused to interpret."[38] The unit's first research student, Hugh Huxley, found "the terrible chore with Beevers-Lipson strips" dishearteningly dull.[39] Unlike so many others who suffered through quantitative toil while pining for more stimulating work, however, Huxley was in a rare environment in which he could complain to somebody who had the means to reduce the crystallographers' workload—somebody who had access to an electronic digital computer.

On the receiving end of Huxley's lament about working with Beevers-Lipson strips was his friend John Makepeace Bennett (1921–2010), an Australian engineer-mathematician who was responsible for programming Cambridge's Electronic Delay Storage Automatic Calculator (EDSAC), one of the earliest examples of a stored-program electronic digital computer. Inspired by John von Neumann's 1945 "First Draft of a Report on the EDVAC," in which von Neumann outlined the architecture of a digital computer that could store programs, EDSAC was built by Maurice Wilkes from 1947 to 1949.[40] Using some 3,000 vacuum tubes and consuming roughly 12 kilowatts of electric power, EDSAC physically dwarfed today's machines. Though it occupied the better part of a large room, EDSAC was considerably less powerful than modern desktop computers. Its memory was built out of mercury delay lines that had been developed during the war as a means to cancel radar echoes.[41] Each line was about 5 [per

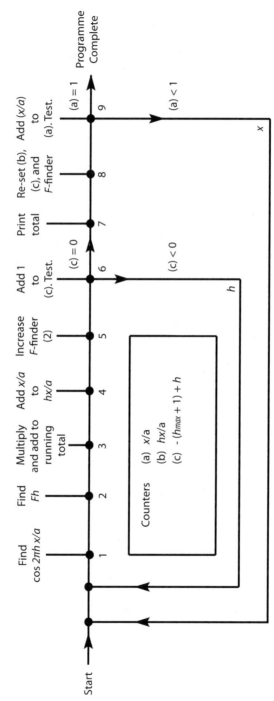

Fig. 1.2. Bennett and Kendrew's 1952 "scheme for computing one-dimensional Fourier synthesis." This program carries out the same kind of one-dimensional Beevers-Lipson summation as one would perform with the strips pictured in fig. 1.1. John M. Bennett and John C. Kendrew, "The Computation of Fourier Synthesis With a Digital Electronic Calculating Machine," *Acta Crystallographica* 5 (1952): 109. By permission of the International Union of Crystallography, journals.iucr.org

jm]feet long and could store 576 ultrasonic binary pulses. Martin Campbell-Kelly notes that "the contents of a delay line were constantly re-circulated with a cycle time of approximately 1 ms; this determined the basic speed of the machine—which averaged about 600 operations per second."[42] Furthermore, although Wilkes designed EDSAC to hold 32 delay lines, he could only manage to get 16 of the lines to work for the machine's first two years of existence, giving a total of "512 'short-storage locations' each capable of retaining 17 binary digits [bits]," that is, 512 17-bit words, or 8,704 bits, which is 512 bits more than a modern kilobyte (8,192 bits, or 1,024 8-bit words).[43] By comparison, the typical desktop computer today has processor cycle speeds in the range of billions per second and the capacity to store billions of bits in its memory. That translates to thousands of times faster and more powerful than EDSAC.

Consequently, EDSAC could outperform human calculators and adding machines but was incapable of carrying out complex calculations without their being parsed into simpler problems first. As Bennett later explained, "The machine can carry out directly only the simplest arithmetical operations—addition, subtraction, multiplication, and 'shift' (equivalent to multiplication or division by an integral power of 2; e.g. the number 24 in binary form is 11000—a right shift of two places give 00110 or 6, i.e. $24/(2^2)$, and similar left shift gives 1100000 or 96, i.e. $24 * (2^2)$; more complex operations are carried out by using appropriate combinations of the simple ones." These simple arithmetic operations EDSAC could execute relatively quickly. "Addition and subtraction are carried out in a mere 1.5 milliseconds, and multiplication in 6 milliseconds." Once Bennett understood that working with Beevers-Lipson strips amounted to nothing more than performing thousands of simple arithmetic operations (addition and subtraction) he realized that the entire task could be automated by EDSAC.[44] Within weeks, Bennett created a program that enabled EDSAC to perform two weeks' worth of Huxley's calculations in a mere 30 minutes, plus another 30 minutes to print the results (fig. 1.2).

When Bennett informed Kendrew of his program, Kendrew immediately saw the implications and with Bennett's help began to learn how to program EDSAC himself. Thus marked, in Kendrew's words, "the beginning of a fruitful collaboration between Cambridge crystallographers and the Mathematical Laboratory."[45] This collaboration allowed Kendrew and Perutz to perform the calculations that other crystallographers could not, such as those necessary to determine the highly complex structures of hemoglobin and myoglobin. Compared to mental or mechanical calculation, EDSAC was indeed speedy. As

Bennett and Kendrew explained in a 1952 *Acta Crystallograhica* article, "A two-dimensional summation of about 400 independent terms for about 2000 points takes [EDSAC] 1.5 hours; a three-dimensional summation of 2000 terms for 18,000 points takes 9 hours."[46]

Getting EDSAC to actually carry out these calculations presented a host of new problems. In today's parlance, one would call EDSAC a batch processor; that is, the user entered the program into the computer, let the computer run, and then received the results. There was no real-time interaction or feedback to allow the users to gauge whether or not they had made any errors while entering the data. Thus, using the computer required extraordinary attention to detail and patience. After EDSAC's programmers converted the Beevers-Lipson summations into an algorithm the machine could process, the crystallographers faced the tedious challenge of encoding their program onto EDSAC's input medium, a perforated paper tape that had to be punched *perfectly* using a special typewriter. The cosmologist Fred Hoyle, who had less-than-fond memories of the EDSAC's successor, EDSAC 2, captured the frustrations of this process in his science fiction novel *Black Cloud*. He complained, "Not one single hole among many thousands could be out of its proper place, otherwise the machine would compute incorrectly. The typing had to be done with meticulous accuracy, with literally one hundred per cent accuracy."[47]

Once the tapes were punched, there was the hurdle of EDSAC's unreliability. As Kendrew noted, "If you did your programming correctly, everything was checked, double checked, there couldn't be a mistake in the final result, but you could spend an immense time arriving at the result because the machine could go wrong."[48] EDSAC's lead programmer, David Wheeler, recalled that "the average time between machine errors was about half an hour. However, this is deceptive as there were 'good' and 'bad' days, and most faults were intermittent."[49] To get a sense of the number of errors Kendrew faced, one should bear in mind that his EDSAC calculations often spanned entire weekends.

With EDSAC at his disposal, Kendrew believed that the discouragingly enormous burden of the myoglobin labor could be borne. To prove the concept, he set EDSAC to work on running the calculations that would let him compare the diffraction patterns of several myoglobin crystals. Each crystal had a diffraction pattern consisting of over 25,000 reflection points, which translates to at least 12 hours of error-free runtime on EDSAC per crystal. However, by ignoring all but a few hundred of these reflections, Kendrew was able to optimize the problem to the point where he could reduce EDSAC's processing time from days to hours. By taking just the inner 400 reflections, Kendrew revealed (to a resolution of 6 angstroms) the basic structure of each of myoglobin's four polypeptide (protein) chains, and of the iron-holding, disk-like heme groups they were wrapped around.[50]

Besides automating the Beevers-Lipson summations, EDSAC proved instrumental in translating those summations into a 2-D and then 3-D model of myoglobin. To do this, EDSAC was employed to plot Patterson projections of electron density contours. Moreover, EDSAC could be programmed to plot such contours at whatever intervals (within reason) the crystallographers wanted. After they were plotted by EDSAC, the contours were translated into actual contour maps that contained "altitude lines." By stacking the maps, Kendrew and Perutz arrived at their 3-D model of myoglobin.[51] After several months of nights and weekends with EDSAC, Kendrew had coaxed the computer into running enough Beevers-Lipson summations that he could start to build a 3-D model of myoglobin. For this work, Kendrew and Perutz received the Nobel Prize in Chemistry in 1962; Kendrew was knighted in 1974.

Kendrew later reminisced: "Without that computer we would certainly have been simply unable, I mean, the amount of calculation by hand, it would have been impossible, even if you had money to hire twenty, fifty people."[52] Moreover, Kendrew regarded access to EDSAC as a necessary component of his and Perutz's crystallography success: "Supposing the Cambridge computer had not existed, until ten years later say. Well, we would not have got the result until ten years later. It would have been impossible without it."[53]

Pointing to EDSAC's role in the myoglobin triumph, Bennett and Kendrew predicted crystallography's broader computerization: "We anticipate little difficulty in applying similar methods to other problems, especially since nearly all crystallographic computations can easily be reduced to Fourier summations."[54] Over the next decade the proliferation of electronic computers in crystallography indeed came to pass—though perhaps not with the ease Bennett and Kendrew foresaw—first in the UK and then spreading to the United States (table 1). Clearly Cambridge had a head start, which contributed greatly to its later prominence in the field.[55]

That Kendrew was so enthusiastic about computers at such an early date was the consequence not merely of EDSAC's speed but also of Kendrew's background in OR. During World War II, the mathematical education and mechanical training and organizational proclivities that would enable Kendrew to adapt so quickly to the novel demands of digital computing had drawn him to opera-

Table 1   Crystallography Projects Using Electronic Computers (before 1960)

Institution(s)	Computer(s)	Year
Penn State*	X-RAC	1949
Cambridge University	EDSAC 1	1950
	EDSAC 2	1959
Leeds University	Ferranti Mark I	1951
	Ferranti Pegasus I	1952
Glasgow University	RUFUS	1954
Oxford University	DEUCE	1954
UCLA	SWAC	1956
	IBM 709	1958
University of Pittsburgh and University of Washington	IBM 650	1957
University of Manchester	Ferranti Mercury	1958
	Ferranti Muse	1959
University College, Cardiff	Stantec ZEBRA	1959

Source: Conference on Computing Methods and the Phase Problem in X-Ray Crystal Analysis. Report. University of Glasgow, 1960.
    *Penn State's X-RAC was an analog computer.

tions research. Already, Soraya de Chadarevian has made a compelling case that there was a strong relationship between Kendrew's wartime activities and his use of EDSAC. She observes that years before he encountered EDSAC, Kendrew was already conceptualizing the challenges that crystallography posed as problems that could be overcome by "effective methods of information storage and retrieval."[56] Furthermore, de Chadarevian characterizes Kendrew's preoccupation with information as an "obsession" that had also manifested itself in the course of his wartime work optimizing air patrols.[57]

Kendrew's analysis work also likely prepared him for the task of troubleshooting EDSAC. When a program did not work, Kendrew, an experienced operations researcher, could be confident that his program was at least conceptually sound, namely that he had formulated the problem to be solved by the program in such a way that it could indeed be expressed to the computer. Consequently, he could devote his energy to the more pragmatic challenges EDSAC operations posed. As has been illustrated, employing EDSAC—even casually—required intimate knowledge of its electronic components. When a program failed to execute as planned, the likely cause could have been: 1) a typographical or syntactic error in the program's code; 2) a fault in the program's logic; or 3) a failure of one or more of the machine's electronic components.[58] Only those who were familiar with the program's language, logic, and the hardware it utilized would effectively be able to use EDSAC. Did the program fail because of an input error, an illogical algorithm, or a blown-out vacuum tube?

In the first year of World War II, Kendrew was assigned to the Air Ministry Research Establishment (later known as the Telecommunications Research Establishment) as a "Radio Operational Research Officer," where he collaborated closely with military and civilian engineers and scientists to develop Britain's then-secret air-defense radar network.[59] After the Battle of Britain in 1940, Kendrew was put in charge of organizing and analyzing data collected by British coastal air patrols. To better coordinate the data provided by the air patrols, Kendrew designed a mechanical punched card indexing system for use by aircrews to record data from their operations in a comprehensive and uniform way in order to make it amenable to mechanical statistical analysis.[60] Kendrew and his colleagues treated the challenges they faced as ones of organization, and they strove to synthesize the particulars of protecting fleets from German U-boats into a general organizational scheme that could be applied to any military problem.

It was especially Kendrew's work with the air patrols that stoked his postwar enthusiasm for applying computer technology to solving protein crystallography problems. In interviews with de Chadarevian, Kendrew "explicitly stressed the 'close analogies' of the problems regarding the organization of scientific manpower with those 'studied in OR sections.'" For the air patrols and later for crystallography, Kendrew not only wanted a means of automating calculations but also sought to use computers to build a "comprehensive indexing system," which seemed to him the only possible way to "keep abreast of the vast literature of most of biochemistry and much of physiology and physics" that pertained to his newly chosen line of research. Based on her discussions with him, de Chadarevian concluded that "Kendrew may well have viewed EDSAC not just as a fast calculating machine but as a system to handle and retrieve large amounts of data,"[61] adding that she sensed that Kendrew "viewed the whole myoglobin project as a huge data operation system."[62] Looking at Kendrew's work from a broad perspective, she proposed that Kendrew "from the beginning viewed protein structure analysis as a huge data handling problem and approached it in operational terms, that is, assessing the efficiency of the single steps and devices involved as well as the operation of the whole. This general attitude would also determine his approach to the new electronic computer."[63]

Kendrew's treatment of the myoglobin work as a data-management operation was most evident in two areas: first, the data-collection system he devised to measure intensities in diffraction pictures; and second, his readiness to adopt protein sequencing as a means to determine protein structure—even at the cost of abandoning crystallography. Before Kendrew arrived at the Cavendish, Max Perutz personally estimated by eye the intensities used to interpret diffraction spots produced when X-rays were shone through crystals of hemoglobin. Kendrew, however, deskilled this labor. First, he found a densitometer (initially used at Kings College London to measure the density of cell sections) to help him perform the same task without needing Perutz's tacit knowledge of the idiosyncrasies of the interaction of complex crystals and X-rays. When the machine was commercially produced starting in the 1950s, Kendrew got one for the Cavendish and set up a small team of women clerical workers to take measurements of tens of thousands of reflections. The women would work all week on the measurements, which Kendrew then checked over the weekend. Workers who erred more than 5 percent more than once were summarily dismissed.[64]

Kendrew and Perutz's computerized triumph may be considered a legacy of the development of OR, but the connection between OR and the scientific breakthroughs of its practitioners did not translate into much institutional support for OR in Britain after the war. In large part, OR was the victim of the excitement surrounding it. In the postwar years, when some prominent operations researchers cast their work not only as an alternative to traditional military decision making but also to traditional economic regulatory mechanisms, OR came to be viewed by the British scientific and political establishments with skepticism and even alarm.[65] Although a case can be made that OR methods spread quietly into peacetime business practices and into efforts to manage Britain's struggling economy (particularly in the construction of the British welfare state), only to a limited degree did it penetrate British university-based scientific research. Already hostile to the hubristic claims of prominent OR figures, the British scientific establishment rejected OR's use as a full-fledged intellectual tool, dismissing it as "an exceedingly practical matter," one that was "not so much a science as a scientific attitude of mind on the part of its practitioners."[66] Without access to classroom instruction, those who wanted to master OR methods would need to do so through on-the-job training. In the postwar environment, where the development of complex technical systems was scaled back, few opportunities existed to recreate the experience of operations researchers during the war. Thus, computational methods associated with OR did not become a major part of postwar British scientific training in any major area, and the practices like those found in Kendrew's laboratory remained exceptional.

Considerable debate continues over why OR was resisted by British scientific institutions following the war.[67] Nevertheless, that British computer use in science was confined to a small number of institutions during the 1950s and 1960s can certainly be traced to the austere conditions in the country following the war. Although a handful of British crystallographers brought computers to bear on their own research during those decades, as late as 1967 the UK Ministry of Health's David E. Clark, fresh from touring over seventy US laboratories and hospitals that were employing computers, would complain that "as far as medical computing is concerned, England is in the dark ages."[68] While US-based researchers enjoyed generous—and growing—support for computing projects, their British counterparts worked within a system that was impoverished by the war. Given that Britons were still on some food rations almost a decade after the war's end, it should not be surprising that the integration of costly computers into biology and medicine was a low national priority. Tellingly, just to secure the most basic funding for molecular biology research in Britain, Kendrew had to personally lobby Parliament, where he adroitly broadcast support of the new field as necessary to stem the "brain drain" to the United States.[69] Due to this lean funding climate, Eric Rau notes, "the center of the OR world soon shifted from Britain to the United States, where the bonds of the Cold War's iron triangle—military, industry, and the academy—continued to provide an abundant source of patronage." As the center of OR moved to the United States, so did the use of computers in the study of life.[70]

DNA and the Number of the Beast

It took a few years longer for OR to catch on in the United States than it did in the UK. Intrigued by the work of operations researchers on Chain Home, and facing catastrophic losses from German submarine attacks in the North Atlantic, American military planners sought to emulate the British model by building an OR group of their own. Established by physicist Philip Morse in 1942, the Anti-Submarine Warfare Operations Research Group (ASWORG), based in Boston, quickly grew into a large, prestigious project that brought the expertise of dozens of civilian analysts to bear on military problems. Using statistical methods and new technologies and techniques modeled after British OR antisubmarine work, ASWORG became an integral part of the Navy's fight against submarines. For instance, after being lobbied by ASWORG analysts, the US Navy took a much more aggressive approach to countering the U-boat threat in the North Atlantic. Guided by ASWORG advice, the Navy shifted its strategy from supplying trans-Atlantic fleets with escorts to actively seeking out and destroying submarines.[71]

As was the case in Britain, American operations researchers enjoyed a privileged interaction with the military during the war. As John Krige shows, Morse—quite tellingly of his and other American operation researchers' view of both their own status and that of those who sought their input—cast the relationship between ASWORG and the Navy as being analogous to that of a doctor and patient. In Morse's asymmetrical scheme, the Navy was the "patient" while the OR worker was the "doctor." As a "doctor," the operations researcher required access to all the facts of the Navy's problem at hand, while he also "had to be outside the usual chain of command, in order to maintain an impersonal point of view . . . [and be] free to use [his] own methods of analysis, to reach a diagnosis."[72] After the war, the strong bonds between operations researchers and the military held, with operations researchers becoming crucial actors in the growing military-industrial complex. In contrast to its use in Britain, OR in the United States openly flourished in the postwar years. The Operations Research Society of America (ORSA), founded by Morse in 1952, had over five hundred members within its first year of existence and by the mid-1950s had its own major peer-refereed journal, *Operations Research*.

The story of how OR and also computers came to American biology begins back in England, just down the hall from Kendrew and Perutz. While they were investigating the structure of oxygen-transport proteins, two of their colleagues at the Cavendish, a precocious American visitor named James Watson and the considerably older but similarly flamboyant Cambridge graduate student Francis Crick were teaming up in an effort to determine the structure of deoxyribonucleic acid (DNA). Watson, who had been trained by Delbrück's collaborator Salvador Luria, was, along with Crick, pursuing the questions Delbrück had initially raised about the molecular mechanisms of heredity and development. In 1953, after making extensive use of X-ray crystallographic data provided by Rosalind Franklin and Maurice Wilkins of King's College London, Watson and Crick elucidated the now well-known double-helix structure of DNA, proposing that the molecule's two long strands of complementary nucleotide bases could both store an organism's genetic information and serve as the template used by the organism to build proteins.

In late 1953, fresh from the double helix breakthrough, Watson journeyed to California to begin working with members of the Phage Group to determine how, precisely, DNA worked. This proved to be quite challenging. When Watson arrived, his welcome by Caltech phage workers was icy, the mood set by Delbrück, who was "dissatisfied" with the double helix model on the grounds that there was no basis for "Watson and Crick's optimistic belief that the two strands [composing DNA] could somehow untwist."[73] Besides that fundamental problem, which was not resolved until the 1958 Meselson-Stahl experiment, there was the matter of how DNA generated proteins. In attempting to solve the problem of protein synthesis, the scientists who surrounded Watson and Crick in the mid-1950s would treat DNA as if it transmitted information, and some would take rudimentary steps, employing the methods of OR, toward using electronic computers to study both DNA's workings and the content of its nucleotide sequence.

A major preliminary step toward using computers to study DNA was Crick's "Central Dogma," his notion that there was an irreversible process of DNA being transcribed into RNA, which in turn encoded proteins, and that understanding this process would show how DNA related to the rest of an organism.[74] To paraphrase Crick, his Central Dogma model held that that once "information" has passed into protein it could not ever return again. In this model, the transfer of information from nucleic acid to nucleic acid, that is, DNA → DNA or DNA → RNA or even RNA → DNA was possible, but the transfer of information from protein to protein or from protein to nucleic acid was impossible. The information around which living things were built, therefore, could be found in the precise sequence of bases of nucleic acids or their products, the sequences of amino acids that built proteins.[75] Crick's idea had at its core the precepts of Delbrück and Schrödinger's earlier conceptions of the gene. All life could be reduced to a string of letters, which could, in turn, be treated like any other form of information.[76]

Having settled on what would become the Central Dogma, it remained for Crick, Watson, and their Phage Group colleagues to determine the mechanism by which RNA converted DNA's information into proteins. This turned out to be a far greater challenge than they anticipated. Frederic Lawrence Holmes observed that Watson had bet that the strategies that led him and Crick to their DNA triumph could also be transferred to the chemically similar RNA.[77]

Watson lost that bet, and in the long process of trying to figure out how RNA worked, some of his collaborators, led by "Big Bang" cosmologist George Gamow, who attached himself to Delbrück's circle in 1954, took tentative steps toward bringing information technology to bear on the study of DNA and RNA transcription and translation.

To rally other elite scientists to the mission of determining how RNA translated DNA's four bases into twenty amino acids, the building blocks of proteins, the gregarious Gamow established an informal but exclusive group called the RNA Tie Club.[78] Gamow whimsically assigned to each member of the club a moniker based on the name of one of these amino acids; each member also received a necktie—to be worn at scientific gatherings—bearing the name of his amino acid. Beyond Gamow, Watson, and Crick, RNA Tie Club members included phage researchers like Delbrück and Stent as well as the prominent physicists Edward Teller and Richard Feynman.

At the time Gamow established the Tie Club, he was working as an analyst at the Operations Research Office at Johns Hopkins University, in Baltimore, Maryland. Among his colleagues there was Robert Ledley, a twenty-eight-year-old whose official job was related to using computers in military research but who also hoped to apply OR methods and computer technology to the study of life. Impressed by Ledley's knowledge of computers and biology, Gamow invited Ledley to join the RNA Tie Club in December 1954, with the hope that electronic computers would carry out the arithmetic operations he believed were necessary to crack the code of life. After asking James Watson if he thought Ledley should be allowed to join, Gamow inducted Ledley as "ASN," for asparagine.[79]

Ledley's involvement in the RNA Tie Club was largely confined to working with Gamow, but among the early investigators of DNA Ledley and Gamow were the closest semblance to a group dedicated to treating genetic molecules as if they actually carried information. As Francis Crick explained to Horace Judson in 1970, it was Gamow who provided the impetus to articulate the nature of DNA as an encoding scheme: "The importance of Gamow's idea . . . was that it was really an abstract theory of coding, and was not cluttered up with a lot of unnecessary chemical details." Judson concluded, "Gamow disentangled the problem, stating it for the first time in its modern form." What Gamow specifically had in mind was to express DNA as a number, or in his colorful words, "the number of the beast." Given that DNA consisted of side-by-side complementary chains, formed and joined by only four kinds of nucleotide bases, "It follows that all hereditary properties of any living organism can be characterized by a long number . . . written in a four-digit system, and containing many thousands of consecutive digits."[80] To explain how the code of DNA was translated into amino acids (which then went on to build proteins) Gamow proposed the "diamond-slot" model whereby consecutive bases along the double helix formed diamond-shaped slots into which a particular amino acid would fit, depending on the configuration of the diamond.

It did not take long for the Tie Club to reject the diamond-slot model, and while other mechanisms of encoding were being debated, Gamow chose to ignore the particulars of chemistry and treat the problem of how the DNA bases translated into the twenty amino acids that form all proteins as one purely of code-breaking or "deciphering." Gamow began with the assumption that each amino acid was encoded by a series of three consecutive, non-overlapping bases, or "triplets." Given the sheer number of possible correspondences between the twenty amino acids and the sixty-four hypothetical triplets of bases, a brute-force computation of possible correspondences was impossible. Thus, Gamow turned to Ledley for help in streamlining the protein-decoding problem so that it could be processed in a reasonable amount of time by the fastest digital computers of the time.

Robert Ledley and the Roots of US Biomedical Computing

Like so many others who would be instrumental in facilitating the computerization of the life sciences, Robert Ledley (fig. 1.3) arrived at the endeavor in the course of trying to find a career that would bring together an unconventional combination of skills and knowledge. By 1957, when Ledley stood before the National Academy of Sciences–National Research Council (NAS-NRC) Committee on Medical Uses of Computers, he described himself as "an engineer who was interested in biology and medicine, and [who] incidentally also was knowledgeable in the new, hot, engineering field of digital computer design."[81] At this point, however, Ledley was also considered an expert in operations research, was a member of George Gamow's elite RNA Tie Club, and was a licensed dentist.

Ledley's interest in computers at this early date was the product of a long, circuitous process of "finding himself," a journey that would produce a CV that stood out as chimerical even in postwar America. Ledley began his undergraduate career at Columbia University in 1943 as a physics major with a strong

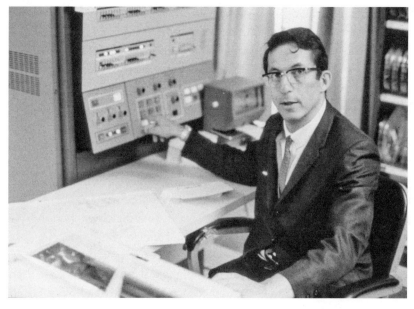

Fig. 1.3. Robert S. Ledley posing in front of an IBM 360 console in 1966. By permission of the National Biomedical Research Foundation

interest in mathematics and engineering. As a freshman, he observed that mathematics and science did not always interface smoothly when it came to applying mathematical concepts to specific problems in science, and he expressed interest in looking for ways to overcome this challenge. His teenage dreams of uniting mathematics and science, however, were postponed by his parents, who convinced him that "physics was not feasible, because in those days . . . everyone knew that physicists were either independently wealthy gentlemen or starving dedicated scientists, and I was neither."[82] Thus, in order to pursue a career in physics and remain reasonably comfortable, Ledley believed he would first need a substantial amount of money, which he intended to acquire by taking up the family tradition of practicing dentistry.[83]

For the next few years, Ledley attended New York University's College of Dentistry during the day and took physics and mathematics courses at Columbia at night. Initially these two pursuits had little to do with each other. Dentistry was his vocation but physics was his passion. Moreover, Ledley was not alone in sensing the incongruity of his educational pursuits. He recalled that one of his Columbia teachers, the physicist Isidor I. Rabi, "would poke fun at me saying I was the only physics student he knew who could pull a tooth."[84] By the time he completed dental school in 1948, Ledley had exhausted most of Columbia's rich offerings in mathematics and physics; when he received his MS in 1950, he had taken every available course.[85] Ledley was unsure of what to do with his degree, and from his experience as a dentist he had concluded that mathematizing biological problems was "no small deal—there were too many variables."[86] In the late 1940s, Ledley also caught his first glimpse of the OR methods and computing machines he would later harness to solve problems in biology and medicine. This happened when he visited his childhood friend Margaret Oakley Dayhoff (see chapter 4) while she was training as a graduate student in the Columbia University laboratory of George E. Kimball, a prominent chemist and also, as Morse's second-in-command at ASWORG, one of America's foremost operations researchers.[87]

Ledley was on a track to become a dentist when war intervened. In June 1950, just weeks after he completed his studies at Columbia, war broke out on the Korean Peninsula. That summer a military recruiter gave Ledley, then twenty-four, an ultimatum: volunteer for the Medical Corps as a first lieutenant or face being conscripted as an infantry private.[88] He quickly volunteered. Once in uniform, Ledley spent the vast majority of his time alone and aloof. Socially and intellectually, he felt out of place in the Medical Corps because most of his colleagues had followed a very different trajectory to that point. Typically, they were at least a decade older than him and had served in World War II. Many were bitter that the medical education they had pursued under the GI Bill had made them eligible once again for the draft, this time as physicians. Almost none of the military doctors shared his interest in cutting-edge mathematics or physics.

Ledley was further isolated after basic training, when he drew an especially plum assignment and consequently was ostracized by envious Medical Corps colleagues.[89] The Medical Corps, it turned out, was looking for a dentist who knew enough physics to help improve dentures in order to alleviate the military's chronic—and massively expensive—problems related to dental health. Hence, instead of being sent to Asia, Ledley was stationed at Walter Reed Hospital in Washington, DC, where he was assigned to help the military build better dentures. His first task there was to determine where contemporary dentures were failing, which he did by devising a two-surface-slope model to measure the "angle of chew." He found that if this angle was not accurately determined in each patient when fitting dentures, then they would loosen under the force of daily chewing.[90] He also built several models of dental pressure (that is, tooth grinding and gnashing). Ledley's models were a hit at Walter Reed because they were accurate and effectively conveyed information about the problem at hand. His work even caught the attention of the Associated Press. The *Los Angeles Times*, which carried the AP article under the title "Mathematics Now Protects False Teeth," reported that "Lt. R.S. Ledley . . . had worked out a mathematical formula expressing the direction of chewing forces" and hailed the breakthrough as a boon to the dentists who were "fitting approximately 1,500,000 sets of false teeth every year."[91] This success led to other modeling assignments related to medical prosthetics, including an attempt to create an artificial heart valve.[92] Much of his time at Walter Reed (1950–52), however, Ledley idled, sitting at an empty desk, fastidiously avoiding new assignments—"in the Army you learned never to volunteer," Ledley explained. He passed the days reading physics and mathematics journals, and he retrospectively noted that the voluminous bibliographies that accompanied many of his early articles and textbooks owed their existence to two years of devoting his entire workweek to almost nothing but reading.[93]

After being discharged from the Army in 1952, Ledley found a research job at the Dental Materials Section of the National Bureau of Standards (now the National Institute of Standards and Technology), in Maryland, where he began working with computers. While at the NBS, Ledley became interested in the organization's new electronic digital computer, the Standards Eastern Automatic Computer (SEAC), which like EDSAC had been modeled after the plans for EDVAC. Ledley's arrival at the NBS was fortuitously timed because in the early 1950s the NBS was uniquely situated to serve as a hub for the development of computers and techniques for their use. Further, the NBS, under pressure to implement and make good use of SEAC and under limited oversight, was also a place where mobility was high.[94] Seeking to get his foot in the already somewhat open door of the SEAC operation, Ledley secured a programming job for his wife of several years, Terry, who had a master's degree in mathematics from Queens College. Once employed, she made a habit of bringing home programs (in the form of perforated paper tapes) and manuals for her husband to study.[95] After teaching himself the basics of SEAC's operations from the materials his wife had brought to him, Ledley began to spend more and more time in the building that housed SEAC under the pretext of learning new methods to improve his dental models. He quickly proved an adept programmer and troubleshooter and soon found himself working with SEAC almost full time and on a wide variety of tasks. Many of these tasks had nothing to do with dentistry—his first major project was to develop a remote-controlled aircraft guidance system.

For Ledley, few routes to mastering the operations of modern digital computing could have been more effective than to have undertaken the programming of the SEAC, one of the earliest high-speed computers in which programs were stored digitally in the machine's memory. Comparable to EDSAC in terms of design, speed, and difficulty to operate, SEAC initially had nothing in the way of a "front-end" of higher-level languages that would allow the user to design and run programs without needing to know the function of most components of the machine's hardware. Thus, as Ledley learned to operate SEAC, he was also becoming intimately familiar with what such a machine could accomplish and the exact limitations of what could be expressed on it.

Ledley began to grasp the unique challenges life sciences problems posed to those who wanted to use digital computers when he tried to use spare run time on SEAC to create simulations of his dental pressure models. He quickly found that the bottleneck lay not so much in encoding the models but in the prerequisite process of conceptualizing the models in such a form that they could be communicated to the machine. Ledley found that any component of the model that could not be expressed as an equation had to be discarded, but he also realized that SEAC's processing power afforded him the luxury of including an enormous volume of simple equations in his model.[96]

In the course of Ledley's struggle to prepare the dental pressure models for computerization, he had an epiphany concerning both the direction of his career and the potential importance of computers to biomedical research. He remembered, "I had previously realized that although, conceptually, physics equations could be written to describe any biomedical phenomenon, such equations would be so complex that they could not feasibly be solved in closed form. Thus SEAC would be my panacea, because the equations would become tractable to numerical methods of solutions. Or so I truly believed at the time. That was to be my field, application of computers to biomedical problems."[97] Ledley had found his calling, but it would be another five years before he would pursue it in earnest.

Following the completion of his dentistry-related work at NBS, Ledley found full-time employment with the SEAC group. There he became interested in the systematic design of logic circuits. In the course of trying to come up with a calculus for logical circuit design, he realized that some of his proposed solutions were also applicable to military intelligence problems.[98] The product of this insight was an article in the journal *Operations Research* on a "digital logic machine" that instructed military planners how to use Boolean algebra to construct truth tables in order to clarify logistics decisions, determine how an enemy would act under certain circumstances, and reduce the writings of military theorists such as Clausewitz to their most precise form: a series of yes or no questions and contingent answers.[99]

Unlike Kendrew, who had been active in the area ten to fifteen years earlier, Ledley was working within OR as a formalized field. Nevertheless, the two men were both preoccupied with organization and both clearly worked under the premise that the military could overcome many of the complexities of war by mathematically formalizing decision-making processes. Moreover, Ledley's analysis echoed Kendrew's in that he called for the military to implement his suggestions to express their planning procedures in such a manner that they could be processed by a "logic machine."[100] It is unclear what the Pentagon made of Ledley's proposal to computerize military planning, but a civilian reviewer, Raymond J. Nelson, writing in *The Journal of Symbolic Logic* in 1955, found "an appallingly wide gap between what, as Ledley says, is computable in principle . . . and what can in fact be done technically." Furthermore, Nelson attacked Ledley's paper for mixing algebraic and logical terms as well as abandoning "mathematical computer theory" for an "algebraically oriented approach," which he found "irrelevant to these problems (except, of course, that the logician is free to use any mathematical conceptions in his metalogic which he explicitly permits himself)."[101]

When the Eisenhower administration cut the budget for the NBS in 1954, Ledley was among the many researchers who lost their jobs there.[102] Most of Ledley's colleagues who were involved in computer design were hired en masse by IBM, but Ledley opted to further pursue his interest in OR, eventually landing a job as an "Operations Research Analyst" at the Strategic Division of the Operations Research Office at Johns Hopkins University.[103] His very military-oriented job description there outlined his responsibilities as including "supervision of mathematical aspects and programming and coding of operation (war) gaming" and the "development of a logical format for operational gaming that aids the formulation of a game and the use of computers of gaming and simulation. Practical application of these methods to Civil Defense games, Defense of the Continental U.S. games, Communication Queuing games, etc."[104]

Ledley did not stay away from the life sciences for long, though. Shortly after arriving at Johns Hopkins, he met George Gamow, who had by then joined up with the Delbrück clique centered at Caltech, and who subsequently brought Ledley into the RNA Tie Club. A close inspection of Ledley's work in this area reveals that he was not so much trying to actually decrypt DNA's code as he was trying to describe it and devise efficient means to work with it given very limited information about its structure and content. In a 1955 *Proceedings of the National Academy of Sciences* article titled "Digital Computational Methods in Symbolic Logic, with Examples in Biochemistry," Ledley described what he saw as the challenge posed by DNA. He began with Gamow's assumption that there was a "one-to-one correspondence between the 20 amino acids and the 20 hypothetical triplets of bases," noting that "since there are 20! = 2.3×10^{17} such one-to-one correspondences (which equals the number of seconds in the age of the universe), the straightforward test of all possibilities is out of the question." As Ledley explained, even the fastest conceivable computers in the early 1950s were not up to the task of trying every possible combination: "To try 20! solutions, a computer put to work in the days of the Roman Empire, at the rate of one million solutions per second, 24 hours a day, all year round, would not yet be close to finishing the job."[105]

The next step, Ledley proposed, would be "to find a systematic and feasible procedure for solving the problem (with the aid of high-speed electronic computing machines)."[106] To reduce the number of possibilities to a number that could reasonably be processed by available equipment, Ledley proposed that scientists create schemes that would only require on the order of a few hundred hours' computation on the best electronic digital computers. Although he suggested no rules of chemistry that could help DNA decoders to eliminate possibilities he did provide a template, based directly on his earlier OR work for the Army, which would allow them to express their schemes in the most succinct manner possible. Just as he instructed the military intelligence analysts and war gamers, Ledley called for DNA decoders to articulate the problem in terms of a series of true/false statements (Boolean algebra). Given the complexity of the coding problem, traditional approaches to thinking about scientific problems would not suffice. He explained, "In such a complex situation the ordinary simple logical analysis usually used in experimental science is found inadequate. In these cases the logical computational methods . . . can be extremely useful for evaluating experimental results as well as for planning future experiments to yield the maximum information."[107]

After setting forth his OR-inspired approach to studying DNA, Ledley

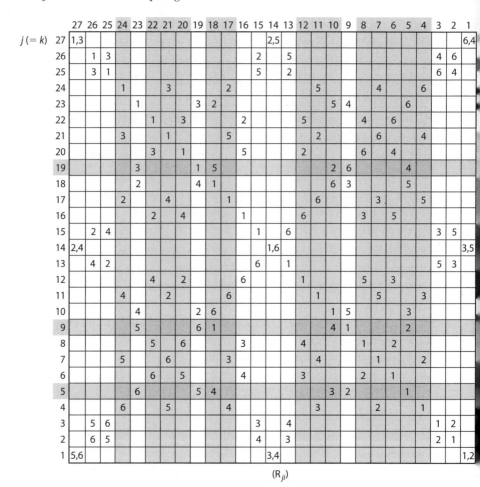

(R_{ji})

Fig. 1.4. Ledley's RNA encoding matrix. This matrix could just as easily be used to describe contingencies in war games. Robert S. Ledley, "Digital Computational Methods in Symbolic Logic, with Examples in Biochemistry," *Proceedings of the National Academy of Sciences* 41 (July 1955): 505 (fig. 2). By permission of the National Biomedical Research Foundation

devoted the bulk of his article to explaining the processes by which scientists could translate their proposed RNA encoding schemes into arrays modeled after the one shown in figure 1.4. The matrix represents how $3^3 = 27$ conditions (that is, amino acids) could be generated from $3! = 6$ possible configurations of a triplet in a simplified world where there were only three types of bases, which, in turn, generated only three types of amino acids. One advantage of the array, Ledley argued, was that it treated data just as computers could readily be prepared to do. All combinations, including those impossibly generated by one or two bases instead of the required three, were entertained, and were only eliminated if the user explicitly instructed the computer to do so.

The other advantage Ledley saw in employing such arrays is that it would be no more difficult to consider coding problems if it transpired that amino acids were not generated by the proposed scheme involving contiguous triplets. The Boolean approach would seem onerous for those who wanted to catalog the possibilities of the standard triplet encoding scheme:

$$-\underbrace{1-3-4}_{E}-\underbrace{3-2-3}_{M}-$$

but it could just as easily work with less straightforward schemes whereby amino acids were generated by overlapping triplets:

$$-\underbrace{1-3-4}_{E}-\underbrace{3}_{A}-\underbrace{2-3-3}_{M}-$$

or restrictive schemes where certain combinations (N) were not allowed:

$$-\underbrace{1-3}_{E}\overbrace{-4-3}^{N}-\underbrace{2}_{A}$$

or even schemes in which the sequences of triplets that generated amino acids were both overlapping *and* noncontiguous:[108]

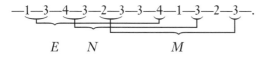

Ledley had provided the Tie Club with a powerful conceptual tool, but it is likely that much of his intended audience of biophysicists could not surmount the prerequisite knowledge of symbolic logic (and the Boolean algebraic methods needed to work with that logic). Gamow, at least, did not seriously entertain many of the possible encoding schemes Ledley proposed and instructed him to proceed as if the simple, non-overlapping, consecutive triplet scheme reflected how nature worked.[109] Consequently, Ledley wrote a program that would generate a list of possible base/amino-acid combinations depending on which amino acids the user paired with particular sets of triplets. In the fall of 1954, Gamow reported to Watson that Ledley had "completed the details of [an] automatic decoding procedure, by means of symbolic logic equations," which Gamow sent to Los Alamos to be run on MANIAC (Mathematical Analyzer, Numerical Integrator, and Computer), an early electronic digital computer based on von Neumann's plans that was primarily used to carry out calculations related to the development of the hydrogen bomb.[110] The program required several days of continuous running, but it did not provide Gamow the means to decipher the genetic code.

In 1955 Gamow and Ledley drifted apart. After Ledley's program failed to crack the genetic code, Gamow gave up on operations research techniques in favor of a statistically oriented approach to using computers to crack the code of life. Having accepted the premise that the Tie Club was working with a comma-less, non-overlapping code, Gamow now faced the problem of distinguishing consecutive triplets that occurred consecutively along the sequence of nucleic acid bases. Working with Martin Yčas, Gamow again turned to Los Alamos, conducting thousands of runs on MANIAC to determine whether or not patterns of nucleotide triplets could be distinguished statistically from randomness.[111] This approach too failed, and the code was not deciphered until the early 1960s, when Marshall Nirenberg, working with Heinrich Matthaei at the National Institutes of Health, used radioactive labels to identify which RNA triplets coded for particular amino acids. Nirenberg and Matthaei used traditional experimental laboratory techniques, not computers.

After Ledley parted ways with the RNA Tie Club, he maintained his interest in applying computer technology to problems in molecular biology. In 1959, Ledley requested a grant from the National Institutes of Health to use two of SEAC's descendents, the Florida Automatic Computer (FLAC) I and II, to set up a "Computational Center" at George Washington University. Part of the center's mission, he proposed, would be to "explore the application of digital-computer techniques as a significant aid for determining the amino acids and sequences of proteins." Ledley's plan was to examine and optimize Frederick Sanger's painstaking methods of determining the amino acid sequence of the protein insulin—Sanger had just been awarded the Nobel Prize in 1958 for his work on insulin at Cambridge University. As Ledley saw it, Sanger's method had two components: "(1) the chemical identification of peptides isolated from various hydrolyzed fractions of the protein in is question, and (2) the logical analysis of such results to piece together the entire sequence of amino acids in the protein." Ledley believed that computers could be used to "simplify the chemical methods by making the logical analysis bear more of the burden, and to expedite the analysis of proteins."[112]

From Ledley's perspective, as researchers examined ever-larger proteins, the logical component of amino acid sequencing was growing too complex for them to handle. With each additional amino acid the number of possible configurations increased geometrically. This, in turn, produced more possible models than could ever be chemically tested in a reasonable amount of time and with a reasonable amount of money. The largest protein sequenced at the time, ribonuclease, had 124 amino acids, but the bulk of proteins of significant biological and medical interest were considerably larger.

Ledley's solution to this problem was to relieve humans of the logical analysis component of protein sequencing. This entailed studying Sanger's logical methods for determining sequence order and reducing them to a set of rules and procedures that could be expressed as a computer program. The process had three stages. First, "Previous work on protein analysis will be studied, and rules for analysis of the experimental results will be extracted in a form precise enough for computer programming." Second, he proposed, "These rules will be tested on the computer, by means of experimental data already reported in the literature, to determine if they are adequate. If they are not, further analysis of previous work will be carried out." Finally, "When a set of adequate rules is produced, it will be tried on the analysis of proteins not previously reported on, and on proteins of which only fragmentary knowledge exists. It is expected that as more experience is gained, more details and subtleties can be incorporated into the computer program."[113]

Besides automating logical analysis, computerization would, according to Ledley, help to improve the benchwork component of sequencing. He explained, "The use of a computer to analyze results may allow for significant simplification and further systematization of the chemical laboratory procedures by placing more of the burden on the analysis of the chemical results and less on the experimental processes required."[114] The fruits of computerization would be twofold. In the near term, it would enable researchers to "extend the current chemical analytic methods of determining amino-acid sequences of proteins to much larger proteins than have presently been approached." More broadly, by expressing the analytic methods of successful sequencers as computer code, these methods could be reproduced anywhere a compatible computer was available. Indeed Ledley saw the computerization of sequencing as a world-changing project, predicting, "If the computer aid proves successful, the computer program developed by this study can then be used by investigators throughout the nation and the world."[115]

As it turned out, in late 1959 the NIH rejected Ledley's proposal to build a computing center, and therefore Ledley's plans to computerize amino acid sequencing went unfunded. Mostly this seems to have been a consequence of bad timing. At that point, the NIH remained divided over the applicability of computers to biomedical problems (see chapter 2), and Ledley's plans to use the only two-of-a-kind FLACs were incompatible with the agency's preference for more widely-used IBM computers.

From War Games to the Ledley-Lusted Vision of Computerized Biomedicine

Ledley's attempts to decode and sequence amino acids, though intimately connected to the major theoretical challenges facing the nascent field of molecular biology, were not his only focus during the mid-1950s. He directed much of his considerable energy to military-related projects related to his job at the Johns Hopkins University's Operations Research Office. There, his official task was to apply OR techniques to military problems, and he published several internal memoranda discussing war gaming and refining logical and mathematical techniques for military uses. Nonclassified examples include "A Systematic Logical Format for Operational Games Requiring Human Decisions," Operations Research Office (Hopkins) Staff Memorandum S-516, 5 May 1955; and "Computational Methods in Symbolic Logic: A New Methodology in Operations Research," *JHU Seminar in Operations Research*, Paper No. 17, 1954–55. Ledley's focus remained on the organization of operational knowledge and information, specifically on the development of simulations as problem-solving tools, and the theme unifying his work was that computers could be used to address problems posed by OR. His goal, as expressed in a 1956 Operations Research Society talk, was to establish that computer-enabled "operational simulation (also called operational gaming or war gaming) appears in many instances to be the only method available for solving certain highly complicated operations-research decision problems." He further claimed that the "simulation" approach "promises to become an important operations research method in many fields of industry, government, and science."[116] He explained that the format of each operational simulation (game) had three objectives: (1) "help the translation of an intuitive game concept into specific events;" (2) "aid the formulation of each event by isolating from other events;" and (3) "present the completely compiled game in a format best suited for playing on a high-speed computer."[117] He also coauthored several papers related to war gaming that were classified.

Ledley's preoccupation, however, was still to apply operations research techniques to biology and medicine. In June 1956, he gave two papers in this area at the Operations Research Society's Fourth Annual Meeting in Washington, DC.[118] The first conference talk, "Operational Simulation in Medicine," was a general pitch to encourage others to bring operational research methods, particularly operational simulations, to bear on life science problems. In this case, he argued that the same kinds of simulations he had proposed to the military for war gaming were appropriate for life sciences as well: "The methodology of operational simulation seems ideally suited for application to the analysis of many complicated and highly involved phenomena that occur so frequently in medicine and biology."[119] Pointing to the "regulation of the heart and circulation of the blood" as an example of a complex biological phenomenon that had eluded comprehensive modeling, Ledley argued that "when the formulation of such a simulation is aided by a systematic format . . . and the computations are performed on a high-speed electronic computer, the consideration of these phenomena becomes entirely feasible." Thus, Ledley continued, by coupling OR techniques with computers, "these complicated biological phenomena with all their detailed feedbacks, interactions, and special considerations can be studied as entire entities."[120]

In his second paper presented at the 1956 ORS annual meeting, "Logical Aid to Systematic Medical Diagnosis," Ledley provided an example of the methods he had proposed by demonstrating a scheme to use McBee needle-sorted edge-notched cards to enable doctors to economize the "logical sorting and combinatorial analysis necessary to deduce the disease associated with a combination of symptoms." His system was straightforward. As he described it, "A McBee sort card is associated with a disease and appropriately punched according to symptoms. By successive sorts on symptoms, a deck of such disease cards can be reduced to one or several cards, thus aiding in proper diagnosis."[121] Ledley described how he "even made a little device for facilitating the shaking and dropping of the cards," and he recalled that "as I carried this deck and my device around the halls . . . it didn't take the physicists"—that is, the physicists who were Ledley's coworkers at the Johns Hopkins Operations Research Office—"more than a fraction of a second to say to me, 'Oh, you're going to automate medical diagnosis, huh?' "[122] Anticipating physicians' fears of being replaced by computers, he cautioned, "It is to be emphasized that such a system is merely an aid to medical diagnosis and is not a mechanical substitute for experience, skill, judgment and insight."[123]

Ledley's talks on OR applications in biomedicine were enthusiastically received but generated no concrete projects. Nevertheless, there emerged at the conference a small core of researchers dedicated to exporting OR to the life sciences. Most exciting to Ledley was a paper by William J. Horvath, of Airborne Instruments Laboratory, Inc. of Mineola, New York, titled "An Operations-Research View of Medicine and Health," in which the author drew a parallel between the military problems OR had been devised to solve and challenges of optimizing medical practices. As Horvath put it, "Strategic problems in medicine, dealing generally with the distribution of effort in different areas, generally suffer from the same uncertainties of sub-optimization and inadequate definition of goals and objectives as the analogous military problems."[124]

Horvath, it transpired, was tremendously excited by Ledley's vision of OR-inspired computerized biology and medicine, but he did not know enough about computers or mathematics to seriously consider making a career of implementing these ideas. Horvath did, however, have a younger colleague at AIL, radiologist Lee B. Lusted, whose interests he believed strongly complemented those of Ledley. Thus, in the summer of 1956, just a few weeks after the ORS conference, Ledley received a telephone call "out of the blue" from Lusted, sparking off a collaboration that would find both men at the center of efforts to computerize biology and medicine for years to come.

Like Kendrew and Ledley, Lee Browning Lusted (1922–1994) came to computing via military research. As an undergraduate at Cornell College, in Mount Vernon, Iowa, during World War II, Lusted participated in an accelerated physics and mathematics program designed for draft-eligible science majors.[125] Upon his graduation in 1943, Lusted was recruited to a team that was developing radar and radar countermeasures at Frederick Terman's Harvard University Radio Research Laboratory (RRL). Prior to joining the RRL, Lusted had no experience in electronics or engineering principles, but by war's end he had acquired considerable expertise through night courses, lectures, and mainly "tutoring at the work bench." His specific tasks included installing radar in P-38 fighter planes to detect rocket launches and reverse-engineering captured German Würzburg FuSE 62 anti-aircraft gun-directing mobile radar units.[126]

When the war concluded, Lusted had trouble finding an outlet for his interdisciplinary interests. The solution, he decided, was medicine, and in 1946 he began his training at Harvard Medical School. At this point, despite his years of conducting research for the military, he remained eligible for the draft. Thus, to ensure that conscription would not interfere with his education he volunteered for a reserve commission in the US Public Health Service (PHS). By the early 1950s, Lusted had become a radiology specialist and was based in the San Francisco area. He was also active in the Institute of Radio Engineers (IRE—now called the Institute of Electrical and Electronic Engineers, or IEEE) Group on Medical Electronics, based in Palo Alto. Although he was keeping abreast of electronics and computer developments, he was still unable to bring these interests together. Looking back on this period from 1987, Lusted recalled, "I felt that medical data could be processed by computer and that medical information could be made more useful to physicians by repackaging it in a more usable form. I wasn't sure how this could be done, but the idea of making information more useful by making it more usable stuck with me."[127]

Lusted planned to pursue a career in academic radiology in California, but as was the case with Ledley, the prospect of conscription forced him to take a new direction. In late 1955, the PHS sent him a letter offering the following choice: he could serve two years on active duty for them or he could give up his commission and be subject to the "doctor draft." Lusted opted to serve the PHS and in so doing found himself on a trajectory that would bring him to the heart of the NIH's efforts to introduce computer technology to the life sciences. Assigned to the Radiation Department at the NIH Clinical Center in Bethesda, Maryland, he had found his official duties to be rather light; it only took him a few hours per day to report on his fluoroscopic examinations, leaving him with ample time "to explore other NIH opportunities." Namely he began talking to people at the NIH about his interest in electronics and computers, and consulting for companies that were trying to build electronic devices for use by NIH clinics and labs.[128]

Lusted began his first major endeavor in biomedical electronics in early 1956, when he served as a consultant for Airborne Instruments Laboratory (AIL), which was developing an instrument called the Cytoanalyzer to perform mass screening of cytological smears for the detection of cervical cancer.[129] AIL was building the device to address a shortfall in the number of clinicians who were trained in the then-esoteric Papanicolaou method of analyzing cytological smears. Lusted and his AIL colleagues believed that by automating much of the arithmetic work of medical workers who could reliably interpret Pap smears, the Cytoanalyzer could potentially save many lives. While helping to develop the Cytoanalyzer, Lusted saw the interface of cutting-edge electronics with cutting-edge science, leading him to think broadly about how computers could improve medicine. Lusted regarded machines like the Cytoanalyzer as a boon, but he found that they did not address what he had conceived as the core problem plaguing medical practice, namely that physicians trying to diagnose a disease were usually unable to implement new research findings and techniques because they were overwhelmed by too much information.[130]

The surfeit of knowledge, Lusted reasoned, was largely responsible for the lack of a comprehensive, universal system of medical diagnosis. Evoking the Rockefeller Foundation's Alan Gregg, Lusted later articulated the problem and its computerized solution. He wrote, "[Gregg] once noted that 'the great task in medicine and public health today is to make use of the immense store of knowledge accumulated in the past eight decades, and particularly in the past two or three. So much more might be done than is being done.' There is good reason to believe that automatic data processing can help the physician with this great task."[131] Essentially, Lusted sought to distill the knowledge of symptoms and diseases that underlay diagnosis—many parts of which were only accessible to or comprehensible by specialists—into a form so basic and general that any physician could use it to assign the logical aspects of the labor of diagnosis to computers.

Lusted shared his thoughts on the potential of computers in medicine with others at the NIH who were interested in computer technology, including the agency's head, James Shannon. But Lusted's ruminations did not lead to action until William Horvath, one of his Cytoanalyzer collaborators at AIL, drew his attention to Robert Ledley's 1956 talks to the Operations Research Society.[132] After making several phone calls, Lusted tracked down Ledley at the Johns Hopkins OR Office and arranged a meeting at the NIH. As Lusted remembered, they immediately recognized each other as kindred sprits: "We found that we had been thinking about similar problems and possible solutions. The problems were caused by the large and increasing volume of medical literature. The possible solutions involved mathematical and computational aids for the physician."[133]

Thus began a decade of intensive collaboration, one that brought both men to center of efforts to formalize medical diagnosis and to computerize the life sciences. In 1957 Lusted and Ledley began their first major joint project: working out the details of computerizing diagnosis. Ledley explains their motivation: "The idea of using computers to assist in medicine had, of course, been discussed from time to time by many people, but a specific idea of how to go about it had not been published."[134] The main challenge they faced was that of how to formalize the process of medical diagnosis to the point where it could be computerized. Broadly, their plan was to develop Lusted's "logic of diagnosis" with the intent of building a computerized medicine around that logical base. To get physicians to work with vast amounts of medical data within the framework of the "logic of diagnosis," Ledley and Lusted sought to equip them with the tools and techniques for information management developed in OR.

After several months of informal discussions, they began with what they believed most fundamental: introducing mathematical rigor to the process of diagnosis. In 1958, Ledley suggested to Lusted that Bayes' theorem, which is used to determine inverse probabilities, for instance, if one knows the conditional probability of B (for example, a disease) given A (for example, a symptom), then what is the conditional probability of A (a symptom) given B (a disease)? The theorem, which had been popular among operations researchers for its utility in establishing posterior possibilities, could be used to transform much of the guesswork in medical diagnosis into formal procedures. In particular, Ledley and Lusted "hoped that Bayes' theorem would be used to study the conditional independence of signs and symptoms for a given disease."[135] In short, they sought to turn on its head the way physicians diagnosed a patient's condition. "We observed," Lusted recollected in a 1991 autobiographical essay, "that medical knowledge was usually presented as symptoms associated with a disease, rather than the reverse, that is the diseases associated with a symptom. In probability terms we said medical knowledge should be expressed as the probability of a disease given the patient's symptoms." "This information," Ledley and Lusted argued, "is what the physician needs to know for the diagnosis of a particular patient's condition, and Bayes' theorem . . . could be used to convert medical textbook knowledge to a form applicable to an individual patient." By "reordering" medical knowledge in this way, Lusted "hoped to make it more useful and more useable to the physician."[136]

For Ledley and Lusted, using Bayes' theorem was but one part of bringing order to "the complicated reasoning processes inherent in medical diagnosis." This, in turn, they saw as a necessary step toward their ultimate goal of computerizing medicine. To give physicians the conceptual tools they needed to break down their diagnostic practices to the point where they could be computerized, Ledley and Lusted attempted to teach them OR techniques for studying complex systems. They published their ideas on the application of OR techniques to medicine in a July 3, 1959, *Science* article, "Reasoning Foundations of Medical Diagnosis," which served as a crash course, grounded in medical examples, in symbolic logic, probability (including Bayes' theorem), and value theory.

As part of building this "reasoning foundation," Ledley and Lusted introduced physicians to operations researchers' mechanical techniques for organizing information. For example, they showed physicians how to make a system of marginal notched cards, modeled after Ledley's 1956 demonstration to the Operations Research Society, to store and sort information on patients and symptoms (fig. 1.5).[137] The exercise showed that when physicians collected enough cards—perhaps as little as a few dozen—they could use their card collections to visualize the probability of a patient having a particular ailment, given some combination of symptoms and circumstances.

Ledley and Lusted's article was, in terms of reprints and citations, a "best-seller."[138] Within months of its publication, reprint requests ran into the thousands; and the article was translated into Russian in 1961. Published reader reactions reveal that the article also generated considerable controversy. The first area of contention involved "the appropriateness and acceptability to the medical profession of computer-aided diagnosis." Ledley and Lusted had been careful in the article to clarify that computers would not supplant physicians, noting "[our] method in no way implies that a computer can take over the physician's duties. Quite the reverse; it implies that the physician's task may become more complicated."[139] Nevertheless, *Science* received letters, such as that by Robert G. Hoffman, complaining that computers represented a threat to the "interpersonal relationship between the physician and patient."[140]

A second "area of controversy" the article generated pertained to the "appropriate use of Bayes' theorem in computer-aided medical diagnosis." While preparing their article, Ledley and Lusted had been undeterred by the widespread criticism of Bayes' theorem as a diagnostic tool. The chief complaint they faced was that the theorem assumes that all variables and parameters are known and fixed.[141] Lusted, retrospectively surveying the crux of the matter, claimed, "Critics pointed out that use of the theorem required that disease attributes should be conditionally independent, that diseases should be mutually exclusive, and that the disease list should be complete."[142] In medical practice such conditions were usually not met, and therefore there were credible fears that using computers could "lead to a perpetuation of errors."[143] Such doubts, according to Edward A. Feigenbaum (see chapter 5), who developed MYCIN, a medical

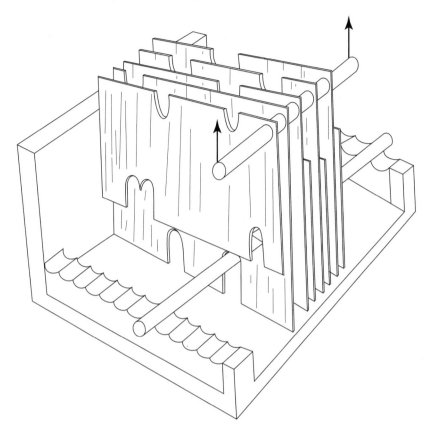

Fig. 1.5. A sketch of Ledley's mechanism for sorting marginal notched cards. Robert S. Ledley and Lee B. Lusted, "Reasoning Foundations of Medical Diagnosis," *Science* 130 (July 1959): 20 (fig. 13). By permission of the National Biomedical Research
Foundation

diagnosis expert system based on backward-chaining logic, likely prevented the
proliferation of computerized Bayesian diagnostic systems in clinical settings.[144]

Despite the criticism, the 1960s and 1970s brought several prominent studies—ones with access to relatively complete sets of data—that implemented
systems following Ledley and Lusted's suggestions. The best known was led by
Homer R. Warner, a University of Utah physician and cardiology researcher,
who used Ledley and Lusted's Bayesian methods to devise a scheme for diagnosing congenital heart disease.[145] Warner recalled, "I read an article in *Science*
by Ledley and Lusted that suggested using a conditional probability approach

to modeling the way a physician thinks. At the time, we [at the Latter Day Saints Hospital, Salt Lake City] had lots of patients coming through our laboratory who had congenital heart disease, and we began systematically collecting data on the incidence of history and physical findings that were obtained before catheterization revealed the ultimate diagnosis."

Emulating the models Ledley and Lusted had shown in their article, Warner's group "accumulated a data matrix by asking each physician who referred a case for study to fill out a checklist as to what the manifestations were." Once they had accumulated enough data to perform robust statistical analyses, Warner and his colleagues compared the "computer diagnosis using Bayes's theorem to what the physicians thought the diagnosis was before they sent the case in." The remarkable outcome was that "the computer outperformed all but one of the physicians, most of whom only occasionally saw a patient with congenital heart disease."[146]

Within a few years, Warner implemented a history-taking Bayesian diagnostic system, which was used on almost every patient entering the hospital for elective surgery. For elective surgery patients, the primary problem was already known, but Warner hoped the computerized screening would "pick up secondary problems."[147] By the mid-1960s, following the success of the system at Latter-Day Saints Hospital in Salt Lake City, a similar Bayesian system was set up in at a children's hospital in Kiel, Germany. Another study, which did not come to fruition until the early 1970s but that generated widely used computer diagnostic programs in Latin America, was led by a Brazilian researcher, F. T. de Dombal, and concerned the diagnosis of abdominal pain.[148]

Ledley and Lusted's work also drew popular attention. In July 1959, the *New York Times* ran an article about the authors' understanding of how medical diagnosis worked and could be improved. "Many doctors," the *Times* reported, "now believe that most errors in diagnosis result from omission rather than any other source. That is, the doctor simply overlooks a possibility." According to the *Times*, Ledley and Lusted's solution to this problem was to devise a scheme, "which could assure the doctor that every possibility will be dug out of the 'metal brains' of the computer. The machine would eliminate all diseases that are unrelated to the unknown disease." The logic behind their plan, the paper relayed, was grounded in their belief that "medical diagnosis consists of three ingredients: medical knowledge, signs and symptoms from the patient himself, and logical reasoning." The "medical knowledge" and the "logical reasoning" components of diagnosis, Ledley and Lusted argued, could be managed by electronic computers. In the face of the prospect of computers performing two-thirds of diagnosis, the article assured its readers that Ledley and Lusted did not envision to replacing doctors with computers. Instead, the two men saw computerized diagnostics as a way of "leaving the doctor free to concentrate on the important intangible decisions concerning the patient's condition."[149]

To convey his and Lusted's ideas about diagnosis, Ledley built a demonstration device that one reporter from the *New York World Telegram* called "A Metal Brain for Diagnosis."[150] The electromechanical "brain," which was built into a two-by-five-foot plywood and glass box, enabled users to diagnose diseases of the tongue by choosing combinations of symptoms. To enter a symptom, the user would press a cash-register key that corresponded to the symptom. Depending on which combination of symptoms was entered—that is, which combination of keys were pressed—the light boxes corresponding to various tongue-related maladies would turn on or off. When several symptoms were entered, usually just one light—one disease—out of the 48 possibilities would be offered as a possible diagnosis. When an "impossible" combination of diseases was selected, a special box with the message "THIS CONDITION IS NOT CLINI-CALLY POSSIBLE" would light up.

Even more widespread media attention came in November 1959, when the Associated Press, while covering the annual meeting of the Operations Research Society in Pasadena, California, highlighted Ledley and Lusted's talk there on computerized medicine. The *New York Post*'s rather sensational version of the article, titled, "Dr. Univac Wanted in Surgery," began, "The day will come sooner than you think when improper diagnosis and treatment of human ills will be virtually impossible. The latest research, which now sifts down through scientific journals to doctors who sometimes are too busy to read them, will be at your physician's fingertips." Pointing to Ledley and Lusted's talk, the *Post* predicted that "this Utopian world will come about through the use of the 'black boxes' known popularly as electronic brains."[151] Ledley and Lusted explained that "you will walk into your doctor's office and tell him your symptoms. He will feed this information, plus all he knows about you into an electronic data coding machine." In the future, read the article, "He [the physician] must learn how to communicate with the computer and how to evaluate the information obtained from it." The article's only caveat was that when it came to the question of when such a system would be ready, "No one is ready to pin down the date."[152]

Within the medical press, Ledley and Lusted's analysis of the future role of computers in medicine took a more sober tone. In the same month as the AP coverage of Ledley and Lusted that led to the *New York Post* article, November 1959, the *American Medical Association News* reported that "the optimistic view on cost cutting with computers is not shared in full by Robert S. Ledley." Rather, quoting Ledley, the AMA noted that "[computers'] prime advantage is that they can make possible advances in medical research and application that would otherwise have been impossible. It is certain that computers will bring better and more uniform medical care to more people."[153] Also in 1959, *Scope Weekly*, a newspaper produced by the Physicians News Service, ran a piece about Ledley and Lusted titled, "Electronic Computer to Complicate Task of MD," pointing out the immense amount of training most physicians would need in order to effectively use computers. "In addition to the knowledge he presently needs," Ledley was quoted as saying, "the physician will have to know more about the methods and techniques of computing mathematical probabilities and the laws of logic before he can make full use of the electronic gadgets."[154]

As professional and popular interest in "Reasoning Foundations" grew, so did Ledley and Lusted's ambitions to introduce more OR techniques to biology and medicine. Thus far, they had neglected a crucial aspect of OR, optimizing communication, but that changed in early 1960 when they issued a call in the journal *Operations Research* to build a "health computing system" for the purpose of coordinating medical care and research at the national level. Outlining a "network," (fig. 1.6) they imagined a system that would first gather data from healthcare locales nationwide via regional computers and then relay the data to a massive computer at a central research facility. Within a local network, "each computer would communicate with individual physicians and hospitals within its area, receiving, transmitting, and computing medical information as required." Each of the local networks had at its hub a large computer, which they called an "area computer," that would serve as a clearinghouse for medical information. However, the local networks were not isolated, because potential patients living in a highly mobile society do not confine themselves to a particular region at all times—Ledley and Lusted noted that "20% of the American public change address each year and probably almost all of us go on at least one extended trip each year." Thus, to pass information from one local network to another, the area computers would link together to form a national network, so that the data could follow people all around the country. Besides providing nationally accessible medical records, the information gathered by the network

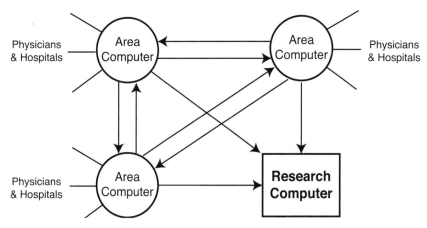

Fig. 1.6. "Outline of a computer network." In Ledley and Lusted's scheme, "each area computer serves the physicians and hospitals in the area and supplies information to other areas and to a central research computer." Robert S. Ledley and Lee B. Lusted, "Computers in Medical Data Processing," *Operations Research* 8, no. 3 (May–June 1960): 309. By permission of the National Biomedical Research Foundation

could be harvested by "a special research computer that can sample data as required, for various research and public-health investigations."[155]

Unfazed by the circumstance that "much research and planning will be necessary before this health computer network can be a reality," Ledley and Lusted argued forcefully that linking health providers' computers would not only be good for science but also the nation and indeed humanity. They insisted that "the great significance of such a health network cannot be overestimated, both as an aid to increasing individual good health and longevity (leading to per capita productivity corresponding to a greater gross national product), and as a vast new source of medical information concerning mankind."[156] To this they added waggishly, "Someone recently observed that we would indeed be living in J. K. Galbraith's 'Affluent Society' if we had a complete central charge service—and this before a central health records service."[157]

Translating the *Operations Research* article for an audience of physicians in 1962, Lusted attempted via an editorial in *Annals of Internal Medicine* to promote among medical practitioners the computer use he advocated. He portrayed computers as weapons to be wielded against what the eminent Mayo Clinic psychiatrist Howard P. Rome had earlier cast as the "four horsemen [who] constantly threaten the practice of a superior type of medicine." These "horse-men," which would later be quite recognizable to anyone following twenty-first-century efforts to reform US healthcare, were: (1) "the relentless pressure of the time available for a complete examination"; (2) "the spiraling tower of cost in money and effort"; (3) "the large number of dependent variables that have to be recognized and then examined for significance"; and (4) "the waning tolerance of the patient's endurance for all of this."[158] By way of addressing these problems, Lusted argued that computer technology could enable physicians to devote more time and resources to patients by automating many aspects of medical diagnosis. As an example he pointed to a pilot study conducted by Hubert V. Pipberger for the Veterans Administration that demonstrated that "automatic analysis of the electrocardiogram is superior to the analysis by conventional means"—in other words, the machines at once outperformed physicians at a routine task and freed their time for challenges that required a human touch.[159]

While Ledley and Lusted were promoting OR techniques in biology and medicine, OR itself was enjoying a golden age of sorts. Its methods were being adopted widely in business and especially by the military. However, by the early 1960s OR came to be overshadowed by the rise of new fields that had adopted many of its techniques, particularly computer science and management consulting.[160] As computing grew in its own right, computer experts and new users alike lost sight of many of the assumptions and ways of thinking in which early electronic computing was grounded. OR's reductive methods and quantitative simulations, two major tools used for recasting a problem in such a way that computers could be brought to bear on it, became standard computing tools. Instead of promoting OR methods themselves, Ledley and Lusted would shift their focus toward promoting the means to pursue those methods: electronic digital computers. In the early 1960s, they would inspire, and in Lusted's case directly lead, the powerful NIH Advisory Committee on Computers in Research (ACCR), steering many millions of federal dollars toward reshaping biology and medicine to realize their vision.

2

Building Tomorrow's Biomedicine

The National Institutes of Health's Early Mission to Computerize Biology and Medicine

To James Shannon, the breakthroughs in Cambridge, England, during the early 1950s were an inspiration. They indicated to him that a productive, new approach to studying life was afoot. At its root, he declared, was "the fact that the research of Watson and Crick on nucleic acid structure and that of Kendrew and Perutz on the three-dimensional structure of proteins had been aided significantly by computational techniques." After becoming director of the NIH in 1955, Shannon made it clear that he hoped the agency would foster similar "computational" triumphs in the United States. Pointing to the digital electronic computer, Shannon voiced his "expectation that this powerful and new technology would not only facilitate the solution of problems as currently formulated, but also, like the telescope, would permit the exploration of phenomena otherwise unapproachable."[1]

During his thirteen-year tenure as director, Shannon would lead the golden age of NIH expansion. From almost the outset, he made computer technology a central component of his ambitious plans for establishing the NIH as the leader of a national push to rationalize and coordinate biomedical research.[2] Within the NIH, however, Shannon's embrace of computers was met with skepticism and hostility. Shannon never overcame the opposition to computing within the NIH but rather circumvented it by drawing resources from beyond the agency. By 1960, the NIH was leading a massive effort to computerize the life sciences notwithstanding the unpopularity of the machines on its main campus. That effort, sponsored by the US Congress and initially led by Lee Lusted, would build on Robert Ledley's operations research approach to using computers to try to propagate a new, mathematized way of investigating life.

The computers in which the NIH initially invested were many orders of magnitude slower than today's computers, and of course they were enormous— often taking up whole buildings and weighing in the tons. They were relatively cumbersome to use because data and instructions had to be prepared on punch cards—output, meanwhile, was printed onto tapes or sheets of paper. Nevertheless, in contrast to the computers used by Kendrew and Ledley, the transistorized "second generation" of general-purpose computers of the late 1950s and early 1960s were significantly faster, more reliable, less expensive, and much easier to program (due to the development of assembly languages and high-level languages like FORTRAN and COBOL) than their vacuum-tube based predecessors.

The computers the NIH purchased or rented starting in the late 1950s were mostly treated as ultra-fast calculators, and were therefore viewed as serving similar functions as adding machines, tabulating machines, and other devices that performed arithmetic operations. This particular approach to using computers opened many avenues of biomedical research but would also for many years restrict most biomedical computing activities to quantitative rather than more broadly logical or symbolic domains. One result, as William F. Raub, who guided NIH efforts to computerize the life sciences during the 1970s, explained during a "confession" he made to a meeting of the Association for Computing Machinery in 1971 was that "too many life scientists associated with our resources hold on to the outdated concept of the computer as a giant calculating device; not enough of them are led to appreciate that it is a powerful symbol manipulator and that arithmetic operations are only one of the many manifestations of this."[3]

It is tempting to regard the NIH's early effort to computerize the life sciences with a knowing smile and attribute to hubris and ignorance its inability, despite the many millions invested in it and despite the zeal with which it was pursued, to bring about the particular transformations its advocates sought. Indeed, by the mid-1960s it was quite evident that the life sciences were not becoming more mathematical and logical just to accommodate computers. However, by introducing computers to so many areas of research and treatment, the NIH would create many opportunities its planners had not foreseen. In trying to realize its vision, the NIH would also profoundly influence the development of computer technology itself, with consequences for almost everyone who has ever used a computer.

Finding a Sponsor for Biomedical Computing

Before 1960, when the NIH became heavily involved in promoting computer technology on its campus and especially among the many external researchers the agency supported, there were very few life scientists using the machines. The work of Kendrew and Perutz or of Ledley and Lusted was exceptional and isolated. Rare attempts to use computers in the life sciences were generally one-off efforts using UNIVACs and a wide variety of one-of-a-kind computers. Most of this research was directly supported by the military, particularly the United States Air Force (USAF), which was also the primary sponsor of the development of computers themselves.

Beyond providing access to computers, the Air Force's role in promoting computer use among life scientists was fairly limited. Nevertheless, as part of its effort to justify its immense research budget, the Air Force did play a significant role in encouraging civilian agencies to invest in biomedical computing. In the mid-1950s, as the USAF came under pressure to economize, it sought to transform its enormous investment in computers into political capital.[4] Its leadership concluded that biomedical computing would be particularly well regarded by the general public. To claim biomedical computing as a success, however, the USAF would need to cultivate its development in the civilian world.

Within the USAF the most vocal agitator for a serious inquiry into "the possibilities of applying computers, or automatic data-rendering machines to medical science" was the Human Factors Division of the Air Research and Development Command (ARDC).[5] As a key sponsor of basic computer research in the United States, the ARDC had by the mid-1950s appropriated "major amounts of national resources for the advancement of computer technology and theory," and its leadership had developed "a conviction" that the Air Force "had an obligation to acquaint the civilian scientific community with information developed for military purposes which would also contribute to the general body of scientific knowledge."[6]

To the ARDC's alarm, there appeared to be few if any life scientists interested in using or even learning how to use computers. Adding to the ARDC's concern was "the enormous rate at which scientific data is piling up," a looming problem that seemingly could only be alleviated by researchers adopting technology that would allow them to manage accumulated data; and there were no signs that life scientists were moving in that direction.[7] ARDC planners attributed biologists' apathy toward computers to their sluggishness to break from the past practices of their discipline, noting that "computers certainly would not have found any application in the traditional descriptive approach to biology." However, as noted in chapter 1, by the mid-1950s the study of life appeared to have reached an unacknowledged junction where computers could be of major utility, one marked by the "increasing use of mathematical concepts such as curve fitting, probability theory, advanced statistics, and model construction."[8] The Air Force also had a political motive to encourage the spread of computers in the life sciences. Wary that the public associated its research with ultimately destructive endeavors like waging nuclear war, the ARDC research directors were, in their own words, "keenly aware of the fact that public funds spent for defense could accrue scientific side-benefits that might have more lasting effect and applications than some of the computer-monitored weapons it has today."[9]

In early 1956 General Thomas S. Power, overall head of the ARDC, directed the Human Factors Division, the group responsible for the health of America's aviators and early astronauts, to set up several informal conferences for the purpose of trying to understand why biologists and medical researchers were so slow to adopt computer technology and to propose means to rectify that situation.[10] The first such conference, described by ARDC researcher Albert W. Hetherington as "a gamble," was held in Baltimore that year and amounted to a speculative discussion between ARDC representatives and Johns Hopkins University researchers on the possibility of introducing biologists to computers. The Air Force's goal in Baltimore was "just to sort of feed the idea into them [biologists] and see how they'd react."[11]

The conference demonstrated that the biologists were enthusiastic about using computers but understood very little about the new technology. Given the amount of effort required to prepare biologists to use computers Hetherington concluded that the Air Force was not equipped for the endeavor of computerizing the life sciences and encouraged the ARDC to muster American civilian institutions interested in the advancement of science. Most willing to help the ARDC was the National Academy of Sciences' National Research

Council (NRC), but the nonprofit group lacked the resources to undertake a major effort. More reluctant, though much more powerful, was the National Institutes of Health.

The NRC and the ARDC attempted to secure NIH support at the January 1957 "Roundtable Conference on a Symposium on the Use of Computers in Biology and Medicine," organized by R. Keith Cannan, head of the NRC's Division of Medical Sciences and the executive director of the NRC's Atomic Bomb Casualty Commission.[12] Far from garnering a commitment from the NIH or even bringing about a conference on biomedical computing, the round-table conference revealed that the NIH was deeply split over the issue of computers. Without a consensus among its leadership, the NIH therefore could not devote any significant funds to promoting computerization.

Faced with the NIH's indecision, the NRC attempted to influence the debate within the NIH by better defining the possibilities electronic computers could offer to biology and medicine. To that end, several weeks after the round-table conference, Cannan established the NRC ad hoc Committee on Medical Uses of Computers, which would conduct a survey of computer use in biology and medicine and generally lead the effort to persuade the federal government to help computerize those fields. To head the committee, Cannan settled on Robert Ledley, then based at the George Washington University Engineering School, in Washington, DC. Ledley, with his experience in engineering, operations research, molecular biology, and dentistry, seemed to Cannan "unusually well qualified, as a biologist, mathematician, and engineer, to undertake this work."[13] After haggling with Ledley's deans at GWU, the NRC hired him on a part-time basis and instructed him to spend the summer of 1957 beginning the survey and establishing a framework for a comprehensive textbook that would introduce life scientists to computers.

As Ledley began his survey, a divisive internal debate at the NIH over whether or not to invest in the new technology intensified. The controversy surrounding computing at the NIH during the late 1950s would probably surprise modern observers. One of the most important things that our thoroughly computerized modes of work and living make us overlook is that fifty years ago it was far from obvious that computers could be useful for scientists and doctors, let alone necessary. There is a parallel in the corporate world. One survey of efforts to sell general-purpose digital electronic computers to businesses between 1954 and 1958 makes clear that there was at the time almost no rational basis for any group to invest in such a machine. The contraptions were extremely difficult to use, unreliable, not very capable (vis-à-vis cheaper human computers or adding machines); worse, they were astronomically expensive. Yet, computers were sold anyway, not on their current merits, but for their potential. Driving irrational computer adoption, historian Thomas Haigh shows, was the seductive claim that computer technology, even though it would take years to master, could rapidly and fundamentally reshape a firm's competitive position. A corollary of this claim was that if a company hesitated to adopt this "disruptive" new technology, it would be left behind by any competitors that had invested in computing.[14] The reception of computers at the NIH in 1956 was similar to that found at the reluctant corporations. Parties seeking to invest major resources into computing were decidedly in the minority at the NIH, but they were fervent in their belief that computers could change biomedicine for the better and that there would be a steep long-term cost associated with not adopting the new technology.

The NIH's first persistent advocate of digital computing was biophysicist Frederick Sumner Brackett (1896–1988), the head of the Laboratory for Physical Biology at the National Institute of Arthritis and Metabolic Diseases (NIAMD—today called the National Institute of Diabetes and Digestive and Kidney Diseases, or NIDDK). By the mid-1950s, when Brackett began to promote computers on the NIH campus, he was considered an expert in the use of electronic equipment in biomedical investigations. Renowned since the 1920s for having designed and built the electronic spectroscopy equipment he used to discover the "Brackett series" of infrared lines in the emission spectrum of hydrogen, he had led major NIH investigations of the effects of radiation on organisms. During World War II, Brackett became familiar with electronic means of managing information while designing bombsights for the US Army Air Corps.[15] Following the war, Brackett expressed interest in applying information technology to biomedical problems.

It is clear from Brackett's correspondence in the late 1950s that he eagerly entertained the nearly earthshaking sales pitches from computer manufacturers like IBM, who promised world-changing returns for those who invested early in electronic data processing. Looking back on such tactics from the mid-1960s, the editors of *Computers in Biomedical Research* (1965) joked, "It is somewhat surprising that someone did not suggest in the late 1950s that the digital computer was capable of everything including resurrecting the dead. Certainly every other claim was made!"[16] Brackett's own claims about computing were no exception to the late-fifties norm of hyperbole. In an April 1956 memo titled, "Electronic Data Processing and Computing Equipment: The Meaning for NIH," he described three new developments in the life sciences that had pushed those fields to the brink of surpassing the traditional bounds of research set by humanity's limited ability to gather and access information. First, he had observed the "growing use of methods requiring mass observations, measurements and manipulations of data both in laboratory work and in clinical trials." Second, he saw an "increasing importance of the physical sciences in their biologically oriented forms to medical research with attendant emphasis upon quantitative and mathematical approaches." And third, he noted, was "the dependence of present-day research and experimental design upon biostatistical and biometrical techniques, and the developing prospect of direct exploration of the dynamics of biological phenomena by means of mathematical models."[17]

Brackett cast in no uncertain terms the importance of these circumstances, pointing out that "the expansion and intensification of medical and biological research over the recent years has been paralleled by developments in methods and approaches transcendent in promise of rapid, meaningful advances but formidable in scope and complexity."[18] Thus, in this potential was a pitfall: researchers could not analyze the bounty of information their new methods had created. The data were there, and so were the techniques to analyze data, but the capacity to manage all that information was lacking. To "transcend," biomedical researchers would, according to Brackett, need to take advantage of the "the tremendous capacity of these machines [computers] for handling masses of quantitative data, the speed with which difficult and extensive calculations can be performed, and the facility with which diverse processes can be carried out simultaneously." In so doing, he believed, biologists could "wipe out the mechanical limitations encountered in expanding the use of newer mathematical and biometrical techniques in the fields of biological and medical research."[19]

Brackett's vision of computerized research resonated with James Shannon (1904–1994), who in 1955 had just been appointed director of the NIH. Shannon was already enthusiastic about using computers as administrative tools, to the point where he had taken a one-week intensive course at IBM Laboratories to become more familiar with the technology.[20] However, after his exchanges with Brackett, Shannon embraced the notion that introducing computers to biomedical research would bring about important and otherwise unobtainable advances in research.

In October 1956, Shannon approved Brackett's request to purchase an IBM 650, IBM's first mass-produced digital electronic computer. The choice of the

650 demonstrates the two men were well aware that their colleagues regarded general-purpose digital computers with trepidation. First, the 650 was about as practical as a mid-1950s computer could be. Launched in 1953, the 650 was significantly more convenient to operate than the earlier generation of computers like EDSAC, SEAC, or the UNIVAC computers. Unlike those older vacuum-tube based machines, the 650's data and instructions were stored as magnetized spots along tracks on the surface of small drum (4 inches in diameter, 16 inches long) that rotated 12,500 times a minute, making data relatively easy to retrieve.[21] Second, the 650 used familiar technology. Data was entered via traditional IBM punch cards, which were already commonly used in mechanical data processing, and results could either be punched onto other cards or stored on magnetic tapes. Third, the 650 was much more powerful than traditional electronic data processing equipment—it could to execute 138,000 logical operations per minute and store 20,000 decimal digits in its memory. Although the 650 was most commonly used to manage accounting information, it could also be used to relatively quickly perform the large numbers of simple calculations required by statistical studies or physical simulations. By 1956, the 650 was a proven success. Hailed by IBM as "the workhorse of modern industry," the 650 was the most popular digital electronic computer produced by any manufacturer in the 1950s, and by 1956 IBM had sold more than three hundred.[22]

Compared to today's computers, which can perform billions of calculations per second, the 650 was slow, but it was also sluggish compared to computers manufactured by IBM's rivals at the time. One opponent to NIH plans to acquire a 650 remarked that "the IBM 650 is not a grown-up computer."[23] However, besides bearing the IBM brand, the 650 was relatively more appealing to Brackett and Shannon, because, "as a 'decimal' machine, it retained, as one wag put it, a proper respect for the human being's comprehension of the base-10 number system. It was not one of those newer, ugly machines that performed arithmetic and other symbol-processing tasks in the binary (base 2), octal (base 8), or hexadecimal (base 16)."[24]

The 650 may have afforded a relatively gentle introduction to digital electronic computing, but the machine and Brackett's plans in general were greeted with hostility on the NIH campus. Brackett had Shannon's support but not that of most of the institute directors, who killed the initial plan to acquire the IBM 650. One in particular, the biostatistician Harold Fred Dorn (1906–1963), personally intervened to ensure that NIH did not devote resources to the 650. The objections of Dorn and other researchers critical of Brackett's plan are important because Brackett and Shannon's response to them would deeply inform later NIH efforts to computerize biomedical research.

Neither Dorn nor the other opponents of acquiring the 650, like protein crystallographer Alexander Rich (b. 1925), were technophobes. Dorn had earlier made ample use of punch card adding machines—which could be classified as electrical accounting machinery (EAM)—to famously make his statistical argument that there was a link between smoking cigarettes and getting lung cancer. As a spin-off of his research, Dorn oversaw operations at the EAM data-processing facility NIH built in 1954, "weld[ing] his small group of biometricians and the production staff into a cohesive, efficient group."[25] Rich, meanwhile, was a regular user of computer programs written especially for crystallographers.

Dorn's objection to Brackett's plan was based on a simple premise: "digital computers—like all other computers—are justified by being kept busy."[26] And Dorn did not see how NIH researchers could keep an IBM 650 busy without spending an enormous amount of money. Dorn observed that machines like the 650 amortized the cost of programming them only when they repeated for long amounts of time a particular program—but this was a rarity in the study of life, where conditions typically did not remain constant. The cost of creating customized programs for each research group would be extraordinary. In a study of potential expenses related to the 650, Dorn found that it would cost over $1 million to purchase and operate a 650 for five years.[27]

On the other hand, Alexander Rich, then chief of the Section on Physical Chemistry in the NIH's National Institute of Mental Health (NIMH), did not see how most biomedical research could be computerized at all.[28] Contrasting his own field, crystallography, with the rest of the life sciences, Rich pointed out that "few problems in biology have been treated mathematically." As he saw it, biologists did not have the mathematical background to make their work quantitative enough to be computerized, and—unlike crystallography work—those few projects that were quantitative involved equations sufficiently complex that programming would be difficult. Instead of buying a computer, Rich suggested that "a mathematician trained in biology might look through the projects and do some good." He further held that most biological problems were far too complex for the IBM 650, on which "only limited mathematical operations can be carried out."[29] Rich's doubts were confirmed in an informal survey of a group of NIH cancer researchers who were investigating the effectiveness of various forms of chemotherapy. Among these researchers there was universal enthusiasm for employing computers but also universal ignorance concerning how to go about using them.[30]

Brackett's plan to acquire a 650 was stymied, but he still saw computers in the NIH's future. In November 1956, he defiantly declared that "the computer's presence and use at the NIH is one of form and timing rather than acceptance or rejection."[31] To overcome the institute directors' doubts, Brackett formed the NIH Mathematics Panel, the aim of which was to encourage researchers to mathematize their work in a way that would let them take advantage of digital computers. To computerize biomedicine Brackett would therefore need to mathematize it first. Mathematization, he believed, entailed training two new types of research personnel to serve as interlocutors between computing and biology. "First," he explained, there would be "a mathematician whose specialty is numerical analysis and with an extensive knowledge of computing equipment and its applications. Such an individual would face toward the computer and have the function of producing solutions to more or less well-defined computational problems." That mathematician would work in conjunction with "a person with classical training in applied mathematics and strong orientation toward biological research. Such an individual would face away from the computer toward the biological research problems. His responsibility would be the mathematical formulation of biological problems."[32]

Brackett's call to mathematize biomedical research as part of computerizing it appealed greatly to Shannon, but it did not win over Dorn. In January 1957, the Brackett-Dorn dispute spilled over into the round-table conference the USAF and the NRC had organized to persuade civilian agencies to devote resources to developing biomedical computing. Both Brackett and Dorn were active at the round table, each officially representing the NIH. For his part, Dorn declared that he and the rest of the NIH's research leadership were almost unanimous in their skepticism of computers, and suggested that life scientists should be content in the foreseeable future to use the electronic calculators in the NIH's Payroll Office. Expensive computers, like the IBM 650, Dorn insisted, were vastly overrated. He railed, "You don't have to worship these machines. There seems to be a lot of awe about them, they're going to do things you can't do now. This is really a lot of nonsense . . . these machines are just an auxiliary step in here that will perform computations for you more quickly."[33]

In countering Dorn, Brackett found an ally in another attendee, computer pioneer Howard H. Aiken (1900–1973), well known since the 1940s for designing the Mark I, arguably the first fully automated computer.[34] Objecting to confining biologists to using the equipment in "Accounts Payable," Aiken stressed that a biologist could only harness the potential of the digital electronic computer if it were much more flexible than business machines. Drawing a historical analogy, Aiken compared the administrative office to "production lines [that] are equipped with specialized machines and tools" and the biologist's laboratory to "model shops [that] have general-purpose equipment."[35] Thus, reasoned Aiken, general-purpose computers such as the 650 suited biology work and should be acquired in spite of their expense.

After the round table, the NIH Institute Directors grudgingly agreed to purchase the IBM 650 but remained skeptical about its utility as well as the feasibility of mathematizing biomedical research. Consequently, when the 650 was finally installed on the NIH campus in 1958, the machine and its operators were generally held in low regard. Pratt, who set aside his cancer research to run the 650, remembered, "Many senior scientists openly questioned the value of computing in their programs. These attitudes were heard and only partially discounted by the NIH leadership."[36]

The low standing of computers on the NIH campus was strikingly evident in the extremely poor conditions in Building 12, then an animal-storage facility, where the 650 was housed and its operators worked. The space, which reeked of animal odors and gasoline fumes (from a nearby depot), was remembered even decades later by workers as one of the worst environments on campus.[37] The squalid state of Building 12 perpetuated a vicious circle that further slowed the acceptance of computer technology on the NIH campus. In the "turbulent if not chaotic" years following 1958, "the central facility was chronically short of materiel and personnel . . . as a consequence, the users were frequently dissatisfied and discouraged with the services."[38] The poor performance of the group running the 650, in turn, reinforced negative views of computing. Consequently, Shannon was not able to devote major resources to NIH campus computing until the mid-1960s, when he established the Division of Computer Research and Technology (DCRT), which Pratt directed from 1966 to 1990, and which still operates as the NIH Center for Information Technology (CIT). Presently, CIT enjoys strong funding and considerable prestige because expertise in computers has become an essential component of new research—its humble roots long forgotten.

Brackett, meanwhile, made little use of the IBM 650 he had struggled to acquire, and instead devoted his time to mathematizing biomedical research and to his biophysics projects. To follow through with his call to mathematize the

study of life, and to encourage use of the 650, Brackett formed the Mathematical Research Branch (MRB) in 1957. Through the MRB, Brackett's computing
agenda has been quietly pursued by a small group of NIH researchers up to the
present day. Originally the MRB was part of the NIH's Office of the Director
(OD), and was charged with a mission of promoting mathematical techniques
among researchers working in the NIH's various institutes. However, as the
MRB began to "explore theoretical biology without being limited to consulting
as a service to NIH," the group conducted research in its own right. At the time,
no research was permitted in the OD, so out of "administrative convenience"
the MRB joined the NIAMD, the institute that already housed Brackett's Laboratory for Physical Biology.[39]

Over the following decades the MRB received steady if not particularly
generous funding, and it focused on "developing and analyzing mathematical
models of various physiological systems such as neurons, the pancreas, mito-
chondria, human metabolism, cortical circuits." Although the MRB's growth
was limited, researchers working within the group went on to found other informatics and mathematical modeling laboratories at the NIH. Most notable
among these offshoots is the National Library of Medicine's National Center
for Biotechnology Information (NCBI), home to GenBank and PubMed, which
is directed by former MRB post-doc David Lipman (the developer of the widely
used BLAST bioinformatics program). As Arthur Sherman, who became acting
lab chief of the MRB in 1997, put it, "Other ICs [NIH Institutes and Centers]
have computational groups, but we gave birth to NCBI . . . when the genome
project took off it outgrew the lab here. It was time for the cuckoo to leave
the nest, and now it dwarfs its parents."[40] Presently, the MRB is known as the
Laboratory of Biological Modeling (LBM) and is part of the aforementioned
National Institute of Diabetes and Digestive and Kidney Diseases (NIDDK),
the renamed NIAMD. The LBM is housed in NIH's Building 12 along with
CIT, where conditions have improved considerably since the 1960s.

Toward a Mathematized, Computerized Biomedical Future

In stark contrast to the low status of computing on campus during the early
1960s were the extramural effects of Brackett's coupling of mathematization
and computerization. Computers may not have been embraced by most NIH
researchers, but Shannon's enthusiasm for the technology remained unabated
and he began to look beyond NIH's walls to Capitol Hill for others who sub-

scribed to the notion that by computerizing and mathematizing biomedical research it could be fundamentally improved. For the rest of his years as NIH director, Shannon would foster an effort to use computers to transform the whole world of biology and medicine beyond the limits of the NIH campus.

The reaction to the launch of Sputnik in October 1957 provided Shannon with the means to circumvent the institute directors and consolidate control over many aspects of the NIH's budget. Congress, in turn, was receptive to Shannon's lobbying for funding for biomedical computing because several of its members had been persuaded by Robert Ledley's argument that computers, a fairly risky investment, could yield great benefits in terms of advancing science and healthcare. Consequently, the NIH's major, Congress-supported effort to computerize the life sciences during the early 1960s was effectively an attempt to realize Ledley's ambitious vision for biomedical computing.

Like Brackett, Ledley saw computers as the means to radically and quickly transform the study of life. Also like Brackett, Ledley cast mathematization as a preliminary step toward the computerization of biology and medicine, though Ledley went on to portray the very presence of computers as a catalyst for mathematical thinking among their users. Given the similarities between Brackett's and Ledley's mathematization-first approach to computerizing the life sciences, it is unsurprising that under Shannon's leadership the NIH would prove highly receptive to Ledley's plans. Indeed, Shannon's selection of Lee Lusted—Ledley's partner in an attempt to introduce OR techniques to medicine—to lead the NIH's effort to computerize the life sciences, should be regarded as an attempt to ensure that the effort conformed to Ledley's plans.

As Ledley canvassed the nation's laboratories and began to work out what he thought needed to be done in order to computerize the life sciences, his surveying caught the attention of Capitol Hill. Most receptive was the Minnesota Democrat Senator Hubert H. Humphrey (1911–1978), who came to devote much time and energy to the cause of introducing computer technology to biology and medicine. A political progressive, Humphrey had long encouraged many levels of government to harness new scientific techniques and technologies to improve society. Starting in June 1958, he began offering Ledley both financial and bureaucratic support in his endeavors. The Senator's help ranged from writing letters of introduction to securing funds for biomedical research utilizing computer technology.[41] In his capacities as chairman of both the Subcommittee on Reorganization and International Organizations (part of the Senate Committee on Government Operations) and the International

Health Study, Humphrey also commissioned the publication of Ledley's survey in 1960 as an official Senate report titled *Scientific Achievements and Future Possibilities for Computers and Other Electronic Devices in Medicine and Related Biology.*

Without Ledley's survey, it is highly unlikely that enough leading Senators would have become sufficiently excited about biomedical computing to fund its development. As Humphrey explained in a 1959 International Health Study memo addressed to "Individuals, Organizations and Agencies Interested in Electronics and Medicine," the Senate was entertaining several strategies to improve American research and healthcare. But in reaction to Ledley's findings, Humphrey reported, "It is [our] feeling that, just as the science of electronics has revolutionized so much of the life of our own and other peoples, so, the application of electronics and mathematics to medicine offers some of the brightest opportunities for advancing human health."[42]

Humphrey had two major motives for supporting Ledley's work. One was that he saw computers as instrumental in the progress of biomedical research, and therefore a potential boon to Americans' (and the burgeoning Minneapolis computer industry's) well-being. Writing to Atomic Energy Commission chairman John A. McCone on Ledley's behalf in July 1960, Humphrey explained, "I have been deeply interested in stimulating progress through the most creative and imaginative use of computers in the fields of biology and medicine."[43] Ledley's work also resonated with Humphrey's aim of computerizing American science and engineering in general in order to maintain scientific and technological superiority over the USSR.

That Humphrey linked computerization to America's Cold War struggle can be seen clearly in his December 1959 address to students attending the George Washington University Engineering School, which was Ledley's employer at the time. Humphrey began by noting that the USSR was surpassing the United States in the number of scientists and engineers trained each year, and that a consequence of Soviet numerical superiority could be that the USSR would overtake the United States in production strength. What America needed, Humphrey insisted, was for researchers to adopt measures that would allow them to become more efficient. In particular he saw them squandering scientific and technical information because of a lack of coordination and organization. He cautioned: "The rapidly expanding research activities of government agencies, universities and business firms are pouring out a flood of new knowledge, but much of this valuable information is often wasted, because many people who need it simply cannot find out what has been done already by somebody else."

Pointing to what he saw as the core of the problem, Humphrey explained, "A major reason for this inefficiency stems from the lack of effective indexing to coordinate and control scientific information." As a consequence of neglecting information management, he concluded wistfully, "Our stockpile of knowledge has become an embarrassment of riches."[44]

Humphrey proposed two solutions to prevent American researchers from drowning in the "flood of new knowledge" brought about by the rapid postwar growth of science in the United States. In the long run, Humphrey wanted to create a "Department of Science and Technology," which would direct research on a national level and thereby "put more 'horsepower' behind governmental scientific activities." More immediately, however, he wanted to encourage researchers to use computer technology to manage information. Pointing to attempts to computerize indexes, he explained, "This kind of research in electronic indexing may well provide the most fruitful method of organizing and spreading scientific information. Successful indexing of research and information will enable us to exploit our knowledge instead of wasting time and manpower in experiments or investigations made already." Looking to a computerized future, Humphrey predicted, "Our engineers and our scientists will be able to apply existing knowledge more efficiently, and they will be able to push out the frontiers of knowledge more rapidly.[45]

Ledley published his formal survey findings in a widely read November 6, 1959, *Science* article, "Digital Electronic Computers in Biomedical Science," in which he outlined the benefits he believed life scientists would reap if they mastered electronic computers. Likening the information revolution to the industrial revolution, Ledley proclaimed that "we are on the threshold of a new era in the history of mankind, arising from the utilization of electronic computing machines." During that new era, he predicted, "perhaps the greatest utilization of computers will be in biomedical applications."[46] However, having reviewed his survey data, Ledley concluded that there were several "formidable problems" that would prevent biologists from using computers in their research. His plans for overcoming these obstacles amount to a push to change the fundamental way in which biological research was pursued—and he hoped that reformed life sciences could harness the power of the computer. Specifically, by training these scientists to approach their research in a manner that would enable them to use computers to analyze their data, Ledley sought to bridge what he labeled "the gap that frequently exists between the knowledge and training of the biomedical research worker and the knowledge necessary to use the computer."[47]

For Ledley, crossing this gap necessitated biomedical scientists acquiring training in "coding and programming" and "the mathematical methods and techniques that would allow biologists to prepare problems in a form appropriate for the use of a computer." To implement this, Ledley suggested transforming biology curricula into a "severe and formidable course of study" that would emphasize coding and programming skills as well as the mathematical methods and techniques that form the analytical basis for the statement of problems in computer programming languages.[48]

Under Ledley's proposed regimen, students (as early as primary school) interested in pursuing an education in biology would be taught in several subjects that were then absent from life sciences curricula. First would be "basic coding and programming of digital computers." Although much progress had been made developing higher-level languages, computers were far from user-friendly in 1959. If researchers or engineers wanted the computer do something, they often wrote the program from scratch. Computer memory constraints often necessitated writing in machine code. Training coding and programming would be followed by instruction in "sampling methods and techniques for appropriately preparing (that is, digitalizing [*sic*] and interpreting) experimentally-generated data for use on computers." In other words, the object of study must be translated into a form that the computer can process.

Once aspiring life scientists were familiar how to write programs for and prepare data for computers, they would undertake the third component of Ledley's course of study, learning the "minimum basic electronics" so they could overcome hardware problems "involved in analog-to-digital and digital-to-analog conversions." His illustration of this process is pictured in figure 2.1.

Ledley hoped that while preparing to use computers biology and medical students would also receive rigorous training in "basic mathematics: the origins of numbers, the meaning of significant figures and their relation to relative arithmetic operations." Here he was reacting to what he viewed as the sorry state of mathematical aptitude among life scientists. A survey of L. J. Hale's standard 1957 bench-side reference book for biologists, *Biological Laboratory Data*, demonstrates that even established practitioners of quantitative biology generally were not expected to be familiar with proofs of the formulas they employed. Furthermore, a 1961 study by C. E. Hopkins and V. B. Berry of mathematical literacy among medical students concluded that "medical students generally, though sufficiently apt and scholarly in quantitative relations,

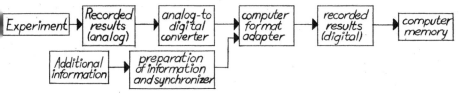

Fig. 2.1. Ledley's illustration of how biological data is entered into the computer's memory. Robert S. Ledley and Lee B. Lusted, "Reasoning Foundations of Medical Diagnosis," *Science* 130 (July 1959): 1230. By permission of the National Biomedical Research Foundation

are not sufficiently equipped with basic mathematics to master an introductory course in statistical methods." Hopkins and Berry went on to suggest that this "deficiency" stood in the way of "mastery of the fundamental philosophy and techniques of science."[49]

Ledley also sought to introduce life sciences students to "higher mathematics with focus on the function concept. Instruction in the classification of functions by analytic properties, the approximation of functions by series, and numerical techniques for function evaluation." Here too, Hale's book illustrates the challenge Ledley faced. Limited to the most basic arithmetic and statistical operations, the book contained almost no calculus and no Boolean algebra (or any other means of working with symbolic logic).

Finally, and perhaps most ambitiously, Ledley wanted to train students in "critical analysis of techniques of the scientific method, such as model building, testing of hypotheses, the problem of overdetermined and underdetermined systems."[50] His thinking was that in the event that biomedical research managed to reorient itself away from observation and toward experimentation via computer-generated models, there could arise a new danger, that of being seduced by those models. Thus, Ledley wanted scientists to be critical of the assumptions behind the models they were building. If, after all, a model was based on faulty premises, then the knowledge it generated could be quite misleading.

Besides biologists' lack of intellectual training for computer work, Ledley held that another barrier to computer use could be found in the individualistic, small-scale approach biologists took to conducting research. Ledley had found that even the typical biologist eager to use computers "carries through almost all phases of the research himself, frequently with little or no assistance."[51] Such practices could not, he feared, be reconciled with the scale of biomedical computing projects. Given that "the number of man-hours required to construct a complicated computer program is often much too large for any single individual to accomplish alone, in any reasonable time" he concluded that "in many instances biological scientists may find orientation toward individual research incompatible with the use of computers."[52] Therefore, to use computers biologists would need to take what Ledley termed the "staff approach" to their research, which "involv[ed] the partition of problems into smaller parts among the members of an integrated group." Such an approach went against deeply ingrained norms of mid-twentieth-century American biology, where researchers typically worked independently or in small groups, usually unsupervised. Furthermore, the vast majority of life sciences researchers conducted the analytical aspect of their work alone, and therefore dividing their intellectual labor would be new to most of them, but Ledley believed that researchers with sufficient mathematical training could plan experiments that could indeed be partitioned.

There was also the matter of expense. Ledley acknowledged that "projects utilizing computers in biomedical science will frequently become more costly than heretofore," noting that processing time on the advanced computers cost $200–300 per hour ($1.00 in 1959 = $7.58 in 2011). But such costs would be more than offset, he declared, by "the vastly increased capabilities such computer usage presents for the exploration of the complicated and intricate biophysical and physicochemical basis of biological systems."[53] To address this issue, Ledley called for biologists to reorganize themselves in institutions that could afford computers. This idea Ledley got from Lee Lusted. In a forward to the NAS-NRC's widely circulated monograph version of Ledley's article, Lusted proposed establishing "biomedical computer research centers" for the purpose of scaling-up biology so that it could harness computers. Lusted explained that "the purpose of these centers would be to cooperate in large-scale biomedical research projects that utilize computers as a necessary adjunct and to make computer facilities available for the use of biomedical research workers from other institutions." Pointing to the (then forming) Stanford Linear Accelerator Center and Brookhaven National Laboratory as examples, Lusted stated, "Precedents for such large-scale cooperative efforts have already been set in basic physics and other areas of science."[54] Essentially, Lusted envisioned large, centralized computing facilities as biology's counterparts to successful "big" physics projects. In place of a linear accelerator or cyclotron as the institution's instrumental centerpiece, there would be a large computer shared by hundreds or even thousands of biomedical researchers. In the early 1960s the NIH would devote considerable resources to establishing such centers at UCLA, MIT, and several other large research universities.

The response to Ledley's 1959 "Digital Electronic Computers in Biomedical Science" was mixed but generally enthusiastic. According to Ledley reprint requests numbered in the thousands, though not nearly so many as "The Reasoning Foundations of Medical Diagnosis," the "bestseller" article coauthored that year with Lusted. Ledley's most eager readers were federal administrators. For instance, Frederick L. Stone and Jack Harold Upton Brown, both leading NIH administrators, based their 1965 *BioScience* essay, "Technology in Medicine" on Ledley's article, echoing his calls to establish biomedical computing centers. Also stressing that computers (and new technology generally) had enabled the "merging of the physical and life sciences," Stone and Brown encouraged biologists to apply for NIH grants to support their adoption of computers and other advanced instruments.[55]

Individual reaction among researchers varied widely. On the one hand, MIT neurophysiologist Nelson Y. S. Kiang, who was already working with analog and digital computers in the late 1950s, remembered that Ledley's arguments validated his own informal thoughts on the matter even if believed the article to be short on specifics.[56] On the other hand, geneticist (and, as noted Nobel laureate) Joshua Lederberg, who happened across the article by accident, was inspired to take his first computer programming course and then to devote a substantial portion of his career to computerizing biology. (For more on Lederberg's work with computers, see chapter 5.)[57] Computer architect Wesley Clark, who developed the Laboratory Instrument (LINC) in the early 1960s, recalls that many of the biologists he met had been galvanized by Ledley's piece, and were eager to use computers even if they were not sure how to approach the issue.[58]

As interest in his ideas swelled, Ledley faced mounting resistance from two camps: scientists who opposed his call to mathematize biology and scientists who disagreed with his approach to mathematization. The first group is exemplified by physicist (and RNA Tie Club member) Richard Feynman, who called for biologists to engage with the small scale rather than mathematize their work. Feynman clarified his position in his 1960 talk, "There's Plenty of Room at the Bottom," which is now popularly hailed as the founding manifesto of nanotechnology.[59] Feynman's famous speech illustrates that he viewed working directly with molecular biological objects as a superior alternative to mathematizing the life sciences:

> We have friends in other fields—in biology, for instance. We physicists often look at them and say "You know the reason you fellows are making so little progress?" (Actually I don't know any field where they are making more rapid progress than they are in biology today.) "You should use more mathematics, like we do." They could answer us—but they're polite, so I'll answer for them: It is very easy to answer many . . . fundamental biological questions; you just *look at the thing!* You will see the order of bases in the chain; you will see the structure of the microsome. . . . Make the microscope one hundred times more powerful, and many problems of biology would be made very much easier. I exaggerate, of course, but the biologists would surely be very thankful to you—and they would prefer that to the criticism that they should use more mathematics.[60]

In Feynman's vision of the future of the life sciences, biologists would use tools to manipulate molecules, and they would take advantage of the very small machines nature had already provided. In a sense, they would become like engineers, building or working with artifacts. That vision has enjoyed a renaissance since 2000, as demonstrated by the NIH's multimillion-dollar investment in nanotechnology. Nevertheless, for forty years mathematization and computerization were the NIH's chosen means to the end of fundamentally improving the life sciences.

Compared to those who opposed the whole notion that the study of life ought to be mathematized, those who disagreed with Ledley's particular approach to mathematization proved much more disruptive to his plans, and in 1959 and 1960 they derailed Ledley's attempt to quickly publish a textbook, *Use of Computers in Biology and Medicine*, supported by the NRC and contracted with McGraw Hill, that he hoped would prepare researchers to use computers. The main point of contention was that of how to convey the information necessary to bring biologists up to speed on mathematics in the short space of a single volume. For instance, in December 1960, J. Barkley Rosser (1907–1989), the NRC's chief mathematician, panned Ledley's manuscript draft, raising the question of whether Ledley possessed the knowledge to write a serious study of mathematics. Rosser found Ledley's writing at once insufficiently expert and rambling. He remarked, "The discussion is naïve in many places . . . and some of the mathematical discussions are quite unsatisfactory. With stringent editing, the length of the book could have been considerably reduced and the value of the book increased."[61]

Rosser also took issue with Ledley's descriptions of where computers would fit into the processes through which biologists constructed experiments, calling them "oversimplifications to the point of being an insult to the intelligence of the reader." He concluded that without substantial revisions, the NAS-NRC would have no choice but to distance itself from Ledley's book.[62] Looking back on Rosser's criticism from 2006, Ledley contended that Rosser was nitpicking, probably at the behest of Princeton mathematician Alonzo Church, Rosser's mentor. Church, Ledley recalls, was upset because Ledley had not sufficiently emphasized to biologists the importance of Church's lambda calculus in computer programming. Rosser also took issue with Ledley's "old-fashioned" definitions of basic concepts such as lines, points, and sets.[63]

Compounding Rosser's criticisms of the mathematics discussion were MIT neurophysiologist John S. Barlow's comments on Ledley's discussion of neurophysiology. Barlow found so many basic errors in the neurophysiology section that he recommended Ledley drop the entire discussion and simply refer interested readers directly to Barlow's own MIT Technical Report on processing neuroelectric data.[64] Other reviewers consulted by NAS-NRC sympathized with Ledley's predicament of trying to squeeze so much mathematics into so little space without straying from clear language, but they too cautioned that substantial revisions would be required in order for the book to become an effective teaching tool.[65]

In reaction to these trenchant criticisms, the NAS-NRC officially decided in January 1961 to abandon Ledley's textbook unless he made major revisions to the mathematics section. Their plans for the revised mathematics section amounted to a Herculean task for Ledley. For each concept covered, they wanted Ledley to seek out "competent mathematicians" to provide the instruction. Despite these misgivings and demands, however, the NAS-NRC maintained that biologists could benefit from Ledley's book, because there was great demand for—as made evident by the survey—and no supply of a textbook for biomedical researchers who wanted to introduce themselves to computing.

With little progress being made on the book, the relationship between Ledley and the NAS-NRC deteriorated. Ledley had also grown dissatisfied with his employer, George Washington University, blaming administrators for not letting him "put significant resources into such applications [biomedical] of computers, and therefore I was unable to initiate my own research in this field."[66] Other universities that tried to recruit Ledley, such as Cornell University, also balked at the prospect of investing heavily in digital computers, leading Ledley to the conclusion that he would need to leave academics to pursue his plans to develop biomedical computing. To help Ledley realize his ideas—and also to hasten his parting from the NAS-NRC—Cannan encouraged him to start an independent, nonprofit organization devoted exclusively to developing computers for use in biology and medicine.[67] To this end, Cannan gave Ledley free use of the entire second floor of a Dupont Circle, Washington, DC, office building for a year. Ledley jumped at the opportunity, and chartered the National Biomedical Research Foundation (NBRF) in 1960. For the next fifty years, he would devote his career to directing the NBRF, pursuing projects there and editing journals related to computers in biology and medicine. Ledley would henceforth *build* computers for biology and medicine, rather than just agitate for computer use in these areas (for a detailed discussion of the NBRF, see chapter 4). However, as Ledley turned away from advocacy and toward development, his 1950s calls for computerization began to bear fruit.

A Grand Plan for American Biomedical Computing

The most significant legacy of Ledley's advocacy work in the late 1950s would be found at the NIH. Seeking to capitalize on the Senate's positive reaction to Ledley's survey, Shannon turned legislative attempts to reform research into a boon for biomedical computing. Much of the NIH's other leadership, however, was still not enthusiastic about computers. On paper, Shannon had the Senate's backing, which the institute directors treated as a political obstacle, to be perfunctorily addressed or waited out. Bruce D. Waxman, a young statistician who would become a leader of the NIH's computerization effort, recalled that the institute directors had created "the impression that NIH was really serious and wanted to spend a lot of money to find out what could be done with computers. In fact, they weren't that motivated at all. They wanted to spend a few hundred thousand dollars just to maintain an impression."[68]

Seeking to change this state of affairs and thereby enabling enormous expenditures on computing, Shannon established in 1960 a quasi-independent subdivision of the Division of Research Grants (DRG, now named the Center for Scientific Review) called the Advisory Committee on Computers in Research (ACCR) for the express purpose of facilitating computer use among biomedical researchers.[69] To help the ACCR achieve its goals, Shannon granted the committee extraordinary power. Among DRG grant evaluation sections, the ACCR was unique because it could both choose the projects to cultivate *and* direct money toward those projects through the grant review process. Lusted recalled, "Normally the programming or stimulation activity is separate from the evaluation of grant applications."[70]

Drawing directly from the monies Congress had apportioned to the NIH and therefore unbound by many of the rules governing traditional DRG sections, the ACCR would evaluate and directly fund computer-related research. Nominally, each of the projects the ACCR chose to fund was associated with a particular NIH institute, and the money was channeled through that institute, but the institute could not interfere with the funding process. Effectively, the ACCR had been handed a blank check, and this lack of oversight would provide the ACCR an enormous amount of leeway in spending decisions and therefore in pursuing a very particular intellectual agenda.

The ACCR gathered in one place a large portion of the few people knowledgeable about both biomedical research and computer technology. The committee's composition further reveals Shannon's ambitions for computers in the life sciences as well as his unwillingness to accept computerization as anything but revolutionary. Initially, Shannon had wanted Ledley himself to head up the ACCR, but Ledley declined all appointments on the grounds that he was busy setting up the NBRF, and offered instead to serve as a consultant.[71] Shannon then turned to Ledley's collaborative partner, Lee Lusted, who accepted the position as the committee's chairman. Committee members included biomedical computing pioneers whose work basically conformed to Ledley's call for the development of a mathematized, computerized approach to studying life. Among them were William Ross Adey of UCLA, William Papian of the Lincoln Laboratory (see chapter 3), George A. Sacher of the Argonne National Laboratory, Ralph Stacy of the University of Ohio, and Otto H. Schmitt of the University of Minnesota. Shannon appointed Fay M. Hemphill, chief of the NIH Statistical Design and Analysis Section, as the ACCR's first executive secretary, in which position he served from 1960 to 1961, when he was replaced by a newcomer, Bruce Waxman, whose ambitions for the changes computers could bring to biomedicine arguably surpassed even those of Ledley and Lusted.

Shannon presided over the first official meeting of the ACCR on September 20, 1960. According to Lusted's notes from that day, Shannon made it clear from the beginning that he expected the ACCR to govern the computerization of biomedical research. At the meeting, Shannon proposed three major areas of responsibility for the ACCR. First, the ACCR would "Study . . . the needs of computers in medical and related biological research," advising Shannon "as to the proper role the NIH should play in the support of computer centers and of other research involving the use of computers." Second, the committee was to be responsible for "reviewing applications for research grants involving computer adaptation or utilization and making recommendations to the NIH Advisory Councils." And third, the group would "Survey . . . the status of research in this general field in order to point out areas in which research activities should be initiated or expanded."[72] Implicit in these instructions, Lusted added, was Shannon's understanding that the ACCR would "plan broadly, and look to long-range gains for medical research through the use of computers. He assumed that as individuals we would encourage and stimulate activities in the broad field he had outlined."[73] Thus, the ACCR would not only encourage computer use by expediting grant requests, it would actively proselytize biomedical researchers to adopt computer technology.

In the ACCR's first two years, as it began to offer computers to scientists, its agenda grew both more precise and radical. During this time, the revolution the committee intended to create evolved from a far-off idea into a well-defined plan that could be implemented by following a specific set of directions. Though it is clear in retrospect that the ACCR did not manage to change the life sciences on its own terms, this was not for a lack of effort or resources. The ACCR, in short, sought to refine Ledley's claim that "we are on the threshold of a new era in the history of mankind" into a program of computer use that would involve enough researchers to generate the momentum needed to cross that threshold. The primary challenge the committee faced at its inception was that the vast majority of life scientists were simply uninterested in adopting information technology or changing the way they worked. To overcome this circumstance, the ACCR cast computers as instruments that would greatly accelerate a historical transformation of the study of life in which most researchers were already participating and of which most were unaware.

Though the ACCR would "plan broadly," its initial approach to stimulating computer use focused almost exclusively on reforming research institutions. The consensus among its original members was that to meet its goals the ACCR would concentrate on promoting institutional norms that would foster computer use. This amounted to encouraging researchers to aggregate their projects into centralized "biomedical computer research centers." In the committee's first twelve months (1960–61) ACCR members made numerous "stimulation visits" to universities, medical schools, and hospitals around the United States in order to "discuss local problems dealing with biomedical computing and to determine how NIH could help the investigators or institutions with their needs." Along with the visits, the ACCR provided many of these institutions with small "planning grants" to give them the resources they needed to plan the specifics of computer use and to consult with computer manufacturers.[74]

As they took stock of the landscape they sought to transform, members of the ACCR were dismayed to discover that the Ledley survey of computer use in the life sciences was not just representative but almost comprehensive. Rather than representing the tip of the iceberg of demand for computing among life scientists, Ledley's survey had solicited input from almost everyone in the field even remotely interested in computing. Thus, the overwhelming majority of researchers remained uninterested in the technology.

Writing in the January 1962 *IRE Transactions on Bio-Medical Electronics*, which he edited, Lusted reported, "I had a rather sobering experience while helping to stimulate interest in the field of biomedical computing for the NIH ACCR." As he explained, "I hoped to find in my travels around the country many scientists eagerly waiting to get computer equipment to help solve problems. Instead, I found a few investigators who were already using automatic data processing in the research and a few more investigators who were eager to learn." This left a troublesome question: "Where were all of the investigators who needed electronic instrumentation and computers for their research?"[75] In answering that question, Lusted concluded that what was needed "to build up the biomedical computing capability of the country [was] a large education effort," one that would make the relevance of computers apparent to researchers. However, Lusted still sought a way to engage the multitudes of researchers he and Ledley had not been able to reach via their widely circulated explanations of the benefits of computerization and mathematization in the 1959 issues of *Science*.

While puzzling over this problem, Lusted happened across the June 1961 issue of the history of science journal *Isis*, which contained papers from the November 1959 "Conference on the History of Quantification in the Sciences." The conference surveyed the development and spread of quantitative research methods in the physical and life sciences. Reading this analysis, Lusted found "a new perspective on the current activity in biomedical electronics and biomedical automatic data processing," one that allowed him to both pinpoint the historical significance of the ACCR's effort and craft an argument for computing that was broadly appealing. It should be noted that this is a rare documented example of historians and philosophers of science directly influencing science policy.

Lusted was so taken with what he saw in the June 1961 *Isis* that he encouraged ACCR members and the audience for his *IRE Transactions on Bio-Medical Electronics* to read it immediately. Lusted wanted his colleagues and readers to come away from reading the journal issue with a sense that biology and medicine were transforming into quantitative sciences and that computers would speed up and solidify the gains of that process. He outlined the big picture for them: "An observer of the biomedical scene is struck by the change which is taking place in biomedical science. This change is one of the most important ever to take place in biology and medicine because the qualitative and descriptive effort is being replaced by a quantitative biomedical science. In part this change is represented by the current effort in the field of biomedical computing."[76]

Using the *Isis* issue as a framework, Lusted laid out the challenges and consequences of the process of quantification. The particular model of the process of quantification that captured his imagination was proposed by Ralph W. Gerard, of the Mental Health Institute at the University of Michigan, who stated that "the most salient point about quantification in science . . . is that it must follow not precede, adequate qualification. Measurement can be helpful only when the proper things have been found to measure." He continued that quantification "derives from, feeds into, sharpens and clarifies, and discriminates between alternative descriptions and models. It cannot generate them. The statement underlines Kuhn's remark that 'The road from scientific law to scientific measurement can rarely be traveled in the reverse direction.'"[77]

Lusted himself evoked Thomas Kuhn to explain the benefits of quantification. The passage of Kuhn's conference contribution that Lusted shared with his colleagues began with the claim that "physicists as a group have displayed since about 1840 a greater ability to concentrate their attention on a few key areas of research than have their colleagues in less completely quantified fields." To explain this circumstance, Kuhn wrote (and Lusted repeated to his own readers), "I believe that the nineteenth century mathematization of physical science produced vastly refined professional criteria for problem selection and . . . simultaneously very much increased the effectiveness of professional verifications procedures."[78] Pointing to Kuhn, Lusted expressed hopes for the formation of a similar concentration and consensus in the life sciences. He was encouraged that there was "some agreement" in molecular biology about important problems but noted that in the vast tracts of life science that overlapped social science research "most areas are still characterized by fundamental disagreements about the definition of the field, the problems to be solved, and the models to be used."[79]

Drawing from what he read in A. C. Crombie's "Quantification in Medieval Physics," Lusted painted a picture of the evolution of physics into a quantitative science and drew a parallel to twentieth-century life sciences. "In medieval physics," he began, "there was an incomplete dialogue, or an inability to communicate, between the theoretical concepts and procedures on the one hand, and practical quantifying procedures in contact with the data of observation on the other." Between 1600 and 1700, Lusted maintained, several major transformations took place, most notably "the establishment of a complete dialogue developed as a result of intellectual, professional, and practical pressures, all of which demanded a quantified study of nature." Pointing to twentieth-century biology, he concluded, "Can we find similar pressures developing today which augur for the continued progress in quantification of the life sciences? I believe we can." To support his claim, Lusted pointed to the growing interest in developing a theoretical biology, which he believed would be inconceivable without quantification.[80]

After setting forth a historical model on which to base the mathematization of the life sciences, Lusted then prescribed measures to bring about the changes he sought. Quoting Gerard, Lusted explained that scientists seeking to quantify their work "must choose, digitalize, normalize, code and manipulate to get meaningful relationships from the welter of possibilities." First, the scientist had to decide whether his work was ready for quantification, and, noted Lusted, "He might even ask himself whether the amount of qualitative information already available offers sufficient background to support the quantification he intends to introduce." Once those conditions were met, "the scientist must carefully select his problem, the right units with which to work, the ordering criteria, etc, for he is confronted with a vast excess of information."[81]

What was needed in all areas of the study of life, Lusted implored, was standardization. In his view, those areas of the life sciences that were best prepared for quantification already had implemented relatively strict standards. Electrocardiography and electroencelegraphy, for instance, with their heavy reliance on precisely calibrated equipment and standardized measurements, were fields that seemed to be progressing toward quantification. The much broader field of diagnostic medicine, in contrast, had a long way to go, given the numerous and mostly irreconcilable disagreements over the significance of physical indicators of disease and the "intangibles of mental illness." Without standardization, Lusted argued, "the best methodology of data analysis and the fastest computers will be of little use if we are working with poorly defined signs, symptoms and laboratory data."[82]

Given that there were hundreds of independent subfields and specialties within the life sciences, the task of finding a common, quantitative language would be immense. Complicating the matter further was the reality that in many areas, the object of study was not objectively measurable. Measuring a symptom like pain, for instance, is an almost wholly subjective process. In the face of such challenges, Lusted argued that once a consensus was reached to standardize—he insisted that "the standard has little intrinsic worth in itself; it is the agreement to use the standard which is important"—a culture would be put into place that would have the means to overcome the diversity, complexity, and subjectivity of medical information.[83]

Lusted believed quantification would proceed quickly, precisely because of the dearth of mathematical methods in the life sciences. Ignorance of math obscured many commonalities that could be easily found with rudimentary mathematical training of the type he and Ledley had suggested in 1959. Furthermore, researchers' failure to use electronic equipment had severely limited the amount of data they had gathered and therefore had restricted the growth of the pool of information to be quantified. Lusted saw, however, a silver lining of biology's slowness to adopt new technologies, noting, "I suspect that the biomedical scientists may have shown wisdom in not pushing the development of instrumentation before automatic data processing equipment became available because the instrumentation would have greatly increased the amount of data to be handled, and the task of data analysis would have been unreasonably time consuming."[84] Lusted concluded that the set of data produced by the life sciences was sufficiently small that it could be rendered quantitative in a reasonable amount of time if only the resources of a large government agency or corporation were concentrated on the problem. He estimated that five hundred to six hundred man-years of labor would be required to standardize medical signs and symptoms so that medicine could reach its quantitative stage.[85]

In Lusted's terms, there were two forces outside of the life sciences that were pushing forward the quantification of the field: industry and the general public. By industry, Lusted meant commercial manufacturers of equipment used by researchers and doctors. Increasingly, this equipment, particularly electronic equipment, was becoming standardized, in order for its manufacturers to take

advantage of economies of scale. Lusted deplored the NIH's previously restrictive policies when it came to dealing with for-profit enterprises, but he hailed
a new system of providing contracts rather than grants to these organizations.
This he called "one of the most significant steps NIH has taken to help develop
the biomedical-electronics field and it has important implications for speeding
quantification in all of the life sciences."[86]

Meanwhile, the American general public, the NIH's ultimate patron, was
increasingly demanding more and better health services, and "the circles of
influence spreading from this demand will reach out to stimulate quantification in most of the life sciences." As Lusted saw it, the United States had by
1959 reached the point where simply adding physicians, nurses, and technicians
would not improve the quality of healthcare. The problem was that America's
"$25,000,000,000 health system" was too complicated to accommodate new per-
sonnel: "Medical care and health services are now so complex and sophisticated
that adding people or increasing the length of training often adds to the clutter
and makes the situation more unmanageable." The solution to the problem of
meeting rising expectations while drawing on fairly limited resources, Lusted
argued, was to introduce information technology to healthcare. He explained,
"Electronic instrumentation and automatic data processing systems . . . must be
developed and used extensively if we are to receive the optimum benefit of the
money spent on health and medical care."[87] Or as William Raub put it in 1971
when he reflected on the early days of the ACCR, "Life scientists then as now,
were becoming increasing aware that computers and other techniques derived
from the physical sciences, mathematics, and engineering must become part of
their own repertoire if the world's health problems are to be solved."[88]

In both research and healthcare, those who wanted to actively participate
in—rather than be dragged along by—the process of quantification, would, according to Lusted, become familiar with and acquire digital electronic computers. The ACCR's role would be to provide those computers to as many life
scientists as possible. Lusted explained that "biologists will need ready access to
computing equipment, and I feel very strongly that a computing facility should
be available in the laboratory of the biomedical scientist for his teaching and
his research." He added that "for problems too large for the laboratory size
computer, the scientist should have access to the machines in a computing center.[89] The particular computers, namely the IBM 1400 series, Lusted envisioned
placing inside laboratories were bulky machines—room-sized when fully con-
figured—that would take up most of the space in the typical biology laboratory

of the early 1960s. Thus, by laboratory Lusted meant the large research facilities that he believed would form as part of biology's evolution into a science resembling physics. This was consistent with his and Ledley's 1959 calls for biomedical researchers to model their computerized facilities after the large physics laboratories that had been built around cyclotrons. Meanwhile, the "computing center" he hoped researchers would use would not be a facility shared by many departments at a university, as was the norm then, but rather a regional, multi-institution facility shared by many life sciences labs and research hospitals.

Lusted later defined a regional computing facility: "These centers each must include, in varying degree, three basic functional parts: (a) computer facilities; (b) biomedical research projects; (c) computer research and development projects."[90] By allowing—or requiring—biologists to work together, he believed that the laboratory computers and regional computing facilities could mold biology into a science that would institutionally resemble a quantified field like physics. While elaborating his own plans to build such a center in Washington, DC, Robert Ledley predicted the center's very presence would change the surrounding scientific environment. Writing to the NIH, he "anticipated that cross-disciplined trained scientists who have gained an appreciation of the applicability of computers to the problems of biology and medicine through contact with or participation in the Research Center, would gradually penetrate the ranks of other academic or similar institutions, perhaps changing the entire climate of opinion and knowledge regarding this kind of interdisciplinary scientific activity."[91]

Computerization of biomedical research, Lusted believed, would be rapid, comprehensive, and irreversible. As of 1960, Lusted reported, "not more than one project in 20 is seriously utilizing computers (5%) and the funds allocated to such work are probably less than 2–3% of the biomedical research funds." However, he expected that as the quantification of the field progressed, computers that allowed scientists to manage vast quantities of quantified data would become a central component of research. Once computers were installed, there would be no going back to the "qualitative and descriptive" mode of research. Within a decade, he predicted, most biomedical research projects would have some mathematical component and would be dependent on computers. "Projecting ahead," he elaborated, "it is more than likely that in 5–10 years, the use of automatic data processing and mathematical analysis will have influenced biomedical research so that as many as 75% of the biomedical research projects will be using mathematics and data processing, and at least 50% of all research projects will require automatic computation."[92] These figures were repeated publicly by James Shannon.[93] Lusted's predictions were not just fodder for speculation. As chairman of the ACCR, he would indeed attempt through computerization to accelerate the quantification or mathematization of both biology and medicine. This would be evident not only in the ACCR's choice of projects to fund and computer equipment to purchase, but also in its members' reactions when their efforts did not go according to plan.

Planting the Seeds: The ACCR's First Generation of Biomedical Computers

Between 1960 and 1963 the ACCR received 307 grant applications, of which it approved 178 (58 percent). As part of evaluating those applications ACCR members conducted about two hundred site visits. Both the rate of approvals and site visits were considerably above the NIH's norm during the 1950s. By the end of 1963, the committee had given $17,873,263 to grantees, and had committed another $23,081,114 to them for the years 1964 and 1965, bringing its total expenditure on grants to almost $42 million. It also received a one-time $2 million authorization from Congress in 1962, explicitly for establishing centers that would "foster the sciences of biomathematics and biomedical electronics, with particular emphasis on the application of computers to biomedical problems."[94]

Almost without exception these grant applications were shepherded through the review process by Bruce D. Waxman (1930–1998), who served as the ACCR's executive secretary starting in early 1961. Tremendously powerful behind the scenes in that era, the executive secretary was an individual selected from within the NIH to oversee a study section or committee (like the ACCR). That person's responsibilities included selecting committee members from outside the NIH, encouraging researchers to apply for grants, assigning grant applications and project reviews to particular committee members, and negotiating for funds within and beyond the NIH. By determining the composition of a grant-review committee an executive secretary could wield considerable influence over how NIH money was spent in a particular area, and effectively could steer the group's overall agenda.

Waxman was a University of Chicago–trained Ph.D. statistician specializing in demographics.[95] He first became interested in using computers in 1956 while visiting Pennsylvania State University, where he heard mathematician and scientist Grace Hopper deliver a lecture in which she described the computer's "enormous power to process data and study relationships." During the late 1950s, Waxman became further interesting in computers while working as a consultant for Ruth Whitmore, a pediatric cardiologist at Yale University. As the only such specialist in Connecticut at the time, Whitmore's unique skills were in great demand, and to Waxman, "finding a mechanism for more broadly sharing her particular expertise was very tempting." Recalling Hopper's lecture on the computer's capability, Waxman noted that "it seemed feasible at a minimum to automate her skills at EKG interpretation . . . to imitate Ruth Whitmore's skills, to capture in a computer program the expertise fundamental to scarce and time-consuming tasks."[96]

Waxman's first significant work using a computer came shortly after he joined the NIH in 1960 as a statistician, when he got access to the IBM 650 Shannon and Brackett brought to the campus. During his first year at the NIH, he also became familiar with the work of Ledley and Lusted. By late 1961, at just thirty years of age, Waxman was personally chosen by Shannon to replace Hemphill as the committee's executive secretary. Though the appointment of someone so young to such a position was unusual, it was clear that Waxman's thoughts about computing resonated with those of Shannon as well as Ledley and Lusted. Driving Waxman's push to computerize biology and medicine was a desire to mathematize them along the lines proposed by Ledley and Lusted. As historian Timothy Lenoir argues, Waxman—like Ledley and Lusted—envisioned a transformed epistemology that would also engender significant institutional changes: "The view of the biologist as an individual scientist, personally carrying through each step of his investigation and his data-reduction processes, was rapidly broadened to include the biologist as a part of an intricate organizational chart that partitions scientific, technical, and administrative responsibilities."[97]

Though Waxman had little in the way of computing or government experience, he proved adroit at maneuvering biomedical computing projects through the NIH's often Byzantine bureaucracy. In numerous publications and interviews, life scientists and computer scientists cast Waxman as a highly effective manager of the NIH effort to computerize biology and medicine. Following Waxman's death in 1998, G. Octo Barnett, director of the NIH-sponsored Laboratory of Computer Science at Massachusetts General Hospital, eulogized Waxman's "unusual ability to envision what might be done with computer technology, to identify individuals who showed promise in information technology research and development, and to persist, sometimes against formidable odds, to guide the national government efforts and to provide funding for promising research activities." Also commenting at the time of Waxman's death, Donald A.B. Lindberg, more recently the director of the National Library of Medicine (located on the NIH campus in Bethesda), recalled, "In the formative early years of NIH-sponsored computing, Bruce was a splendid and encouraging guide to many a young investigator testing the waters of the complex NIH grants system."[98]

Other scientists and computer experts appreciated Waxman's abilities as a "backstage actor." Homer Warner, the University of Utah physician who was an early computer adopter, who worked closely with Waxman in the mid-1960s, remembered Waxman as the "'Oliver North' of the medical informatics field. I mean, he found a way to get things done. If he believed in something, he made it happen, and it didn't really matter what kind of gyrations he had to go through."[99] One often-repeated anecdote relates that in his effort to secure NASA support for an ACCR-initiated project Waxman purposefully lost a late-night poker game to a NASA official in order to improve NASA's disposition toward that project.[100] More formal accounts establish Waxman as a crucial contact for those seeking NIH cooperation or support. For instance, due to his "rapport with Waxman," Frank Heart, a Bolt Beranek and Newman engineer, enabled the Cambridge firm to participate in many biomedical computing research and development projects during the 1960s.[101] Additionally, artificial intelligence (AI) pioneers Herbert Simon and Allen Newell were able to secure $1.2 million to build a computing center for the Carnegie Institute of Technology's Psychology Department starting in 1962 after they "had an informal talk with Dr. Bruce Waxman of the NIH and Dr. Lee Lusted."[102]

While serving as the ACCR's executive secretary, Waxman oversaw the distribution of more than $40 million of NIH funds. A survey of the sites the ACCR chose to computerize and of the computers the ACCR purchased or rented reveals that the committee's actions did not deviate far from Ledley, Lusted, and (later) Waxman's rhetoric. Consistent with its calls for standardization, the ACCR funded the use of a narrow variety of electronic computers, considering the diversity of equipment available at the time. The committee did not fund any analog computers, and the majority of the machines ACCR grantees purchased or rented were from four well-established lines of transistorized digital electronic computers: the IBM 7000, the IBM 1400, the IBM 1620, and the CDC 160. Exceptions to this rule, such as a vacuum-tube based Bendix G-15 the ACCR purchased for Pacific State Hospital in Pomona, or the

Packard Bell 440 that went to the University of Washington, were generally the consequence of the ACCR reconciling its mission with local preferences or preexisting facilities. Only when these established machines proved inadequate as analog-to-digital converters did the committee support the development and purchase of a new machine, the Laboratory Instrument Computer (LINC).

In most cases, the recipients of ACCR funds were located in large universities or hospitals.[103] State-supported research universities were clearly favored, though a sizeable minority of funds was directed to private, research-oriented universities. Geographically, ACCR-funded computers were distributed fairly evenly, though a slightly disproportionate number were installed in the Northeast. The ACCR was after all Senate-sponsored, and great care was therefore taken to ensure that most states were represented and that regional computing facilities could indeed be found in each major region. By 1964, the only area that did not have a regional computing facility was the Northeast, despite the concentration of computing resources there—a consequence of the disarray after MIT rejected a plan to put such a facility on its campus (see chapter 3).

Keeping with its goal to provide biomedical researchers unfettered access to computers, the ACCR wholly funded the purchase or rental of the machines for most of its grantees. However, in some cases where it supported the use of a larger computer (for example, a $3 million IBM 7090), the ACCR shared sponsorship of the machine with other large federal agencies (such as NASA) or with the host university or hospital itself.

The largest—and most costly—computers funded by the ACCR were those that served as the centerpieces of the regional facilities Lusted had envisioned. All of these facilities were equipped with a computer from the IBM 7000 family. Even the IBM 7040, the smallest example of the 7000 "scientific" variants, was by any measure a very expensive machine. Its purchase price was almost $1.9 million, while monthly rental costs approached $30,000.[104] Released in 1959, the 7000 family consisted of fully transistorized, cutting-edge computers "designed with special attention to the needs of engineers and scientists, who find computation demands increasing rapidly." The top-of-the-line 7090 boasted a 32 kilobyte (16-bit words) memory and a cycle speed of over 500 kHz, making it considerably faster than first-generation computers like EDSAC or early commercial products like UNIVAC. Data was generally not entered into IBM 7000s directly. Rather, a magnetic tape was prepared on another computer (usually an IBM 1400-series machine) that could process punch cards and then transferred to the 7000-series machine. To facilitate programming, the

7000-series computers came with a FORTRAN compiler, which IBM boasted, "greatly reduces the coding burden by having the machine prepare its own program from combined algebraic and logical statements of the problem solution procedure."[105] Though FORTRAN is far removed from the natural language of everyday speech, using it required considerably less knowledge of mathematics and computer hardware than did programming methods of the early 1950s.

Installing a 7000-series computer was a major undertaking. Weighing in at twenty tons and up, a 7000 required a large room (starting at eight hundred square feet, though usually much more) to accommodate its components and operators. Its central processing unit, logic circuits, and memory were mounted on metal frames, which were housed in refrigerator-sized cabinets—this arrangement is likely the reason computers like the 7000s were referred to as "mainframes."[106] The facility had to be climate-controlled and wired to handle high-voltage equipment. IBM encouraged 7000 users to install raised "false floors" in these facilities to spread the system's weight and to keep its wiring out of the way. Besides the 7094 and 7040 at UCLA, ACCR regional computing facilities included a fully supported center at the University of Cincinnati's College of Medicine (7040) and partially supported centers at the University of Chicago (7090), Duke University (7072), the University of Kansas (7040), and the University of California, Davis (7040).

Keeping with its desire to promote standardization, the ACCR's choice of the IBM 7000 series precluded the use of similarly powerful systems. In 1960, the committee even rejected Robert Ledley's proposal to build a regional biomedical computing center around two Florida Automatic Computers (FLAC I and FLAC II) he had acquired the previous year as surplus from the Air Force. Built along the same architectural lines as the SEAC, the early stored-program machine that introduced Ledley to digital computers, the FLACs were almost completely incompatible with the IBM computers. A program written for a FLAC, which used a three-address system, would need to be entirely rewritten to work on a 2-address IBM computer. Compared to running a 7090, though, the FLAC center was cheap. Ledley had asked only for $300,000 annually to maintain the machines, which he owned outright.[107] The NIH also rejected requests, such as that of Stanford University's George Forsythe (see chapter 5), to install 7000-series computers if the agency was not convinced applicants were sufficiently aggressive in promoting its priorities.

To give researchers a way to prepare data for processing at the regional facilities, the ACCR provided a dozen IBM 1400-series computers. Released simultaneously with the 7000, the 1401 (the earliest member of the family) could be operated as a stand-alone computer or as auxiliary equipment for a 7000. As an independent computer, the 1401 was not powerful by the standards of 1960. Like the IBM 650, the 1401 was a decimal computer, and depending on which model was purchased its memory ranged from fourteen hundred to sixteen thousand words. The most basic model (punch card input) cost $125,600 or rented for $2,500 per month; adding magnetic tape units raised the price by at least 20 percent. Compared to the 7000 series, the physical footprint of the 1401 was quite small, though still massive by today's standards: it weighed over seven tons—IBM suggested investing in a specially rated floor—and required an air-conditioned room of about 350 square feet.[108]

Large, expensive, and difficult to use, the 1401 held little advantage for biologists over a punch card adding machine, but for researchers preparing data for processing on a 7000 series, the 1401 was indispensable. Even without immediate access to a 7090, having a 1401 allowed researchers to write and (slowly) test programs to run on the 7000. It also let its users transfer data stored on punch cards to the magnetic tapes that would be read by the 7000. Given the 1401's impracticality as a stand-alone computer, using one made sense only if it were part of a system associated with a regional computing facility equipped with a 7000.

ACCR and the Travails of Large-Scale Computing in Biology

The ACCR's experience with the first computing centers that it funded, both located at UCLA and both equipped with IBM 7000-series and IBM 1400-series computers, illustrate the reasons the committee began to invest in very small computers as well as very large ones. As the first recipients of multimillion-dollar ACCR grants, special scrutiny was placed on the statistics-oriented Health Sciences Computing Facility (HSCF) and the Brain Research Institute (BRI) Data Processing Laboratory, a computerized neurophysiology research unit. Both programs were highly productive, even in their early years, but neither produced the fundamental epistemological or institutional changes the ACCR hoped to bring to the life sciences. Pointing to the UCLA projects, Ledley reminisced, "It seemed that this was the panacea. Well, it was a panacea but not as tremendous as I had thought. It didn't work out as fast as I thought it would; it didn't solve all the problems immediately."[109] To understand why the

ACCR reacted to this disappointment by promoting small-scale computing, a brief look at the experiences of the UCLA computing centers is warranted.

The HSCF was established in 1959 by Wilfrid J. Dixon, a UCLA biostatistician who wanted to develop "package" programs to enable biologists who did not know how to program computers to nevertheless computerize the arithmetic components of their statistical analyses. Already, there existed several basic statistical programs, but none that accounted for the "missing data and bad data [that] are a fact of life in biology, a fact largely ignored by traditional statistics."[110] In 1960, Dixon approached the ACCR with an ambitious plan to form a regional biostatistics facility at UCLA. There, biologists would have access to dedicated machines, specially modified to meet their needs as opposed to those of physicists, who then comprised the vast majority of scientific computer users. As Dixon and his collaborator Patricia M. Britt put it, "Most scientific computing resources were designed for the physical scientist, and lacked the hardware (especially storage) and applications software (especially statistics) to support biology. Even where assistance was provided, the consultants rarely spoke the language of the biologist. HSCF was established to remedy these deficiencies."[111]

Toward this end, the ACCR paid more than $3 million for HSCF to purchase two major pieces of computer equipment: an IBM 1410 data processing system, used primarily for managing information stored on millions of punch cards and transferring that data to magnetic tapes; and an IBM 7094, a large-scale, transistorized, "scientific computer" capable of running complex programs that analyzed data on tapes prepared by the 1410. Both systems can been seen in figure 2.2. The ACCR also supported the costs of maintaining a staff of about twenty to operate the computers and help the biologists use them. Finally, the ACCR funded the biologists who sought to use the HSCF resources. In 1961, for instance, the ACCR sponsored about thirty non-UCLA biologists (mostly based in California) who used the HSCF, though this number was disappointingly low for the ACCR.

In terms of generating published research and useful software, the HSCF was remarkably productive. In its early years, dozens of West Coast biologists and medical investigators used the facility to process their statistical work. Furthermore, Dixon and the HSCF staff developed the BioMedical Data Packages (BMDP), which were collections of algorithms and small programs that allowed biologists to refine their analyses by, for instance, making it easy to

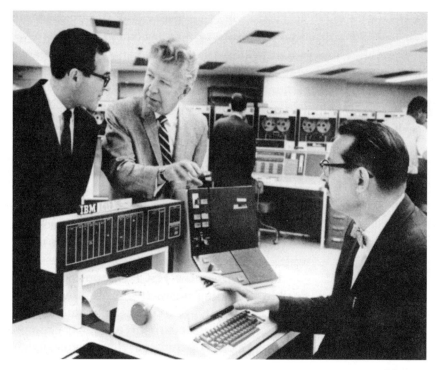

Fig. 2.2. The keyboard console of the Health Sciences Computing Facility's IBM 1410 data processing system (a more powerful variant of the 1401), in July 1963. A small part of the even larger (and more expensive) IBM 7094 is in the background. Neither machine would today be regarded as "interactive." Programs and data were entered into the 1410 via punch cards, stored on magnetic tape, and executed on the 7094; results were then sent back to the 1410, which printed them out on paper or punch cards. Wilfrid J. Dixon is seated on the right. At the left and center are Sherman M. Melinkoff, Dean of the UCLA School of Medicine, and Foster Sherwood, UCLA Vice-Chancellor. "Photo of HSCF," Accession Number 102650886. Courtesy of IBM Corporate Archives

eliminate outliers or apply techniques that accounted for missing data. The UCLA BMDP software enjoyed considerable popularity among biomedical researchers during the 1960s. Decades later, the now widely used Statistical Package for Social Scientists (SPSS) "began as a direct copy of our [the HSCF's] statistical algorithms with modifications to the control language used to specify the analysis."[112] Despite these accomplishments, the HSCF had not transformed the practice of biology to the degree the ACCR had hoped.

Meanwhile, at UCLA's new School of Medicine—its first graduating class was that of 1955—the ACCR had funded the purchase of another IBM 7090 (and support facility) for the Brain Research Institute (BRI). Conceived in the late 1950s primarily by anatomists Horace Winchell Magoun and William Ross Adey (a founding ACCR member) as well as the neurophysiologist Mary A. B. Brazier who had just relocated from Massachusetts General Hospital, the BRI was initially not computerized but was rather an interdisciplinary umbrella organization for several large research laboratories that investigated the brain. Around 1960, Adey, who was an avid ham radio operator, had become convinced of the great potential of digital electronic computers, and after attending the initial meetings of the ACCR he persuaded the BRI planners to approach the NIH for support.[113] Brazier, who had worked with computers designed specifically for neurophysiologists in Cambridge, Massachusetts, in the 1950s, was also eager to bring such technology to UCLA.

The ACCR became involved with the BRI before it was even built. In 1961, as it was being planned, the BRI received a $290,000 ACCR seed grant titled, "The Application of Computing Techniques to Brain Function," in order to "develop new computer methods for treating data derived from brain study."[114] In 1961–62, the BRI received several million dollars from the ACCR to install and operate the 7090. Unlike the HSCF's use of computers, the BRI's use of the equipment was tailored to meet explicit research aims. As retired BRI electrical engineer Thelma Estrin[115] explains, the ACCR grant was provided toward improving several specific areas of EEG analysis, including: "monitoring electrical events in order to map pathways in the nervous system," "correlating EEG changes in electrical activity with different behavioral of physiological states," and "monitoring electrical activity during different stages of sleep, conditioning, and learning." Estrin notes, "All of these experiments, were characterized by great masses of data that were largely assessed by the naked eye."[116] Indeed, the BRI's justification for acquiring its own machine was that life sciences computational work, which frequently taxed UCLA's existing facilities, was criticized by researchers in other disciplines for its seeming inefficiency. Estrin describes the tensions faced by both the BRI and the HSCF: "I recall from conversations with Dr. Dixon that the campus mainframe providers were very disturbed by the vast quantities of input and output data the biologists and medical people used. They believed that only small amounts of input or output were required by scientists, assuming that the computer's speed and sophistication made use of clever algorithms."[117]

With their own computing facility, named the Data Processing Laboratory in 1962, BRI neurophysiologists pursued several EEG-related projects. The largest group within the BRI was the Space Biology Laboratory, which aimed to study the effect of environmental stresses likely to be encountered in spaceflight on the brains on humans and animals.[118] Mary Brazier's Clinical Neurophysiology Unit used the BRI computer both to automatically collect and to analyze data from patients and test subjects staying at the unit's ten-bed clinic. Not only were the patients' implanted electrodes transmitting information to the 7090 (via an Airborne Instrumentations Laboratory analog-digital converter that Estrin modified for the purpose), but their records were entirely computerized.

As with the HSCF, the BRI's 7090 did not bring about a transformation of how biologists approached their subject matter but rather let them proceed with larger studies more quickly. In her 1964 historical survey for *Science*, "The Electrical Activity of the Nervous System," Brazier pointed out that only electronic computers had allowed her group of neurophysiologists to grapple with the large volume of electrical data produced by the brain. For at least a century before she wrote, neurphysiologists recognized that "the nerve impulse is identifiable with an electrical charge" and for just as long most neurophysiologists believed they could only make headway by examining living subjects. With access to computers, she argued, she and her colleagues had been able to refine these old ideas and move beyond them.[119] She regarded the computer as enabling a hitherto impractical "statistical viewpoint," which she "defined as the 'probabilistic' model in contrast to a 'deterministic' one in which a given stimulus elicits a stereotyped response irrespective of the likelihood of its occurrence." She explained that "such a viewpoint releases the investigator from seeking the rigidity of arithmetic relationships and adds another dimension to the neural code."[120] What Brazier could not point to as of 1964, however, was any profound new insight generated by this approach. Furthermore, there was no evidence that the BRI's computer had transformed neurophysiologists' institutional behavior. Even though hundreds of researchers used the computer, they retained their affiliation with their respective laboratories and clinics, few of which housed more than a dozen scientists. In modern terms, using computers did not bring scientists out of their respective "silos."

As early as mid-1961, it was evident to the ACCR that the HSCF was not living up to expectations as a regional computing facility. The computing facility was being managed well by Dixon and significant work was being done on its equipment, but the anticipated throngs of scientists from around the region clamoring to use the facility had not materialized. In its attempt to get researchers to use the regional computing centers it was building, the ACCR would foster the development of small-scale, real-time interactive computers. Ironically, the little machines would in later decades come to be seen as the antithesis of the giant computing centers the ACCR wanted to build, rather than, as the ACCR intended, intermediary devices to make those very centers more usable.

As the ACCR began to draw up plans for a group of regional computing facilities to build around the United States, its members took stock of the reasons for which its existing facilities were not attracting researchers from beyond the universities or even the departments in which they were located. They concluded that biology had unique computing needs because of its lack of an "underlying theory" and its practitioners' unfamiliarity with mathematics. In 1990, Dixon recalled this line of thinking: "Because the underlying theory available to biologists was often less extensive than in the physical sciences, the need for graphical representations, interactive methods, and effective data handling was greater. Finally, being less comfortable with the technical aspects of computing, our research community required specialized assistance in using the tools."[121] Getting outside help to run computers further alienated biologists from the machines because having technical problems solved by others led many users to regard computers with an almost superstitious awe. After observing the way biologists discussed computers, ACCR member Max Woodbury reported, only somewhat in jest, that going to a computing center conjured images of "the rigid rituals of ancient magicians—the precise drawing of cabalistic symbols, the careful attention to proper obeisances and the fabled results attendant upon any errors are hauntingly reminiscent of the procedure of preparing parameter cards just so for complex programs." Woodbury, who was himself a computer expert, warned the committee that it was enabling a "priesthood" of technicians to form around computers and that there was a danger of the mystique surrounding computers becoming institutionalized.[122]

The practical consequence of biology's apparent incompatibility with computing centers was simple. Very few life scientists, it turned out, had data that was compatible with the ACCR-sponsored computers at its regional computing facilities, and few had the means to quickly convert that data into a form that was compatible. Computers like the IBM 7000 series needed digital data to process, and the researchers did not have much. Instead, they had enormous amounts of analog data, that is, continuous signals such as EEG ("brainwave") or EKG (heartbeat) recordings. Looking back on this circumstance from 1964, Lusted singled out the ACCR-sponsored "Conference on Special Aspects of

Electronic and Computer-Assisted Studies of Bio-Medical Problems" held in Washington, DC, on September 14 to 16, 1961, as the point where the ACCR began see analog-to-digital conversion as the central impediment to computerization of the study of life. At the conference, ACCR members concluded that the committee's priority should be providing the means for researchers to digitize enough of their work that they could use the facilities the ACCR was building for them. Without enough digital data to keep computers busy, the efficiency one gained by using state-of-the-art equipment appeared not to be worth its enormous expense. As Lusted put it, "The gains in shorter processing time from a large machine are probably not commensurate with the increase in cost of a large machine." The reason for this, he explained, was that "many immediate biomedical computing problems are data reduction in type and require minimal computation. These types of problems are often input-output limited and require several cycles of human and machine processing" (Lusted, "Guidelines," 14).

To address the shortage of digital data, the ACCR sought to quickly provide life scientists with the means to produce such data. Specifically, the committee supplied researchers with small-scale computers that they hoped would allow laboratories to convert the analog data they were producing into a digital form that could be processed by the large IBM computers the NIH had already purchased. By placing computers directly in the laboratory, the ACCR hoped to avoid another major pitfall of using the centralized computers, their inflexibility: "In the present state of computer technology, the small computer still excels in its versatility of application over a wide range of problems from the treatment of unit record data to the conversion and processing of real time information" (14).

In the face of growing doubts about the effectiveness of regional computing centers, the ACCR increasingly funded the acquisition of small, self-contained, general-purpose computers. The capabilities, size, and expense of these machines fell between those of the 7090 and the 1401. The most popular were variants of the IBM 1620. By late 1963, the ACCR had fully sponsored the rental or purchase of fifteen and partially sponsored acquisition of another six. First produced in 1959, the fully transistorized 1620 was marketed by IBM as a general-purpose computer for small businesses and individual departments of large companies or universities. It was also a popular teaching computer because it performed arithmetic with decimal numbers (rather than binary numbers), and its variable-length words (rather than fixed-length 8- or 16-bit words) made the machine more approachable to first-time users. With a cycle speed of 50 kHz, the 1620 was only a tenth as fast as the 7090, while the machine's memory held 20,000 decimal digits (5-digit addresses). Physically the 1620 measured 22 square feet—it came packaged in 3 large office-style "desks"—and weighed 1,210 pounds, making it difficult, though not impossible, to install in a typical biologist's laboratory.[123]

Generally, the 1620 was programmed via punch card or paper tape, and users received output on paper tapes as well. The 1620 also had a teletype keyboard that allowed limited real-time interaction with the computer as it ran programs. Machine feedback was printed on paper, rather than displayed on an electronic monitor. Programs for the 1620 were typically written in FORTRAN, thus providing a degree of compatibility with other computers also programmed in that language. However, transferring a program written in FORTRAN on a 1620 to a different kind of computer that could compile and execute FOR-TRAN programs, such as a 7000-series machine, was usually not a smooth process due to the architectural differences between these two computer systems.[124]

Though the majority of ACCR computer acquisitions were of IBM computers, the committee also fully sponsored the use of half a dozen "small" (700 pound, 10 square feet) computers produced by IBM's rival, Control Data Corporation (CDC). Hoping to expand its business into the biomedical sector, CDC responded to the ACCR's efforts to computerize the life sciences by including biomedical researchers in its market target for the 160-A line. Like the IBM computers, the CDC 160-A was a stored-program general-purpose computer. Its memory held between 8 and 32 kilobytes of 12-bit words, and its cycle speed was 6.4 microseconds (156 kHz), or triple that of the IBM 1620. Data was generally entered via punch card or paper tape, storage was on magnetic tapes, and output was printed on paper. Programming was usually done in FORTRAN, although 160-A programs were not readily compatible with programs in the same language on IBM computers.

In a 1962 advertising brochure, CDC demonstrated that it was familiar with the ACCR's new misgivings concerning large computing centers as well as the committee's new preference for small, real-time computers. It read: "Today's biomedical research is confronted with the need for a small, real-time, inexpensive, powerful, 'hands-on,' data acquisition and data processing system. The 160-A meets these needs and more." For the 160-A to be useful to biologists seeking to digitize their data, CDC recommended coupling its machine with "a high-speed analog-to-digital converter system." Once paired with such a converter, the 160-A would be capable of real-time processing of biotechnical signals (such as EKG or EEG signals), "averaging evoked-response physiologic signals," statistical analysis, surveillance of vital signs in patients (for example, pulse, blood pressure, respiratory rate, temperature, or oxygen saturation). By real time, CDC meant that console lights would flash immediately in response to an unexpected value, prompting the user to stop the program and make changes to the paper tape being fed into the computer.[125]

Another solution to the analog-to-digital conversion problem was elucidated by Wesley Clark, an engineer working in ACCR member William Papian's group at MIT's Lincoln Laboratory. Clark, a leading computer architect who had experience building both large-scale general-purpose computers as well as specialized digital machines for life scientists, had been encouraged by Papian to share with the ACCR the insights he had gained by working in these two areas. Clark's report of November 22, 1961, titled, "Data Processing Aspects of Biomedical Computing Centers," pinpointed the computer center itself, where data could not be manipulated in real time as it was acquired, as the key impediment to life scientists who wanted to use computers. Instead, he proposed building a small, self-contained computer that would have a user experience akin to an "oscilloscope" rather than the "desk calculator" that the big, centralized computers resembled.[126] Clark's planned machine, the LINC, was extremely slow compared to the IBM 7000s but it was also highly flexible. Like an oscilloscope, the LINC allowed its users to immediately see the consequences of changing a parameter via a visual display. This made analog-to-digital conversion of dynamic signals (for example, EEG waves or pulses) much less frustrating because the process did not require extra trips to the computing center and repunching programming cards when a parameter needed changing or when the program needed fine-tuning to accommodate the particular idiosyncrasies of the living subject.

Clark's proposal to build the LINC was greeted enthusiastically by the ACCR and funded generously. For Lusted, who had conceded that "no economical solution has been found to the A-D [analog-to-digital conversion] problem for direct input to a large computer," the LINC seemed like a promising solution to this disruptive problem ("Guidelines," 16). Compared to the IBM computers, the LINC was inexpensive, totaling only $50,000 per machine. However, the ACCR also bore most of the costs of the LINC's development and had secured millions of dollars to build a center at MIT to further develop the little computer. By 1963, Clark's group at MIT had produced eighteen LINCs, a dozen of which went to directly to researchers who applied to the ACCR for grants to use the machines. When the MIT faculty revolted against NIH's plans to build a computing center on its campus, the NIH moved the entire LINC operation to Washington University, in St. Louis, where it remained funded for the following two decades.

By demonstrating the effectiveness of small-scale, real-time computing, the LINC brought many important changes to computer design in the 1960s and 1970s (see chapter 3), but for its sponsor, the ACCR, the LINC was foremost a means to getting biologists' data into the computing centers it had built, rather than an end in itself. For Lusted, the LINC's development was a historical breakthrough precisely because it allowed researchers to convert their data into a form compatible with the large IBM computers. Referring to components of the LINC that allowed it to transform analog signals into digital data, he wrote in 1964 that "Good A-D convertors for small computers became available in 1963. These devices make it possible to transmit continuous signals directly from an experiment, or from a tape recorder, to a small digital computer" Looking to a future in which the life sciences were computerized, he concluded, "It seems almost certain that a small computer will be needed to organize converted analog data before entry into a large computer" (16).

A Future Denied: The Post-ACCR Direction of NIH-Sponsored Computing

In March 1964, Lusted surveyed the ACCR's accomplishments and reported to NIH director Shannon that the committee's work was a resounding success. From Lusted's perspective, the mathematized biology and medicine the ACCR had sought to help develop seemed to be emerging. He claimed that computers had played a significant role in this transformation, noting that "biology and medicine are becoming more like the other quantitative or exact sciences in that the role of calculation is emerging as an important investigative procedure." He further explained that "the computer has provided an essential means of exploring the nature of calculations which may become effective tools in biological and medical science. Based on such observations it is apparent that support of computer research materially assists in making biomedical science a more formal discipline" (19). According to Lusted, spreading computers around had hastened that process by enabling or forcing researchers to think in quantitative terms. He concluded, "The most encouraging change in the biomedical computing field in the past three years is than an increasing number of biomedical researchers have come to appreciate the importance of data gathering and data reduction procedures" (1).

In the three and a half years since its inception, that ACCR had also come to recognize the unique challenges biology and medicine posed to computing. The ACCR's frustrating experiences computerizing the work of life scientists convinced members that quantification of the physical sciences was a problematic template for the mathematization of the study of life. The point of departure was that living systems were much more complex than nonliving physical systems. As a consequence, they claimed, "the role of computation and calculation in biological research may one day involve much more complicated calculation procedures than are now prevalent in physical science" (1). Already, in their sponsorship of the development of the LINC, they had demonstrated that the process of mathematizing the life sciences would involve an approach to computing distinct from that taken in the physical sciences.

Diagnostic medicine, the area that according to Lusted had the longest to go to reach quantification, also seemed to be showing significant improvement after the introduction of computers. The ACCR explained that new methods and a new formalism in medicine had rapidly emerged as a consequence of computerization. By way of example, they explained that the computer "enables the investigator to situate complex biological activities and to use the techniques of multivariate analysis," noting that "neither of these methods of investigation was readily available before the introduction of computers." From this, they concluded, "Based upon such observation it is apparent that support of computer research materially assists in making medical science a more formal discipline" (2).

Looking to the future, Lusted called for the NIH to more aggressively pursue data processing projects in the fields of medical records and medical literature. He also warned of an "acute shortage of knowledgeable personnel in biomedical computing" that would undermine future efforts to computerize the life sciences, and urged the NIH leadership to continuously sponsor training programs. The NIH would indeed follow these recommendations throughout the 1960s and 1970s, by devoting many resources to the task of computerizing the National Library of Medicine, and by spending millions on training biomedical researchers to use computers (19). However, for institutional reasons the ACCR's broad mission of creating a new kind of biomedicine by computerizing it would, by 1965, be almost completely abandoned.

The beginning of the end came on January 1, 1964, when the ACCR formally became the NIH Computer Research Study Section (CRSS), which firmly established its presence at the NIH but also stripped it of much of its power. Now an official study section, the ACCR's "dual duties" of stimulating activity and reviewing grant applications came to an end, leaving it to focus solely on grant application evaluation, the traditional domain of NIH study sections.[127] Meanwhile, the ACCR's task of actively promoting computer use among life sciences fell to the newly formed NIH Division of Research Facilities and Resources (DRFR), which would emerge as a major sponsor of biomedical computing in the late 1960s but had a mission that was markedly distinct from that of the ACCR.

Structurally and in terms of its leaders' motivations for introducing computers to biology and medicine, the early CRSS resembled the ACCR. Both consisted of non-NIH members and both were managed by an NIH executive secretary. In adherence to NIH policy, the personnel constituting the group changed. While Bruce Waxman, a full-time NIH employee, remained as executive secretary, the actual members of the group, all of whom were employed outside the NIH, departed. Replacing Lusted as committee chairman was Homer R. Warner, the University of Utah physician and cardiology researcher who in 1961 had used Ledley and Lusted's Bayesian methods to devise a scheme for diagnosing congenital heart disease among patients at Latter-Day Saints Hospital in Salt Lake City.[128] Under Warner, the CRSS quickly emerged as a passage point for young researchers interested in applying computers to biomedical problems. For instance, Edward Feigenbaum, who developed expert systems at Stanford University, recalled that serving on the CRSS "was like getting a second Ph.D."[129] Likewise, Donald A.B. Lindberg, director of the National Library of Medicine since 1984 and a leading developer of medical information systems, who joined the committee in 1967, found that "it was the equivalent of a four-year postdoc fellowship with people who knew much more than I did about computing, mathematics, and engineering."[130]

Warner had enthusiastically implemented Ledley and Lusted's methods, but he could not, because of the CRSS's limits as a study section, attempt to bring about the mathematized biomedicine they had envisioned. Bound by the rules governing study sections, instead of spending money specially reserved for it, the CRSS could only recommend to NIH institutes how they should allocate their resources to projects that would ostensibly make significant use of computers. Between 1965 and 1971 the CRSS advised the NIH's institutes on the distribution of at least $100 million to biomedical computing projects, but it exerted no direct control over the money. If, for instance, the CRSS favorably evaluated a grant application related to using computers in research, the final decision whether or not to actually fund the project fell to one of the NIH's institutes. In effect, the institutes' nominal control over the ACCR's spending between 1960 and 1963 became real, and while the NIH's institutes were eager to put computers to use, they sought to computerize specific domains rather than biomedical science in general. Henceforth, any CRSS-approved request to acquire computers would need to satisfy the agenda of whichever institute was ultimately paying for the project.

Once tasked with aiding particular areas at the various institutes' behest, the CRSS effort to shape the overall direction of the computerization of American biology and medicine came to an end. In 1970, the CRSS reported, "It was apparent that the NIH categorical institute structure was not particularly well suited to the provision of support for research tools that could be useful to all varieties of biological and medical sciences."[131] Instead, they were helping each of the institutes to pursue its own agenda for computer use. As the group put it, "Each of the National Institutes is now involved with the developing discipline we call biomedical computing . . . most notably the National Heart and Lung Institute or the National Institute of General Medical Sciences or the National Institute of Neurological Diseases and Stroke."[132]

Given the passion with which Lusted and other members of the ACCR pursued their vision, it may appear somewhat surprising they that did not more forcefully protest the NIH's new institute-controlled approach to providing computers for biomedical work. This seeming acquiescence can largely be attributed to new circumstances. By late 1964, Lusted and many other early participants in the ACCR had assumed leadership roles in computing projects at their home institutions, and thus they found themselves in the position of trying to acquire NIH support for these projects. Members Jerome Cox and William Papian, for instance, became immersed in the developing the LINC and other computers at NIH-sponsored computing centers at Washington University. William Ross Adey expanded his Space Biology Laboratory to the point that it became the largest component of UCLA's BRI; there, he used computers to study the effects of weightlessness on astronauts' brains. Lusted himself relocated to the University of Rochester, in western New York, where he teamed up with statistician Ward Edwards to further develop the work he and Ledley had conducted in the late 1950s to apply Bayes's theorem to medical problems.

In the course of this—often NIH-sponsored—work, Lusted developed receiver operating characteristic (ROC) analysis techniques, now used commonly in clinical settings as a tool to help medical workers distinguish true positives from false positives (and true negatives from false negatives), most often in X-ray interpretation.

ACCR proponents on the NIH campus, meanwhile, faced a growing consensus that despite its glowing 1964 self-assessment, the group's work had yielded very little in the way of recognizable (that is, published) results. Frustrated by the group's lack of progress and by its loss of autonomy, Bruce Waxman severed ties with the CRSS in 1965. Helen Hofer Gee, Waxman's eventual successor as executive secretary of the CRSS, noted his stinging parting shot: "In 1965, when Bruce Waxman left . . . he said to the committee, in effect, 'It's been great, fellows, starting to fund biomedical computer research and facilities, and getting a new field going, but in all honesty I can't think of a single major contribution biomedical computing has made to the advancement of biomedical research.'"[133] After the ACCR's main patron, James Shannon, retired from his position as NIH director in 1968, hostility toward the ACCR's early activities went unchecked, and the CRSS's ability to direct the overall computerization of biology and medicine on a national scale therefore further diminished. Renamed the Computer and Biomathematical Study Section in 1970, the group evaluated thousands of grant applications, but exerted little direct influence of its own until it was dissolved completely in 1977.

While the CRSS focused on evaluating grants, the ACCR's mission of planting the seeds of computer use in the life sciences fell to the DRFR (today called the National Center for Research Resources, or NCRR). Established in 1962 and led by Frederick L. Stone, the DRFR took responsibility for providing infrastructure resources to biomedical researchers outside the NIH. Besides building and improving facilities, the DRFR sponsored the acquisition of advanced instruments and digital electronic computers. The DRFR's computer-related activities were supervised by its Special Resources Branch, which was initiated in 1964 and headed by Bruce Waxman after he quit the CRSS. Under Waxman, the Special Resources Branch provided additional support to projects initially sponsored by the ACCR, including several of the large computing facilities and the development of the LINC. As computers became increasingly important equipment for life sciences operations, they became more important to the DRFR. By the late 1960s, providing computers had become one of the main activities of the DRFR, and the Special Resources Branch had grown to the point where it managed tens of millions of dollars of grants toward acquiring computer equipment.

In its early years, the DRFR encouraged computer use much as the ACCR had, and arguably continued its original mission for several years. William F. Raub, who replaced Waxman as director of the Special Resources Branch starting in 1968, described his group's mission as follows: "Our computer resources program is . . . concerned almost exclusively with the strengthening of biomedical research institutions *per se* rather than with the direct support of individual categorical research projects."[134] That is, the DRFR would not be beholden to the whims of any of the NIH's institutes but could set its own agenda. Unlike the ACCR, however, the DRFR was mandated to develop research institutions that would be productive and self-sufficient rather than become entities that would transform their surroundings and fields of study. Broadly, the DRFR's policy was, in Raub's words, to "create, nurture, withdraw." That is, the DRFR would provide money for several years to create a computing center, then help that center grow to the point where its use would become "routine," and finally withdraw support when the center became self-sufficient.

As was the case during his tenure as ACCR executive secretary, Waxman continued during his time as director of the DRFR's Special Resources Branch to personally direct money toward particular projects. The *Journal of the American Medical Association* explained in 1966 that "the Bethesda, Maryland desk of Bruce Waxman, Ph.D. is a spot where efforts to incorporate the computer into biomedical research often pause for financial sustenance."[135] By 1966, the Special Resources Branch had an annual budget of at least $8.275 million and sponsored more than forty projects. These included many of the original ACCR-initiated computing centers and new projects, most notably Stanford University's Advanced Computer for Medical Research (ACME). Often, the DRFR would support projects favorably reviewed by the CRSS that were not funded by the categorical Institutes.

In carrying out the "create" phase of its policy, the DRFR's approach to computerizing the life sciences very much resembled that of the ACCR, and it was here that Waxman flourished. As Raub explained in 1971, "Direct institutional support [from the DRFR] can be viewed as means to upgrade and maintain the quality and the vitality of the health research *environment*."[136] Like the ACCR, the early DRFR coupled computerization and mathematization, but the DRFR portrayed the actual *use* of computers as the means by which biomedical researchers could approach their work in a more rational, systematic way. The directions in which the DRFR wanted to propel the biomedical community were presented to the scientific community in 1965 in the form of a glossy booklet published by Waxman. Titled *Special Research Resources for the Biomedical Sciences*, it served to encourage researchers to apply for NIH support in acquiring computer technology.[137] Using computers, the DRFR argued in the booklet, provided the "added incentive for precision of thought, planning and consideration of alternatives in programming data for translation into the unique language of the computer. The very process necessary to meet the precise requirements of computer programming frequently reveals important additional insights" (3). The DRFR further argued that by expressing their problems in a form amenable to computer processing, life sciences workers could create a framework for unifying their disparate fields of study. "Translation of data into such computer languages as Fortran provides a common basis for mathematical and data-handling interchange between widely varied disciplines" (4)

To reap the benefits of computing, the DRFR counseled universities to build "biomedical engineering centers" in which "the engineer joins forces with [the] life scientist," and out of which "a new type of scientist" would emerge. Pointing to the LINC as an "outstanding example of biomedical engineering," the DRFR looked forward to continued growth of medical work in electrical engineering, "a supposedly non-medical field" (5). Echoing Lusted, the DRFR continued to call on biologists to merge their small laboratories in order to cope with the high cost of computing: "To purchase such equipment for one scientist would be prohibitive and impractical, but purchase for use by many scientists in a variety of fields, and by investigators in neighboring institutions and agencies, is sound research economy" (1).

Acknowledging the new capabilities of real-time interactive computers like the LINC, the DRFR also cast computers as means to productively working with complex phenomena without necessarily taking a wholly mathematical approach to studying them. For those who did not want use computers to immediately mathematize their work, the DRFR emphasized conceptual freedom via data processing. The computer would, according to the DRFR, provide the researcher "the capacity to handle large quantities of information, to examine his data for clues to new theories, and to test some of these hypotheses in a short period of time" as well as "the capacity to handle increasingly complex problems involving highly complicated human and animal physiological systems which can now be simulated by computers." Equipped with a computer, life scientists could henceforth circumvent the agony of deciding how to reduce the complexities of the living world to the point where they could be managed by written calculation. As the DRFR put it, "No longer must the scientist over-simplify his research design or mathematical models to avoid time-consuming or virtually impossible calculations. Instead, he can apply his hypotheses to a model which takes into account many more possibilities and variables than former pencil-and-ruler calculations could accommodate" (8). Thus, the main benefit computers offered to biomedical research was not mathematization per se but speed: "With the computer examining his hypotheses and related data, the biomedical scientist gets results in a matter of minutes or hours instead of devoting months or years to following a path which might turn out to be unproductive. He can now swiftly eliminate unproductive effort, turn to new paths, try new hypotheses" (4). Like the ACCR, the DRFR treated using these small computers as an intermediate step toward using larger, centralized computers. Throughout the 1960s, the DRFR's focus would be on building these centers (fig. 2.3), often around IBM's new System/360 line of mainframe computers. The establishment and activities of the largest such center, built at Stanford University, is discussed in chapter 5.

As it initiated computing centers and promoted the technology to biomedical researchers, the DRFR embodied many of the ACCR's aims, not to mention the enthusiasm of its leaders. In the long run, however, the DRFR's "create, nurture, withdraw" policy did not sustain the ACCR's goals and behavior. Once it became clear that the DRFR's leadership did indeed intend to withdraw support for the projects it initiated, Waxman rapidly became discouraged. Searching for yet another environment in which to perpetuate the ACCR's work, Waxman quit the DRFR in August 1968 to become director of the Health Care Technology Program of the National Center for Health Services Research and Development, then part of the Health Services and Mental Health Administration (HSMHA), a Department of Health and Human Services entity outside of the NIH. There, he pursued "the application of computers in public sector medicine: management information, access, costs, quality, and other things that are current [late-1980s] shibboleths."[138]

When Waxman departed, William F. Raub assumed leadership of the Special Resources Branch. In 1965, still in his twenties and fresh from receiving his doctorate in physiology from the University of Pennsylvania, Raub joined Waxman's team at the Special Resources Branch and became an enthusiastic developer and supporter of computer technology. While working for Waxman, Raub had established the PROPHET system, a national network of computers

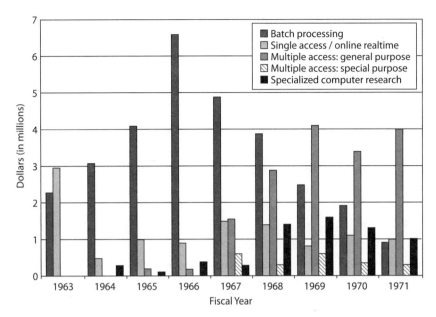

Fig. 2.3. NIH biotechnology computer grants in the USA, 1963–71. This chart shows the different types of computers sponsored by the NIH Advisory Committee on Computers in Research (until 1964) and Division of Research Facilities and Resources. William F. Raub, "The Life Sciences Computer Resources Program of the National Institutes of Health," *Proceedings of the 26th Annual Conference of the Association of Computing Machinery*, 695. © 1971 ACM, Inc. http://doi.acm.org/10.1145/800184.810535

designed to allow researchers to collaborate to "study how chemical substances affect biological activity."[139] As an administrator, however, Raub did not seek to carry on the ACCR's ambitions of transforming the field as a whole.

For Raub, the top priority of the Special Resources Branch was to ensure that computing centers were self-sufficient and productive in terms of generating published research. This new, more pragmatic direction was consistent with the DRFR's mandate, and it was also a reaction among the late 1960s DRFR's leadership to what they regarded as the ACCR's and Waxman's hubris. As Raub put it, the DRFR, "must be prepared to be judged more on our deeds and less on our fantasies, no matter how deep our convictions about the latter."[140] Morris Collen recalled the effects of Raub's more results-oriented and cost-conscious approach to establishing computing centers: "Funding arrangements of these new centers not only affected their economics but also influenced their operational mode. Most of the computing centers soon supplemented their grants with income from user fees."[141] Raising money to cover such user fees usually necessitated restricting that user's research to a domain favored by funding agencies like NIH's categorical institutes, or providing local services. The CRSS regarded the latter as a recipe for the trivialization of the computer centers the NIH had established, predicting that if the centers were left to fend for themselves "an unhealthy state of isolation is likely to occur and result in a mundane, uninspired, technical service operation."[142]

Once the DRFR's support was withdrawn, researchers using the computing centers typically obtained grants to continue their operations—most of the early recipients of ACCR funds were already highly adept at securing grants. By the early 1970s other methods of raising money for computing centers emerged: raising tuition or hospital bills so that students or patients would help to pay to keep the computing centers running. In exchange for direct support by their host institutions, the computing centers would be much more closely controlled by those institutions. Consequently, they began to be heavily used for administrative and teaching tasks, often at the expense of research.[143]

The DRFR ultimately claimed success in its mission to computerize the study of life, whereas the ACCR's goal of creating a mathematized biology akin to the physical sciences quickly fell out of even retrospective sight. For the NIH leadership, it was sufficient that computers were being used productively, and the issue of the broad intellectual and institutional consequences of computer use was dropped. Nevertheless, for Waxman the NIH's new priorities for computing had made working in the life sciences increasingly intolerable. When the HSMHA was abolished in 1973, he left biomedical computing altogether, beginning a twenty-five-year career working with the Department of Defense. Waxman later recalled, "I think the move [from biomedical computing to defense] was motivated largely because I had felt frustration in the inability of computing to show any fundamental impact in basic research."[144]

Following his departure from biomedical computing, Waxman would become one of the few voices of dissent against the way the NIH invested in computers, namely because he believed the agency had not gone far enough in terms of altering biologists' institutional culture. For Waxman, when the NIH had opted not to follow through on calls to change practices and institutions via computerizing the life sciences, it had squandered an enormous opportunity to reform research and save countless lives. Granted, in 1990 Waxman retrospectively took great pride in some aspects of the NIH's work, writing, "Looking back over all this time, it's a tremendous compendium of accomplishments!"

However, he added, "And yet at each point in time, I can't help but remember how disappointed I was that nothing seemed to be happening, which is the sort of parochial view that one has if progress is viewed over too short a time."[145]

Waxman's frustrations were well known to his colleagues and friends, but he did not formally articulate them until the 1980s and 1990s when he gave a number of retrospective talks and self-published a science-fiction novel, *The Venusian Conundrum* (1997). From these sources Waxman's vision for the study of life emerges as thoroughly mathematized, heavily dirigistic, and far removed from today's norms. Looking back on the early 1960s through the lens of *The Venusian Conundrum*, Waxman lamented that the NIH and NSF had spent roughly $35–40 billion on various forms of academic research with "virtually no supervision or planning." The consequence, as one of Waxman's protagonists put it, was that "we spend tens of billions of dollars each year, and at the risk of sounding like a cynic, all we do is keep lots of university professors employed in undirected and unfocused research." He continued, noting, "The idea that one applies systematic planning to decide how to initially proceed in any given area, or to meticulously monitor progress and developments, is an anathema to our research and development bureaucracy."[146]

During the 1960s, Waxman and the ACCR had expected that the exigencies of adapting to computer technology would introduce a degree of discipline to experimental planning and operations, but he later reflected that more drastic institutional changes should have been made to research as well. The main problem was that even computerized research was still organized to seize upon serendipitous events rather than proceed in an entirely managed fashion. In 1987 conference comments titled "A Seed of Dissent," Waxman explained that he believed that "serendipity is only *one* of a large number of possible strategies, and yet it has become so ingrained in our research and bureaucratic culture that it is largely unchallenged. Somehow the idea that scientific and/or technical progress depends entirely on accidental development is counter intuitive!"[147] This approach, Waxman maintained, had proved inadequate to address complex diseases such as cancer. Indeed, the protagonist of Waxman's novel, who is suffering from colon cancer, exclaims, "I'm furious that with all the billions spent there is no real cure in sight. It is appalling to my sense of reason that my doctors are basically guessing how to treat me."[148]

Waxman's novel states the author's argument that the NIH—including entities like the ACCR—was responsible for perpetuating a culture of unplanned, uncoordinated science, even while encouraging researchers to make use of digital computers, which ironically provided unprecedented means to reorganize scientific work. After remarking, "At the NIH planning for biomedical research does not exist," one of his characters lays out how the agency managed to spend so much money so ineffectively. He explains: "The current budget of ten billion dollars is dispensed by study sections, part-time groups of academic consultants that review unsolicited grant proposals and decide which have the greatest scientific efficacy. They are enjoined to only judge scientific merit, not relevance to some major disease, and then advise the NIH staff, who fund the approved proposals until the money runs out." The argument is that only in rare—and highly publicized—cases did such heavy investment generate a serendipitous breakthrough.[149]

To produce the kind of results in biomedical computing that the excited talk of the late 1950s and early 1960s promised, the life sciences research would need to be managed, according to Waxman, "in the same manner as large engineering or industrial projects." The kind of institutional changes advocated by Ledley and Lusted, he argued, did not go nearly far enough. Pointing to the "black world" of military intelligence engineering projects he helped to direct after leaving NIH, he called for a heavily managed "systems engineering" approach to research in which "the number of managers employed, in some cases, equals the number of developers." Such an approach, Waxman predicted, would be vigorously opposed by scientists pursuing "applied" research, a group that includes most scientists working on medical problems: "The scientific community, especially the academic portion, will argue that the problems of astronomy or medicine, for example, are not amenable to so-called engineering solutions. Clearly that is a rationalization to protect their unstructured and unpressured way of life."[150]

In the end, Waxman leaves his readers with only a plaintive question: "Why is so little accomplished?" His uncomfortable answer is that "the medical pundits maintain that biomedical research defies the engineering solutions which have been so successful in the space and intelligence programs." He argued that most researchers, rendered blind to alternatives by the enculturation that comes with university training and therefore adamantly clinging to traditional methods, would "decry the use of organized, systematic, goal-oriented research philosophy appropriate to the entire domain of biomedicine. These views are unsubstantiated by fact or experience." Ultimately, he stresses, the "systems engineering" approach had never been attempted, noting, "The biomedical community has yet to conduct the few controlled experiments which might establish the validity of one form of research management over another."[151]

In 1974, Helen Hofer Gee answered the disappointment Waxman expressed upon leaving the CRSS by boasting, "Just nine years later at this conference, it has taken the better part of a week for our speakers to skim lightly over a wide range of scientific advances in which the computer has played an absolutely critical role. . . . NIH now supports research in which the computer plays a major role at a rate of close to $100 million per year."[152] The "Computers in Life Science Research" NIH conference at which Gee spoke was dominated not by the grand, general visions of what computers would bring to biology and medicine that characterized the ACCR's discourse of the early 1960s but rather by speculations of how computers would transform particular domains and practices.

Absent during the 1970s was talk of the massive intellectual and institutional transformations ACCR leaders like Lusted and Waxman had believed must be part of computerizing biology. As is also evident, Waxman's vision of a heavily directed biology, organized along the lines of military engineering projects, never came to pass. Although access to NIH-sponsored computers had enabled many substantial quantitative projects, such as those at UCLA's HSCF and BRI, the work conducted there brought—at least in the short-term—changes in degree rather than kind. For those who controlled the ACCR's and the CRSS's purse strings, such advances more than justified the enormous expense of purchasing computers, but for Waxman the reality hardly measured up to the ACCR's hopes and expectations. However, by fostering the development of the LINC in trying to achieve the ACCR's goals, Lusted, Waxman, and other participants in the ACCR would help to bring about one of the most significant transformations in the history of computing, one that would, in turn, transform biology, medicine, and indeed computer use in general. It is to the LINC, and the revolutionary development of small-scale, real-time graphical computing that the story now turns.

3

The LINC Revolution

The Forgotten Biomedical Origins of Personal Computing

I n 1961, while the efforts of the National Institutes of Health to mathematize and reform the life sciences faltered, computer designer Wesley Clark was spending time he had taken off from his job at MIT's Lincoln Laboratory to devise ways to turn the problem of biologists' apparent incompatibility with digital computers on its head. Instead of transforming biologists into "computerniks," Clark hoped to transform computers to meet the particular needs of the study of life. In accommodating biologists, Clark would build a machine, the LINC, that defied and subverted the dominant conventions of computer architecture. Clark's MIT colleagues were pushing for ever larger computers to be shared by ever larger numbers of users, while the small LINC put an entire computer at the disposal of a single user. As the first small, programmable computer to combine visual presentation with the ability to manipulate images in real time, and as the first system to employ small, pocketable storage media, the LINC was a progenitor of both the minicomputer and the personal microcomputer.[1]

To understand how efforts to computerize biology and medicine lay at the heart of the development of small, interactive computers, and how those efforts precipitated one of the most important developments in the history of computer design, we must follow Clark from his days as a University of California, Berkeley, dropout to his career as the architect of the enormous TX computers and finally to his break from the world of large-scale computing.[2] During the 1950s and 1960s, biologists' priorities informed Clark's design by providing him insight into the problem of how computers could interface with science. Their work also served to test many of the key concepts underlying real-time interactive computing. Furthermore, biologists and their NIH patrons provided Clark with crucial institutional support when his ambitions to provide researchers complete control over small interactive computers ran counter to the prevailing interest in time-sharing.

A Whirlwind Tour of Early Computing at MIT

The journey of Wesley Allison Clark (b. 1927) to biomedical computing began in 1949, when the young Californian was struggling to find new direction during a leave of absence from the UC Berkeley Department of Physics after "a bruising experience in a seminar with [J. Robert] Oppenheimer." Further impetus for departure from graduate school came when Clark realized that "I really wasn't interested in how the physical world works and how we understand it."[3] Instead of studying for preliminary examinations, he found himself whiling away his days in the department's model shop, where he had developed an interest in machining metal and had even gone so far as to construct a small lathe for himself.[4]

During his leave, Clark used his background in physics to obtain a job as a technician at the Nucleonics Department of the General Electric Company, which ran the Atomic Energy Commission's Hanford Works weapons facility in the desert of eastern Washington state. While waiting for his security clearance, Clark was allowed access only to the site's paltry collection of unclassified reading material, which included a detailed description of Howard Aiken's Mark II (a five-ton electromechanical digital computer built in 1947–48) and Edmund Berkeley's *Scientific American* article on Simon, an extremely simple computer that performed binary additions—it could add 0 + 0, 0 + 1, 1 + 0, and 1 + 1—using magnetic relays.[5] Although Clark devoted most of his spare reading time to the Mark II description, he "became thoughtful" about the tiny Simon, which despite its very limited capacity as calculating machine, broached "serious possibilities" that could be embodied by a machine that was "of a scale significantly smaller than the Mark II."[6]

Upon receiving clearance, Clark found his job at Hanford less than optimal. His work was "concerned principally with the design and analysis of neutron experiments using the Hanford Test Reactor and other critical assemblies."[7] This included nerve-wracking tasks such as monitoring nuclear reactors, and physically dangerous work such as handling enriched uranium. Moreover, after reading about the Mark II and Simon, he was disappointed by the facility's punch card machines.[8] Resolving to learn "computerology," Clark approached the mathematician and numerical analyst Derrick Henry Lehmer to see if he could return to Berkeley to work on his ideas about small computers. Lehmer, however, told him that he should "forget about all that small computer stuff, [and] go with the big boys, that's where the action was."[9]

The action Lehmer spoke of was on the other side of the country at MIT, where Jay Forrester's Digital Computer Laboratory was developing Project Whirlwind, a real-time flight simulator that was to be capable of emulating the in-flight behavior of any airplane. Whirlwind, which was sponsored by the Office of Naval Research, had grown out of the MIT Servomechanism Laboratory's Airplane Stability and Control Analyzer (ASCA), a wartime effort to create an analog computer flight simulator. The ASCA had faltered primarily because of the complexity of implementing so many aeronautical equations on analog machines. In 1946, Forrester, realizing that he had reached a dead end, elected to take a digital approach to the flight simulation project.

Two major factors made Forrester's plans for a digital real-time computer seem far-fetched at the time. First, there was the matter that the earliest digital electronic computers, such as EDSAC or SEAC, did not meet the information storage, or memory, requirements of a real-time computer. Even more important than the lack of sufficient memory was that the early digital computers were not designed to be interactive in real time. As batch processors, first-generation computers could only execute a set of non-interactive jobs serially. In batch processing, as noted, the user introduced the data to the machine's memory, left the machine to process the data, and then received some form of output.[10] This format was inadequate for Forrester's proposal to provide the user a responsive interface. Pointing to the earliest digital electronic computers, Jeffrey S. Young explains that "except for limited self-modifying programming—where interim results could invoke different branches of instructions in a computer program—

it was not possible to vary the operation of the computer once it was started up." Forrester's planned flight simulator, however, would, as Young put it, "need to operate in real time, an entirely different mode of operation. Moving a joystick had to instantly affect the behavior of the equipment, which would then change the next response."[11] Thus, the simulator had to do something digital computers hitherto had not done: interact with the user in real time. In Clark's words, "The machine must be fast enough to do something useful before you forget what it is that you are trying to do."[12]

Nevertheless, Forrester, emboldened by the successful 1945 demonstration of ENIAC at the University of Pennsylvania, managed to convince MIT and the Navy (where his old friend Perry Crawford of the Navy's Office of Research and Inventions had already proclaimed his desire to see the military make greater use of digital computers) that the only major obstacle to developing a digital computer that could run flight simulators in real time was the lack of a medium that could store digital information quickly and reliably. Beyond the Navy, Forrester had garnered support for his project from the US Air Force as well as other organizations and corporations involved in developing aerospace technology.

Forrester first addressed the storage problem by attempting to improve the reliability of Williams-Kilburn cathode ray storage tubes, by devising what he called the "marginal checking technique," which allowed him to detect and remove faulty tubes before they failed. A large memory comprised of electrostatic tubes, all five thousand of which had to be custom built (at the cost of fifteen hundred dollars apiece) for Whirlwind, however, turned out to be prohibitively expensive. Between 1946 and 1949, Project Whirlwind received more than $1 million each year, to pay not only for William-Kilburn tubes but also for thousands of square feet of other hardware, a large staff of engineers, and enough electrical power to run a small city.[13] Meanwhile, many mathematicians and engineers, including John von Neumann, loudly disdained Whirlwind, predicting its failure and calling for the Navy to terminate the project. Granted, by 1949, Forrester had a machine that allowed users to interact with programs in real time and see the consequences of their actions displayed on a cathode-ray oscilloscope, but that was a far cry from the universal flight simulator he had initially proposed.

Facing the budgetary ax, Forrester scrambled for new support, which he received from the USAF. Under the Air Force's patronage, Whirlwind became the heart of a burgeoning project, SAGE (Semi-Automatic Ground Environ-

ment), a computerized radar system that would allow a small group of opera-
tors to monitor and react to Soviet bombers approaching American airspace.
To house this project, and its centerpiece, Whirlwind, MIT built the Lincoln
Laboratory in 1951. Located in Lexington, Massachusetts, near the USAF's
Hanscomb Field rather than on MIT's main campus (some ten miles away in
Cambridge), the Lincoln Lab was generally oriented toward military projects
instead of the research conducted on campus.

As part of planning Whirlwind's new radar mission, Forrester also sought
to develop a new storage medium, and in mid 1949 began working with his
student, William N. Papian, on using small rings, or cores, of ferrite to store
digital information. The cores could be magnetized in one of two directions
(clockwise or counterclockwise), which meant that they could each store one
bit (that is, a 0 or 1). Then Forrester began to create arrays on which he could
store multiple cores. By threading a common wire through all of the cores and
by attaching a unique wire to each core, Forrester could magnetize whichever
cores he chose.[14] Not only did core memory prove much more reliable than the
comparatively expensive Williams-Kilburn tubes, but it allowed any part of the
array of cores to be queried, thus eliminating the need for sequential access.

By 1951, Whirlwind's 2,048-word (16 bits each) memory was housed in
stacks of sheets of the ferrite cores. Even with the core memory, Whirlwind
remained a daunting machine to program. First, there was the challenge of
writing programs directly to the machine's registers, the sections of its memory
where all data must be represented before it is processed. In modern programs,
movement into and out of registers is invisible to users and the vast majority
of programmers.[15] In Whirlwind, however, the programmer entered instructions into the register sixteen bits at a time; five bits were dedicated to the
actual instruction and the remaining eleven pertained to addressing. Besides
the difficulties posed by debugging at the bit level, there was the matter of
being familiar with enough of Whirlwind's twenty-five hundred square feet of
hardware to know how to correctly match—to "address"—various parts of the
program to the hardware it was supposed to manipulate. Familiarity with the
device's operation was also necessary to determine if faults were in the coding
or the machinery.

To operate Whirlwind, Forrester needed a large, mathematically competent,
and energetic staff, and starting in 1950 he had put out advertisements as part
of a staffing drive for the new Lincoln Lab division that comprised his Digital
Computer Laboratory. In 1951, one of Forrester's ads found its way to Wesley

Clark, who lacked an engineering background but who nevertheless applied. On his application, Clark wrote, "Although my formal training in electronics is slight, I believe that I can contribute to the work of the Digital Computing Laboratory in the capacity of applied physicist."[16] Clark was able to compete for a job at Lincoln mainly because Forrester sought bright, young engineers of "doctor's degree caliber" as opposed to engineers who were already experienced and well established.[17] Clark had youth and talent on his side, if not engineering training, and was promptly offered a job as one of Whirlwind's programmers. Within weeks of the offer, Clark, then twenty-four and married with one child, had relocated to Massachusetts, the swift move catalyzed by his already having received top security clearance for his job at Hanford.

Once trained as a programmer, Clark was given a fifteen-minute slot every few days during which he had nearly complete operational control over Whirlwind.[18] As Young relates, running the machine was awe-inspiring for Clark: "All the Whirlwind components were at his disposal. For Clark, it was tantamount to a religious experience. When he was sitting in front of the machine, taking charge of that building's equipment, he felt a power and thrill he had never experienced at Hanford."[19] Clark was captivated, not so much because he could make whole buildings full of equipment move at the flip of a switch but rather because Whirlwind allowed him to interact with it in real time. Instead of waiting for program to run its course and for the computer to produce a printed result, Clark could interact with the program while the computer was running it. He could, for instance, see on Whirlwind's oscilloscope characters he entered by pressing keys on a mechanical typewriter., and he could use various analog input device such as dials to manipulate what appeared on the display.[20]

When Clark arrived in 1952, Whirlwind's memory was still based in the Williams-Kilburn tubes. Having proved adept at troubleshooting the notorious tubes as well as fixing programming errors, Clark was tapped by Forrester and Papian to help develop the Memory Test Computer (MTC), which was built for the purpose of testing the new ferrite core memory that they wanted to implement in Whirlwind. Designed and constructed in 1952–53 by Harlan Andersen and Ken Olsen (who later went on to cofound Digital Equipment Corporation, or DEC), the MTC was, like Whirlwind, a 1 kilobyte (16-bit words) machine with versatile CRT displays, indicator lights, toggle switches, and an audio output. Though many components of the MTC were vacuum-tube driven, the whole device fit into a single (albeit large) room and its maintenance required a much smaller crew.[21] With few users competing for time,

Clark's sessions with the MTC lasted hours rather than minutes. It was during these stretches that his "philosophy of computing" began to gel.

One factor that helped Clark formulate his early thoughts about computing was the interdisciplinary nature of the Lincoln Lab. In building Whirlwind, Forrester had fostered the idea that talented engineers should be allowed to use tools from any disciplines in their work.[22] Consequently, Clark, whose work on the MTC was rather narrowly defined, was able to interact with scientists and engineers who had broad interests. Of these interdisciplinary thinkers, the most influential on Clark was his partner in testing the MTC, Belmont Farley (1920– 2008), a physicist and former wartime radar worker with a strong passion for thinking about how the brain works. Farley was also a regular participant in seminars held at neuroscientist Walter Rosenblith's Communications Biophys- ics Group (CBL) of the Research Laboratory of Electronics, and his enthusiasm for the CBL's work convinced Clark to visit the group.[23] In retrospect, Clark would regard Farley as "my teacher" and one of the major forces that pushed him toward life sciences computing.[24]

When Clark showed up in 1953, the CBL had an agenda that could not be pursued very far with the equipment at its disposal. In the late 1940s, Rosen- blith, then based at Harvard's Psychoacoustic Laboratory (and later at the MIT Acoustics Laboratory), had worked with Norbert Wiener to develop experi- mental studies of the nervous system that tested the applicability to neurophysi- ology of ideas about stochastic processes and techniques in signal processing. Inspired by Wiener's *Cybernetics*, and Warren S. McCulloch and Walter Pitts's "A Logical Calculus of the Ideas Immanent in Nervous Activity," Rosenblith formulated a "thermodynamic" model of nervous activity that related the mac- roscopic aspects of brain function to the "statistical mechanics" of individual neuron activity.[25] Subsequently, Rosenblith's work attracted a following among those who wished to seriously pursue the ideas Wiener raised. "For one whose wartime training experience in electronics had included servomechanisms and their malfunctions," John S. Barlow, who came to the CBL in 1951, remem- bered, "Wiener's discussion in the book on pathophysiological mechanisms of human cerebellar tremor had a particularly strong impact." Barlow added that "exposure at about the same time to the beautifully systematic anatomy of the human cerebellum rendered the prospect of a career of study of the nervous system almost inevitable."[26]

According to Clark's longtime collaborator, Charles Molnar, as of the mid 1950s studying the relationship between neuron firings and higher cognitive processes presented "the need to study ensembles of neural signals, rather than 'typical examples,' which in turn created a need for collection and processing of large quantities of electrophysiological data recorded by gross electrodes." As a consequence of "the rapid development of micro-electrode recording techniques," Molnar explained, "the need to analyze nerve spike discharge patterns as stochastic processes rapidly became apparent as well, creating even more challenging problems in data collections and analysis.[27] To overcome these problems in data management, Rosenblith and Y. W. Lee proposed building digital and analog computers "for carrying out autocorrelation and cross-correlation analysis of signals such as those of speech, music, and random noise."[28] The first such machine, the Analog Electronic Correlator, was built not by Clark's Lincoln group but rather by the MIT Research Laboratory of Electronics, in 1949, as were its successors, the Digital Electronic Correlator created in 1950 and the Analog Correlator System devised in 1955.[29]

All of these computers were dedicated exclusively to correlating EEG signals with evoked signals and could not otherwise be programmed. They were also notoriously cumbersome to use. Looking back on the Analog Correlator System, Barlow remembered, "The system in operation was indeed a spectacle: the points on the correlogram were computed one at a time . . . and after each point had been computed, the magnetic tape was automatically rewound and the magnetic delay drum advanced (usually in a number of steps) to the next delay setting." The reason for this awkward arrangement, Barlow explains, was that "the entire sequence was under the control of a 'recycler' unit (modeled after the control unit for the digital correlator, which itself contributed substantially to the great clicking and chatter, eventually terminated by an equally attention-diverting silence that marked the end of the computation of a given correlogram."[30] To the disappointment of the CBL physiologists, years of correlating EEGs with these machines failed to "provide a Rosetta Stone from which the mysteries of the makeup of the diversity of EEG patterns could be deciphered."[31] Nevertheless, the CBL saw in the interactive Whirlwind and MTC the means to quickly find interesting EEG patterns among all the noise.[32]

For Clark, who had never been particularly intrigued by popular characterizations (by Edmund Berkeley and many journalists) of computers as "giant brains," the work of the CBL neurophysiologists made it seem that brain research could indeed provide something to stimulate computer developers. During a 1953 CBL discussion of inhibition and excitation of cat auditory neurons, physiologist Nelson Yuan-Sheng Kiang introduced Clark to a model of

the neuron developed by the neuroscientist-logician team Warren S. McCulloch and Walter Pitts.[33] Clark was enthused by Kiang's scheme to use a series of
McCulloch-Pitts neurons (also called MCP neurons) to represent the mechanism via which the brain processes sounds detected by the auditory system.[34]
Shortly thereafter, he and Farley attempted to simulate such a network in the
MTC's memory. After all, they may have figured, if they were going to troubleshoot the MTC, they might as well use it to do interesting work.

After a few weeks of debugging, Farley and Clark could consistently evolve
a network that was "initially randomly organized within wide limits" into one
that "organizes itself to perform a simple prescribe task." They published their
findings in the IRE's *Transactions on Information Theory* in 1954. Citing Alan
Turing's 1936 "On Computable Numbers, With an Application to the *Entscheidungsproblem*" and Claude Shannon's "Presentation of a Maze-solving Machine"
(1952) and "Computers and Automata" (1953), Farley and Clark argued that
their network provided a practical example of how one might pursue questions
pertaining to how "information systems whose response to a given class of inputs changes with time in accordance with specified criteria which are chosen
to correspond roughly to the 'self-organizing' concept."[35] Clark and Farley's
emphasis was not on replicating thought or intelligence in a machine but rather
on determining what computers could do with neural networks. Seeking to
avoid discussion of "electronic brains," they purposefully refrained from drawing parallels between their networks and brain activity—even going so far as to
replace *neural* with *neuroidal.* This was largely a consequence of their working
knowledge of neurophysiology; they could see the vast gulf that lay between the
computer's capability and the brain's structures and functions.

As the two men coaxed the "powerful if not yet completely reliable" MTC
into running their neural networks, and incidentally proving the feasibility of
core memory, Clark and Farley spent many hours ruminating over how to bend
computers to the scientific user's will.[36] During his discussions with Farley,
Clark developed many of his "basic attitudes towards computing." Rather than
treating computers as "demigods" or "awe-inspiring golems," the men agreed
on four points: (1) "computers are tools"—ultimately, Clark credited Farley for
introducing him to "the idea of using even a very large computer just as one
would use any laboratory tool"; (2) "convenience of use is the most important
single design factor"—Farley instilled in Clark the notion that anything that
was inconvenient could not be classified as a tool; (3) "separate personal files
are safer than files held in a common shared space"; and (4) "digital computers

should handle analog signals as well."[37] Though Clark and Farley were excited about these ruminations about computer design, their excitement did not initially spread far beyond their own discussion—their ideas were difficult to apply to the Lincoln Lab's main project, building computers for the military.

Real-Time Interactive Computing: Its Development and Divisions

In 1955, Clark made his first attempt at implementing the ideas he and Farley had discussed when he and Ken Olsen (then head of a Lincoln Lab subgroup in advanced engineering development) proposed building a partially transistorized computer to test "very large" (128 kilobytes of 18-bit words) arrays of core and other types of memory.[38] Called the Transistorized Experimental Computer (TX-1), Clark and Olsen's machine was to be capable of providing a user with an interactive experience along the lines of what Forrester had proposed in the late 1940s. Though much smaller and cheaper than Whirlwind, the TX-1 would still be a giant, both physically and in the budgetary sense. Fearing more backlash to expenditure on speculative ventures, Lincoln Lab and its sponsors turned down the TX-1.

The TX-1's demise sent Clark and Olsen on a search for a way to build a computer with a very large memory that also cost substantially less than the TX-1. Olsen found the solution in using transistors in all of the machine's circuits, cutting out vacuum tubes completely.[39] Entirely transistorized, the TX-2 would be much more powerful than Whirlwind, extremely reliable, but still expensive. Once again Lincoln Lab balked at their plans, on the grounds that transistorized circuits were an unproven technology in computer construction. To prove that core memory could interface with the transistorized logic circuits, Clark proposed building a much smaller—merely room-sized—test-bed machine, named TX-0. This time, the project was funded. Clark and Olsen, working under William Papian's supervision in his Advanced Development Group, began construction of the TX-0 in mid 1955.

Built around a then enormous 64K (18-bit words) of core memory, the TX-0 was designed by Clark to facilitate real-time interaction even though its ostensible purpose was really to test whether the combination of transistorized circuits and core memory could be as effective as a vacuum-tube-based machine.[40] Consequently, like Whirlwind and the MTC, the TX-0 was equipped with an interactive display system, specifically, a 12-inch oscilloscope capable of showing 512

× 512 points. As John T. "Jack" Gilmore, who worked as a system programmer on TX-0, recalled, Clark also took pains to make the TX-0 easy to program. He explained, "Wes Clark wrote an assembler called Hark. It was arranged . . . so we could incorporate English-language words, making programs easier to read. We put together one of the first on-line operating systems that could input software in a very easy fashion."[41]

To explore the TX-0's capability as a real-time interactive computer, Clark implemented several programs for use by life scientists. By late 1955, the TX-0 was the only real-time interactive machine to which life scientists had access. Whirlwind and the MTC were mostly committed to USAF projects, leaving the MIT community (that is, non-Lincoln scientists and students) with access mainly to a batch-processing IBM computer that was housed in "a tightly sealed Computation Center."[42] Only a machine like the TX-0 could meet the needs of CBL's research agendas. Namely, CBL researchers wanted to use TX-0 to develop programs that would help them overcome the challenges of reading long, continuous analog signals. For instance, they needed to read hours' worth of EEG output in order to determine if test subjects were truly asleep during sleep studies—all too frequently subjects feigned sleep because they could not relax in the laboratory setting, thus spoiling the tests. In this case, they required a pattern-recognition algorithm capable of distinguishing the "Sleeping Spindle" EEG wave patterns found in sleepers from similar-looking patterns found in people who were awake. As Gilmore explains: "The object of the game was to find spindles and determine the alpha frequency within it. The alpha frequency indicated whether the patient was sleeping or not."[43]

With guidance from Farley, who was then acting as a liaison between the CBL and Lincoln Lab, Clark and Gilmore developed in 1956 the "Moving Window Display Program," which contained the pattern-recognition algorithm as well as an interactive system that would allow the CBL researchers to visually compare sets of wave patterns. The program's name is a clue to its function. Typically, EEG runs for sleep studies produced several hours of data, though the TX-0's 64K of memory could store only about 6 seconds of data at any one time. By using a "moving window," however, the researchers could "run up and down the time axis examining data" by "capturing patterns" from their "data environments."[44] The "captured" patterns were displayed in the bottom half of the monitor while one of thirty-two stored recognized patterns were displayed in the upper half. With this real-time interactive program, researchers could determine the nature of the EEG pattern they were observing while it was being recorded, and could therefore determine on the spot whether or not the subject had truly fallen asleep.[45]

For Clark's supervisors at Lincoln Lab, all of this CBL work was secondary to the TX-0's mission to test the viability of core memory and transistorized circuits. In retrospect, however, TX-0's early users saw the system's most significant legacy as an exemplar of interactive computing. As Gilmore put it in 1989, "What I believe the TX-0 really contributed was an online interactive man-machine communication environment. . . . We were trying to switch from a batch processing orientation to an interactive solution where programmers actually worked at a console and made changes right there on the spot."[46]

After about a year of testing, Lincoln Lab was sufficiently impressed with the TX-0 that it gave the go-ahead to construct the much larger, more powerful TX-2. Building on knowledge acquired from the construction of the TX-0, Clark and his eight-person team put together the TX-2 in about twelve months over 1957 and 1958. With 64K (36-bit words) of memory, the TX-2 was by far the most powerful computer that had ever been built. Like its predecessors, it was designed to make computer use an interactive experience, and it was reliable enough that users who wanted to troubleshoot programs no longer had to be experts in hardware as well. To facilitate human-computer interaction, the TX-2 had a 10-by-10-inch television-like CRT screen on which the user could create and modify images quickly using a light pen that Clark had developed specifically for the purpose.[47]

For Lincoln Lab workers outside of Clark's immediate circle, the TX-2 represented a radical shift from the computer systems they had been using up to that point. Severo Ornstein (b. 1930), who had come to Lincoln Lab in 1955, was struck by the differences between the TX-2 and the air-defense computers he was programming. "In those days," he wrote in his memoir, *Computing in the Middle Ages*, "TX-2 was run totally different from any machine I'd encountered before." He explained, "The difference was much like the difference between taking public transportation and driving one's own car. First, it was operated directly by the programmer rather than by an intermediary operator. Second, you didn't just get a momentary shot at the machine and then carry away a printout to be pored over later, somewhere else." In contrast to the way users of batch-processing computers worked, "TX-2 users simply debugged their programs right at the console, sitting there sometimes for hours at a stretch. . . . This appeared to be a waste of valuable computer time, but it meant that programs could be debugged in a fraction of the calendar time than it would otherwise have taken."[48] What left Ornstein most impressed was the new status the human user had in relation to the machine. As he put it, "This way of using a computer evidenced a profoundly different philosophy: it emphasized optimizing the time of the human beings, rather than the time of the machine; it also looked forward to the day when a few seconds of unused computer time would no longer be so costly."[49]

Another who quickly saw the importance of the TX-2's capability as an interactive computer was Joseph Carl Robnett Licklider, a psycho-acoustician based at Lincoln. During World War II, Licklider had worked to improve electronic voice communication on bombers, and had been captivated in the late 1940s by cybernetics, particularly Norbert Wiener's discussion of human-machine interaction. At Lincoln, to which Licklider was recruited to study the human end of human-machine interaction, he was part of an effort to develop the interface for SAGE. With SAGE, he faced the problem of conveying information obtained from a network of radar dishes to a human operator, which led him to become interested in computer displays, which in turn, brought him into contact with Clark. According to Licklider's biographer, M. Mitchell Waldrop, Licklider and Clark met by accident when Clark wandered into Licklider's laboratory sometime in late 1956 or early 1957, where Clark spied Licklider setting up analog devices for some kind of "psychometric" experiment. The story, which has become a legend of sorts in computing circles, goes that Clark told Licklider that a real-time interactive digital computer could replace every piece of analog equipment he was using, making the work faster, easier, and more enjoyable.[50] Then Clark invited Licklider to see the TX-0 in action.

When Licklider finally took up Clark's offer, the bigger TX-2 was up and running. Licklider was smitten. Waldrop put it thus: "Interactive. Exciting. *Fun.*—JCR Licklider loved it. He absolutely loved it." The concept of real-time interactive computing was hardly new to Licklider, who had worked with Whirlwind for years. However, it was new for him to be sitting at the console of a digital computer that he could program on his own without changing any wires and also be able to watch its responses to his actions appear instantly on the display screen.[51] Working on the TX-2 sparked an epiphany for Licklider reminiscent of Ornstein's analogy that using the TX-2 was like being in the driver's seat of a car after having been a public transportation passenger. For Licklider, it was "like sitting at the controls of a 707 jet aircraft after having been merely an airline passenger for years."[52]

Licklider was not content with just conducting his own experiments on the

TX-2, however. His zeal for real-time computing soon eclipsed his interest in experimental psychology, and in late June 1957, Licklider left MIT for Bolt Beranek and Newman (BBN), a company that provided consultations in human-machine interaction. There he began to think deeply about how humans and computers could divide mental labor, even going so far as to conduct a time study of his own workday to determine where the divisions would occur. In his influential 1960 paper "Man-Computer Symbiosis," which appeared in *IRE Transactions on Human Factors in Electronics*, Licklider shared the result of his personal time study. He found that "about 85 per cent of my 'thinking' time was spent getting into a position to think, to make a decision, to learn something I needed to know" and that "much more time went into finding or obtaining information than into digesting it. Hours went into the plotting of graphs, and other hours into instructing an assistant how to plot." His thinking time was, in short, consumed by "activities that were essentially clerical or mechanical: searching, calculating, plotting, transforming, determining the logical or dynamic consequences of a set of assumptions or hypotheses, preparing the way for a decision or an insight." This led him to the disturbing conclusion that "my choices of what to attempt and what not to attempt were determined to an embarrassingly great extent by considerations of clerical feasibility, not intellectual capability."[53] In trying to work out a solution to the problem of wasted thinking time, Licklider arrived at his "Great Idea," namely, that people and computers would soon form a symbiotic human-machine partnership, thereby freeing humanity from the shackles of mundane mental labor and unlocking its creative potential.[54]

During his years at BBN (1958–62), Licklider became one of the most vocal proponents of real-time interactive computing, and one of Clark's most powerful patrons. But as Licklider's and Clark's plans to implement the "man-machine partnership" each evolved, the two men found themselves champions of antithetical visions of the future of computing. Clark's position, as we will see, was greatly reinforced by his collaboration with life scientists, while Licklider, himself a life scientist, would in his new career as an administrator put institutional and societal needs ahead of the needs of the laboratory.

While Clark was developing the TX-2 his collaborations with the CBL intensified. Besides Clark, Farley, and Gilmore, the group shuttling between Lincoln Lab and the CBL had grown to include several younger engineers and graduate students. Among them was Charles Edwin Molnar (1935–1996, an electrical engineer who arrived in Massachusetts in July 1957, fresh from graduating as valedictorian from Rutgers University. Following a chance encounter with a Lincoln Lab recruiter that spring, Molnar was offered the position of staff associate by two laboratory groups. Flipping a half-dollar coin, he chose Group 63, Papian's Advanced Development Group, where he was placed under Clark's hands-off supervision. In Group 63, Molnar not only became a key member of a team that transformed computing but he became an exemplar of the "bio-engineer" that NIH and other advocates of computerizing the life sciences sought to develop.

Immediately upon arriving at Lincoln Lab, Molnar was intrigued by Clark's collaboration with the CBL, finding it compatible with his own "notion that there might be some relationship of electrical engineering ideas and methods to understanding the nervous system."[55] With little in the way of orders from Clark, Molnar spent so much time at the CBL that he came to be treated as one of Rosenblith's graduate students and "developed a split professional personality." Some days he would attend to his official task of helping Clark build the TX-2, but just as often he could be found at the CBL, helping the researchers there with their older correlation computers. Even when Molnar was at Lincoln, he was frequently programming the TX-0 for CBL work.[56]

As construction of the TX-2 progressed, it became clear that the TX-0 would be superfluous at the Lincoln Lab. To Papian and Clark, it seemed only logical to give the machine to its most enthusiastic users, who were over at the CBL. Rosenblith, much to their surprise, turned down the gift as a white elephant. Clark recalled the rejection as a valuable learning experience, noting, "I therewith gained an important insight about what would work in a small laboratory setting and what would not. It seems in retrospect that the TX-0, small as it was for its time and demonstrably useful in CBL research, was still too much 'the computer' and not sufficiently 'an instrument.'" In other words, "Its care and feeding and the constant need for justification might well have compromised CBL's research objectives." Although Rosenblith was eager to conduct more research using machines like the TX-0, he had noticed that the CBL had become dependent on intermediaries like Molnar, without whose expertise many of the programs required by the experiments could not have been implemented. Furthermore, Rosenblith did not want research agendas built around the TX-0, which he feared would happen when members of his group applied for funds to support the machine. In short, he did not want the computer to take over his laboratory. Eventually the TX-0 found a home in the Electrical Engineering Department where it stayed—and was still heavily used by the CBL— until it was replaced by a donated DEC PDP-1, which was modeled after it.[57]

After the TX-0 was turned down by the CBL, two researchers there, Moise Goldstein and Robert Brown, approached Clark and Molnar to discuss the possibility of building a "next-generation," transistorized auto-correlator. This new machine would be smaller than the TX-0 and would be limited to the task of periodically extracting evoked neuroelectric potentials from a background of unrelated electrical activity by means of response averaging techniques. Appropriately, they called the machine the Average Response Computer (ARC).[58]

To build ARC, Clark and Molnar settled on cobbling together a machine out of spare TX-2 parts. For the new computer's logic circuitry, they used transistor-logic plug-in modules that had been designed by Ken Olsen and Dick Best for the TX-2. These were wired to a 256-word (18 bits each, just like TX-0 and TX-2) ferrite core memory, a mismatch considering the circuitry could operate at a clock speed of about 5 MHz (TX-2's speed), but the memory could only handle about 800 KHz.[59] After some clever stacking and folding, the whole thing fit into a box roughly the dimensions and weight of a large home refrigerator. It also had small wheels, so it could be rolled from one laboratory to another. The final product was, as Clark put it, "a machine of rare ugliness."[60]

Unlike the TX-0 or TX-2, ARC was not programmable; rather its three principal modes of operation, response averaging, amplitude histogram compilation, and time-interval histogram compilation, were wired into the circuitry. Switches on the control panel allowed the user to select from these modes and also to specify values of parameters. The ARC proved to be of great utility to the CBL in a narrow but long-running series of studies correlating EEG response in sleeping humans and anesthetized cats to stimuli. In both the human and cat studies, the ARC was able to average hundreds of responses to produce curves that the researchers would take as stable representatives of the subject's response pattern. Such averaging made it possible to "cancel out" electrical noise generated by recording equipment, be it electrodes placed on the humans' scalps or cochlear microphones implanted in the cats' ears (fig. 3.1).[61]

Looking back on the ARC, Clark claimed that its success "confirmed my belief that there were indeed useful things that small digital computers could do in the laboratory."[62] Still, it struck him that all of the ARC's functions could have easily been programmed on a general-purpose machine like the TX-0 rather than hardwired into control circuits. The neurophysiologists had a use-

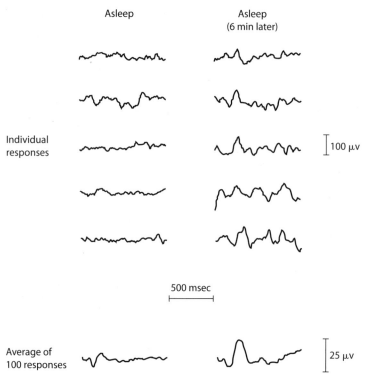

Fig. 3.1. Responses to periodic clicks recorded from a sleeping human subject. "The five traces in the upper left show consecutive responses taken approximately forty minutes after the subject was instructed to sleep. The five traces in the upper right are consecutive responses taken six minutes later. Each of the lower traces is the average of one hundred consecutive responses (computed by ARC-1) and includes the five shown above it. Clicks were presented binaurally at a rate of 0.75 per second. Upward deflection represents positivity of an electrode at the subject's vertex with respect to an occipital electrode (Subject H-432)." Clark et al., "The Average Response Computer (ARC): A Digital Device for Computing Average and Amplitude and Time Histograms of Electrophysiological Response," *IRE Transactions on Bio-Medical Electronics* 35 (1961). © 1961 IEEE

ful machine, but it seemed to Clark that they were not seeing the potential of general-purpose, real-time computing. In a 1960 symposium talk at UCLA's Brain Research Institute, Clark laid out what he saw as the tremendous advantages of using the versatile TX-0 instead of purpose-built machines like the ARC. Comparing the two computers, he noted, "It is quite simple to program the TX-0 to act very much like the ARC; in fact this has been done, requiring an investment of effort measured only in hours. The TX-0 can in addition generate quite varied displays of the data and of results of analysis and can be programmed to carry out exceedingly lengthy and complex operations if desired." However, Clark argued, to realize the full potential of general-purpose computers, institutions would need to change the way they managed computing resources, and "provide for procedural flexibility and easy access to machines of this type. "Ideally," he wrote, "the researcher would have the general-purpose computer in his laboratory for use 'on-line,' enabling him to observe and act on the basis of the calculated results while the experiment is in progress."[63] But by way of a compromise between existing institutional norms and his ideal, Clark expressed hope that "general-purpose machines with a capability somewhere between that of the ARC and the TX-0 will find their way into the laboratory."[64]

Clark recalls that his audience, which included representatives of the NIH-ACCR, was receptive to his speculation, but few believed such a general-purpose computer usable by life scientists would be developed in the near future. Clark, who it must be remembered was working with the CBL on the side of his main job at Lincoln Lab, had only a vague idea of how one could put the functionality of the TX-0 into a package that could fit into a laboratory. There was a practical concern too, namely that Charles Molnar had joined the Air Force. Between 1957 and 1960, Molnar had developed enough expertise in both computer engineering and neurophysiology that he acquired a keen sense of whether or not a particular aspect of a machine would suit the researchers. Clark found himself increasingly dependent on the young man when it came to architectural decisions concerning machines used by the CBL. Fortunately for Clark, strings had been pulled and Molnar was stationed at nearby Hanscom Field, but with his USAF duties Molnar was often too busy to play interlocutor between Clark's design team and the CBL physiologists.[65] Finally, there was the problem that Clark's interest in providing biologists with a small, real-time, interactive computer put him on a trajectory that ran counter to the flow at MIT and to the coalescing plans of Licklider.

The TX-2, it turned out, was overpowered. Sixty-four kilobytes was vastly excessive for most of the programs users were running on the TX-2. As such, there was concern at Lincoln Lab that the computer's resources were going to waste, especially given that with 25 to 40 people wanting daily access to machines like the TX-0 or TX-2 the individual user needed to sign up for a fairly limited time slot days in advance and then, while operating the machine, race against the clock—often with the next user impatiently looking on. This situation precipitated a debate over computer architecture that pitted Clark against most of his colleagues. Almost everyone at Lincoln Lab agreed that the norm of sharing computer resources by having users simply queue up and wait their turns was both inefficient and cumbersome to the point that it precluded inter-active, real-time use. Beyond that basic agreement, however, opinion diverged sharply.

Most Lincoln Lab researchers believed that research should focus on econo-mizing sharing because interactive-capable computers would for the foreseeable future be expensive to build and operate. This group, who Ornstein remembers as the "Big Dealers," comprised the bulk of the Lincoln Lab. During the de-velopment of Whirlwind and subsequent real-time systems, they had noticed that when a person interacted with a computer, the computer spent most of the time waiting for input from the user that is, waiting for the user to make a keystroke or turn a dial. The problem was simple: the computer was working much faster than its human operator. While the fastest human could transfer information—a note to a keyboard—in not much less than a tenth of a second, a computer of the early 1960s could move just as much information in and out of its memory hundreds of times in that same tenth of a second. While waiting for human input, the computer's time was going to waste. "The Big Dealers' solution," Ornstein recalled, "was therefore to divide up the machine's cycles in such a way that many users, sitting at individual terminals remotely connected to it, could use it at essentially the same time." The human operators were not using the computer truly simultaneously, because the computer could only per-form one task at a time, but, as Ornstein explains, a sufficiently fast computer "could switch its attention between users so rapidly that each user would have the illusion of having the entire machine to himself."[66]

During the mid- to late 1950s, numerous Lincoln engineers tinkered with existing computers to try to realize this vision. The most fruitful such effort was that of John McCarthy, a young MIT mathematician interested in computer languages who attempted in 1957 and 1958 to implement a scheme in which computer cycles were parceled out to multiple users of an IBM 704 (and later a transistorized IBM 709). In a now famous memo circulated on January 1, 1959, McCarthy labeled this division of computer cycles "general purpose time sharing."[67] Shortly thereafter, McCarthy proposed building a prototype of a time-sharing computer that would give users access to a rudimentary form of interactive operation via "glass teletype" terminals, or some other serial, text-only medium. During the early 1960s, the Big Dealers aggressively pursued McCarthy's time-sharing scheme, most notably implementing it in Project

MAC (Project on Mathematics and Computation),[68] founded by Robert Fano, Fernando J. Corbató, and Marvin Minsky.[69]

In lonely opposition to the Big Dealers was Clark, who insisted that real-time interactive use required a fast display capable of allowing the user to manipulate programs, data, and images. Thus far, such displays existed only on dedicated machines like Whirlwind, MTC, TX-0, and the TX-2. Even if time-sharing could be implemented, Clark argued, just a few divisions of computer cycles would deprive users of the power necessary to provide an interactive experience involving graphics. With multiple users, each would only have a fraction of the machine's capability at his disposal, thus watering down the interactive experience. Worse, in a time-sharing system many of the computer's fairly limited resources that had been dedicated to displaying an image would be appropriated for managing user access. In 1988, Clark recalled, "[Time-sharing] seemed to me a bad idea and still does, the captive imagination aspect no less than the underlying premise itself. Improved access, yes; thrashing competition and waste, no." Looking back on the development of computers since the 1960s, he opined, "It seems to me that we could have done better than to divert so much of our attention and resources to trying to make good the promise of patently unattainable 'sensible simultaneity' for all."[70] As Thierry Bardini points out, Clark's view of time-sharing was independent of but nevertheless "very close to [Douglas] Engelbart's criticism of the way people become subservient to a big technological system like a steamship or locomotive, instead of being given their autonomy by a technological innovation such as the automobile."[71]

One instance of the debate over time-sharing came in 1960, when the MIT administration organized the Long Term Computation Study Group to make recommendations regarding the future direction of university computers. Within that group was a technical subcommittee, which was chaired by Herbert Teager, and included Clark, McCarthy, Fano, Corbató, Douglass Ross, Jack Dennis, and Minsky.[72] They were charged with the task of bringing real-time interactive computing to the widest possible portion of the university community. With the exception of Clark, the committee settled on time-sharing as the means to that end.[73]

Clark's grounds for casting the dissenting vote was that the proposed time-sharing schemes did not support CRT graphics; that is, they had nothing a modern user would recognize as a monitor. Retrospectively, Clark attributed the gulf between him and his colleagues to his extensive work with graphical displays: "You have to be oriented toward interactive use of machines before you realize that CRT display is the one essential thing that you must have for wide-band presentation of information, no matter what else you have."[74] Pointing to the work of the biologists, Clark noted that "campus-wide time-sharing, so enthusiastically being rationalized as a panacea, would not be able to deal with real-time work such as the CBL's and moreover would inhibit the development of any interactive computing that involved complex displays."[75] The other committee members, who had not worked much with graphical displays, were unsympathetic. Clark recalled that "I tried to point out that it was going to be very hard to do real-time work for displays . . . the image they had in mind was that of a typewriter, or teletype machine actually, as the principal means of interacting with the time-sharing system. And that's very limited."[76]

Clark became even more stubborn when his colleagues asked him to support a proposal to adapt his TX-2 for time-sharing so that it could be accessed from all over campus via a network of teletype terminals. Clark refused, and his colleagues reacted with "disappointment and, as I recall, disgust." As chief architect of the TX-2, Clark would have been a major asset in any attempt to modify it, and without him the effort—which so many at MIT believed was worthwhile—would certainly be more expensive and time-consuming. Worse, from his colleagues' perspective, Clark had violated protocol by declining to submit a minority report explaining his position.[77]

In arguing for the importance of having complete control over a machine, Clark also found himself increasingly at odds with the vision of real-time interactive computing promoted by Licklider.[78] Though captivated by the TX computers, Licklider had, by the time he wrote "Man-Computer Symbosis" in 1960, concluded that there was "a speed mismatch between men and computers," noting that "any present-day large-scale computer is too fast and too costly for real-time cooperative thinking with one man."[79] To address this asymmetry, Licklider proposed that "for the sake of efficiency and economy, the computer must divide its time among many users."[80] Looking back on the early 1960s from 1988, Licklider remembered that he strongly believed at the time that "we needed to have time-sharing systems before we could do man-computer interaction research."[81] Clark's individualistic approach, Licklider argued, was grossly impractical; only time-sharing would provide ordinary people access to interactive computers they otherwise not afford. Thus, if Licklider was an advocate for real-time interactive computing, he was just as fervently advocating time-sharing with it.

Due to the exigencies of the Cold War, Licklider had become considerably more powerful since he had departed Lincoln Lab. In response to Sputnik, the Department of Defense had formed in 1958 the Advanced Research Projects Agency (ARPA) in order to conduct and facilitate the cutting-edge research the Pentagon believed was necessary to stay ahead of the Soviets. Over the next few years as popular sentiment over the "science gap" swelled, ARPA's budget mushroomed, providing it with tens of millions of dollars to spend with few strings attached. Within ARPA, there was a small behavioral science program as well as an intense interest in computers. Not only did Licklider seem like a good choice to head the behavior group, but his "Man-Machine Symbiosis" paper was, as Waldrop put it, "a ready-made research agenda for this whole ARPA program."[82] Consequently, in early 1962, ARPA offered Licklider the opportunity to head its Information Processing Techniques Office (IPTO), thus giving him the means to pursue his vision of time-shared real-time interactive computing.

While running IPTO and, especially after becoming director of Behavioral Sciences Command & Control Research for ARPA in 1963, Licklider generously supported the development of time-sharing computers and networks to allow communication between them. With the resources Licklider provided, MIT's Project MAC and similar endeavors at Stanford, Berkeley, and UCLA flourished. However, Licklider's patronage did not extend to the small group pursuing Clark's more individualistic philosophy of computing. Thus, for all the money ARPA was pouring into developing real-time interactive computing, Clark was seeing none of it. To realize his vision, he would look to the life sciences and its patrons.

A New Approach to Computing for Biologists

As the consensus about time-sharing solidified at MIT, Clark remained adamant that only complete control over the entire computer at all times would yield a truly interactive experience. Throughout 1961 he made the case that his approach to computing was particularly suitable for biology, and that it held the key to overcoming life scientists' reluctance or inability to make good use of digital electronic computers. Though Clark was outspoken at MIT, his supervisor in the Advanced Development Group, William Papian, found an outlet for his ideas at the NIH. Starting in 1960, Papian had been a member of the NIH's Advisory Committee on Computers in Research (ACCR), and was well aware of that group's frustrating experiences trying to get life scientists to use computers. Facilitated by Papian, Clark attempted throughout 1961 to persuade the ACCR to support his approach to computing.

Clark's Lincoln Lab report of November 22, 1961, titled, "Data Processing Aspects of Biomedical Computing Centers," best represents how he framed his vision of computing for the NIH. The report also illustrates the stark contrast between Clark's approach and those of advocates of centralized computing, be it time-shared or traditional batch processing. Though Clark's proposals clashed with the ACCR's preference to build computing centers, a look at his report goes a long way toward explaining why he was so warmly received by that committee. The ACCR's chairman, Lee Lusted, and its executive secretary, Bruce Waxman, both fervent promoters of "biomedical computing centers" quickly endorsed Clark's ideas as crucial to the NIH's agenda of computerizing biology and medicine, and took extraordinary measures to secure funding for Clark's work. The appeal of Clark's vision of computing to the NIH was that he pinpointed a major cause of biologists' reluctance to use computers—and he had proposed a viable solution to that problem too.

Clark started his report by attacking the notion that the "Computing Center," the very type of facility the ACCR was spending millions to establish, was appropriate for the life sciences. He wrote, "In examining the question of what type of computing facilities best meet the needs of biomedical research, it is difficult to escape the conclusion that the present-day Computing Center is an inadequate model." The problem, Clark argued, was that "computing centers are designed primarily to solve mathematically formulated problems arising within the physical sciences, whereas the greater need in the biomedical sciences is for the processing of large volumes of complex data, often without a wholly adequate basis of mathematical theory."[83] Computing centers, Clark acknowledged, "varied in makeup, detail, and administrative procedure" but could all be characterized by a core class of shared problems. Using MIT's various facilities as an example, Clark laid out this class of problems. Typically, the tasks successfully processed by computing centers were mathematically well formulated, relatively small, did not require much input and output, were not strongly dependent on real-time operation, and involved little or no improvisation in equipment or procedure.[84]

Citing Robert Ledley's 1960 NAS-NRC "Report on the Use of Computers in Biology and Medicine," Clark noted that the vast majority of biologists and medical researchers interested in using computers presented a set of problems quite different from those handled at most computing centers. Most biomedical problems, Clark argued, were "characterized by data processing and manipulation rather than by computation. They cannot, in general, be handled well for reasons of volume and complexity of data, the need for special equipment, real-time requirements, and imprecision of statement" (3). The only exceptions, as Clark saw it, were problems being pursued in areas that were essentially applications of physics and chemistry, such as X-ray diffraction analysis and molecular physics of organic molecules. Unlike physicists, most biologists were working in a realm whose governing principles were not understood, where phenomena defied reduction or essentialization, and where breakthroughs were often made via structured guessing that managed—rather than eliminated—the unknown.

Clark had presented a reading of Ledley's report very different from that of the NIH leadership and many members of the ACCR. Like Clark, the ACCR was acutely aware of the incompatibility of biomedical problems with the capabilities of most computing centers, but their solution and Clark's were diametrical opposites. The ACCR, on the one hand, had attempted to remedy this problem by trying to convince biomedical researchers to mathematize their research and to agree on some fundamental standards, so that their work would more closely resemble that of physical scientists, whose work seemed so much more amenable to computing. Clark's solution, on the other hand, was to alter the computers rather than the scientists hoping to use the machines.

The major change Clark proposed was to give researchers a device to digitize their data, that is, to computerize the information they had gathered. This meant giving computing centers the capability of getting the (often nondigital) data into the machines. Whereas the NIH effort called on researchers to reduce phenomena to a digital form before beginning an investigation, Clark wanted to build into the machines themselves the capability of digitally representing existing nondigital biological data. To be useful to those studying life, argued Clark, computing centers would have to be drastically restructured. As he saw it, "The needs of biomedical research for computing facilities include not only the *computation* machinery currently conceived but, more important, *data processing* machinery of considerable flexibility and power." He added that "such data-oriented computers can be expected to differ from the computation-oriented computers in their central logic and organization, in their peripheral equipment capabilities, and in the techniques of their operation" (3).

The hitch in this plan was that "data processing machinery of considerable flexibility and power" did not exist, nor would it exist unless major changes came to computer architecture. Clark characterized what needed to change by way of an analogy: "Most of the world's computers are, in fact, business machines, modeled on the file cabinet. The large-scale computation-oriented machines, in these terms, are based on the desk calculator model. What is urgently required in the biomedical sciences is a family of computers modeled on the laboratory oscilloscope" (4). What Clark liked about the oscilloscope was that, as opposed to a calculator, it allowed its user to adjust signals and ranges in real time via dials. This capability enabled researchers to focus on a particular range of data they found interesting or to quickly recalibrate settings to accommodate unanticipated changes in dynamic objects of study, such as animal or human laboratory subjects.

Clark argued that improving adjustability was the key to making computers more usable to biologists because each group of biologists made unique demands on the computer it used. In an environment in which underlying principles did not exist and standards were impossible to implement, every experiment effectively has its own set of rules, its own world. Each world therefore needed its own computer, or at least one that could be easily adjusted to follow that world's unique rules—that is, the particular needs of those observing particular data in their own particular way. For instance, the kind of data entered into the computer by somebody studying brainwaves would be very different from that input by a cardiologist or a molecular biologist, yet all remained lumped into the same biomedical computing center.

As Clark saw it, the limitations of the traditional digital computers made them incompatible with the reality of biologists' work. To use such a computer effectively in their research, each group of biologists would need full access to a computing center in order to configure it to suit their unique needs. Because constantly and comprehensively reconfiguring shared computers would be grossly impractical, Clark argued that what the biologist—"as yet ill-at-ease with massive mathematical techniques, and in possession of imperfect theoretical 'equipment'"—needed was a way to "realize, on his own terms, the full promise and power of the most important information-handling tool of modern technology" (4). Thus, he called for the NIH to replace or supplement the large batch-processing systems—those modeled after the "desk calculator," such as the IBM 7090—in which the agency had so heavily invested. In their place, Clark called for the development of "computers of several sizes, from small machines for individual laboratory use to extremely large-scale computers of great speed and capability" that embodied the principles of the oscilloscope, namely, "with emphasis on the data-manipulation and flow rather than on computation and precision." Then contradicting what seemed to be the main thrust of the NIH computerization effort, he dropped a bombshell, and bluntly asserted that "biomedical computing centers can best achieve flexibility by, in fact, decentralizing as much of this equipment as is economically feasible in order to simplify problems of special instrumentation and accessibility" (4). In other words, to serve biologists, the biomedical computing center had to cease being an actual centralized facility.

As part of removing the computer from the computing center, Clark also lowered the status of the computer. Rather than being something that scientists would restructure their research and institutions in order to accommodate, computers would, in Clark's conception, become merely a tool that allowed researchers to manipulate data in real time. To the NIH, Clark phrased this idea by quoting Walter Rosenblith: "By emphasizing the use of computers as research tools, there is implied a relationship between scientist and computer that is not unlike that which exists between scientist and microscope" (4). Instead of transforming biology to meet the needs of computers, Clark had suggested the opposite course: transforming computers to serve biology.

Despite Clark's uncompromising assault on the mode of computing in which the ACCR had so heavily invested, the committee received his report quite positively and very quickly provided him with resources to help him build a working computer around his ideas. The ACCR's reports indicate that the committee did not necessarily agree that developing a new type of computer for life scientists was a worthy end unto itself, but it did view the type of system Clark proposed as a promising way to begin computerizing many aspects of biology and medicine. From the committee's perspective, following Clark's advice did not mean letting go of the bigger systems. For instance, ACCR chairman Lee Lusted cast Clark's small, laboratory-based computers as intermediaries—or links—researchers would use in order to ease their transition to using the large, centralized computers.[85] It should also be noted that ACCR members generally did not regard Clark's individualistic computing and time-sharing as mutually exclusive. In late 1962, even after the committee began to fund Clark, member Max Woodbury asserted that "the greatest potentiality in [biologists'] 'creative' directions lies in making small slices of the biggest and best programmed computers available to scientists and creative workers when the inspiration is on them."[86] Throughout the 1960s, the NIH would pursue both Clark's vision and time-sharing.

The ACCR had several other reasons for quickly throwing its weight behind Clark's plans. Foremost, the committee had money to burn, but the money it spent on large computers had not generated much in the way of reportable successes. Second, Clark had by 1961, acquired a reputation as a brilliant computer designer—and it did not hurt that he had been vetted by Papian, a trusted member of the committee. The prestige attached to working with one of MIT's foremost computer developers was considerable. Indeed, ACCR reports on Clark's work almost never fail to mention his affiliation with MIT or the Lincoln Lab; and they often emphasized his prominence in the field of computing. Finally, to the immense satisfaction of grant reviewers, Clark already had by late 1961 a mostly complete blueprint for a system that embodied many of his ideas.

Linc Is Born

As of early 1961, when Clark began to approach the NIH for support, nothing resembling a laboratory-based real-time interactive digital computer had ever been built. As Ornstein recalled, the burden of proof rested on Clark. "Such a vision seemed so implausible at the time, and was so contrary to received wisdom, that the only way to make any headway in promoting it would be to put together a demonstration prototype, and that was precisely what Clark was quietly preparing to do."[87] Looking for a computer that combined the versatility of TX-0 and the analog-to-digital capabilities of the ARC, Clark hoped to give biologists what they needed and to keep the machine's cost to a minimum, cutting out absolutely everything else. Clark ultimately settled on five conditions for biological computing, which he and Molnar reiterated in their "Description of the LINC," a white paper they wrote in 1962 and published in 1965. When taken together, these conditions for life sciences computing had a "principal underlying objective," which was "to maximize the degree of control over the instrument by the individual researcher." "Only in this way," Clark argued, "can the power of the computer be usefully employed without compromising scientific objectives."[88]

For Clark, a useful machine to biologists would have the five following characteristics. First, it needed to be "small enough in scale so that the individual research worker or small laboratory group can assume complete responsibility." He wanted a computer that would be small enough to fit in a typical laboratory, which was already cramped. Moreover, he wanted no interlocutors in the computer's management: individual researchers or small laboratory groups would assume complete responsibility for "all aspects of the machine's administration, operation, programming, and maintenance." Second, the computer would "provide direct, simple, effective means whereby the experimenter can control the machine from its console with immediate displays of data and results for viewing or photographing." It had to be convenient to program and operate. Remembering the ease with which programs could be modified—in real time—on the TX-0, he wanted the computer to be programmable from a console located near, or preferably on, the laboratory bench. This removed the need for batch processing at a centralized computing center, the bane of so many attempts to computerize work with living subjects. Also, given that researchers would prefer to interact with and modify programs during the course of an experiment, Clark wanted them to have complete access to all the computer's resources on demand, so time-sharing was out of the question.

The third characteristic of Clark's computer for biologists was that it would be "fast enough for simple data processing 'on-line' while the experiment is in progress, and logically powerful enough to permit more complex calculations later if required." The biologists' machine, like the TX computers, had to be fast enough to provide immediate displays of data and results for experiments in progress in real time. To help researchers digitize analog data, this machine would need to simulate the oscilloscope and oscilloscope-like instruments that allowed users to make necessary adjustments to data ranges and outputs instantly. At the same time, the computer would also need to be logically powerful enough to allow researchers to conduct more complex calculations offline. After all, the digitized data was only useful if it could be analyzed without too much trouble.

Fourth, the computer Clark envisioned had to be "flexible enough in physical arrangement and electrical characteristics to permit convenient interconnection with a variety of other laboratory apparatus—both digital and analog—such as amplifiers, timers, transducers, plotters, special digital equipment, etc." In order to easily process biotechnical signals, the machine had to be readily compatible with the devices that generated the signals. Perhaps the one operational advantage the inflexible ARC had over the general-purpose TX-0 was that the ARC interfaced smoothly with a variety of analog laboratory equipment such as electrode amplifiers and EEGs. The point here was that the computer would augment existing laboratory equipment rather than require accommodations to equipment.

Fifth and finally, Clark's optimal computer for biologists would "include features of design which facilitate the training of persons unfamiliar with the use of digital computers."[89] It had to be accessible to new users. More than anything else, using the TX-0 and ARC had been a humbling experience for the CBL researchers. When it was necessary to modify hardware or a program, they almost always needed the intervention of a computer specialist. While Molnar's expertise had allowed them to write programs and implement changes quickly, they were still dependent on outsiders to get much use out of the computer. If they were going to tailor their computer to meet their experimental agendas, they would need to set up the machine so as to make the task feasible without much or any help.

Clark had a vague idea of how to reconcile such needs but was blocked in terms of finding a specific solution. Besides the problem of control, he had to contend with the biologists' other circumstances. Could a computer really be made small enough to fit into a laboratory but also powerful enough to support real-time interaction? Overcoming such quandaries took considerable time and energy. As he later explained, "It seemed to me that I now had most of the keys to the design process; a firm belief in the soundness of the goals and a good sense of the functional requirements; the general technology to be used; and the bounds of acceptable size, complexity, and cost." In the first three months of 1961, he "increasingly began to sketch and doodle on various handy sur-faces," but his efforts remained informal and disorganized because he found he lacked "a gimmick, some architectural idea to start the process off in a promising direction."[90]

In April 1961, Clark explained his "block" to Farley, Molnar, and Ornstein. They encouraged him to see how far he could work toward building the biolo-gists' dream machine simply by rearranging existing technology. In late May Clark found his "starting gimmick:" building a large part of the machine's logic out of a new family of plug-in-circuit modules that was being produced by DEC. By using these modules instead of building the logic from scratch, Clark saw that he could drastically reduce the machine's cost without compromising its speed.[91]

Around that insight, Clark's rudimentary design for a real-time interactive computer for biologists came together quickly. Working at home, he drew up plans for a machine in about six weeks (May 24 to July 4, 1961), most of which time he spent drafting plans to cobble the machine's parallel architecture out of the DEC modules and devising an appropriate set of machine instructions. The memory, he decided, would be limited to 1 kilobyte of 12-bit words—enough to run a fully interactive environment in real time but not so much that it would be prohibitively expensive. To address biologists' need for easy analog-to-digital conversion, Clark dedicated a large portion of the memory to analog-to-digital channels. For the interactive display, he used one of the smaller CRT monitors (a 5 × 5 inch 512 × 512 point array) that had been developed for the Lincoln machines. At Belmont Farley's suggestion, Clark added to the interface a special knob that when turned allowed users to modify continuous variables (for example, a user could turn the knob to change the order of magnitude of an axis of a graph on the display). For biologists' information storage needs Clark proposed a scaled-down version of the TX-2's magnetic tape unit. To ensure that the machine would be physically suited for storage in ordinary laboratories, Clark decided that it should be mounted onto standard nineteen-inch laboratory racks. Finally, he set a target price of $25,000 for each machine, which was about what a department head could authorize for equipment without approval of higher management.[92]

Still, without having produced much in the way of a specific blueprint, Clark gave his machine a generic name, Linc, in reference to its Lincoln Laboratory origins. By June 1961, Clark had presented his rudimentary sketch of the Linc to the CBL scientists, who received it warmly. His Lincoln colleagues were excited too; Ornstein and especially Molnar began to devote considerable time and energy helping Clark with the particulars of the Linc's design. Molnar and others at the CBL were attracted to Linc primarily because it manifested an ideal. As Molnar put it, "Technologically, the LINC was no great shakes; certainly the most important component of its success was the clarity and logic of the conception that Wes had of what was needed and possible. Once the vision was presented, a great many people became believers and committed themselves without reservation to making it happen."[93]

The biggest stumbling block turned out to be the storage unit. Clark wanted for each user to own tapes that would contain the programs and experimental data necessary to customize the machine to suit that user's particular needs. However, there were no small, reliable, and easy-to-use magnetic storage media circa 1961. The TX-2's tapes were the size of film reels, and frequently snapped during search operations because the inertial velocity of the spinning reels was upwards of sixty miles per hour. Worse, the room shook when the tapes were being spun—not something tolerable around recording equipment sensitive to vibrations. Clark's solution was a simple read/write unit onto which one could mount tapes that could store 1.5 million bits. At 840 bits per inch, the tape measured 0.74 inches by 150 feet and could be wound onto a reel 4 inches in diameter.[94] To reduce cost, Clark stripped Linc's tape unit of most equipment governing the speed of the tape; to compensate, each storage block on the tape was marked with a unique address.

The task of creating a programming environment on Linc that could be used by neophytes fell to a newcomer to the Lincoln Lab, Mary Allen Wilkes, a philosophy major freshly graduated from Wellesley College. Starting in September 1961, Wilkes began to write a Linc system emulator for the TX-2. Using this emulator, Wilkes wrote several small demonstration programs as well as the Linc Assembly Program (LAP), which served both as an operating system and a code assembler for the Linc. With LAP, the user could choose to write programs in an assembly language developed for the Linc or in machine code.

Between July 1961 and March 1962, Clark and his core team of Molnar and Ornstein translated Clark's sketches into a functional prototype. The plan was to have the machine ready in time for demonstration in Washington, DC, at the late-March 1962 NIH-ACCR-sponsored National Academy of Sciences Conference on Engineering and the Life Sciences, which both Walter Rosenblith and William Papian (an ACCR member) regarded as "an excellent way to introduce the machine to a broad scientific and technical audience."[95] In its final form, the Linc consisted of four suitcase-sized modules (seen clockwise in fig. 3.2, starting from the module under Clark's left hand): 1) *display scope*: this housed the 5-inch monitor and controls to manipulate images and text; 2) *magnetic tape unit*: with two read-write units, tapes could be duplicated easily; 3) *terminal:* this contained the jacks for analog input as well as potentienometer knobs; 4) *console*: a mostly empty module that contained indicator lights (to let users know which part of the memory was being accessed) as well as the a speaker that let users eavesdrop on the machine's circuits so that they could get a gross idea of whether their program was behaving as expected or perhaps looping.[96]

As planned, all four modules could be mounted on standard 19-inch laboratory racks; if stacked, their base was less than two feet by two feet. The wiring for the logic circuitry, however, was so extensive that it had to be housed, along with the core memory and the power supply, in a refrigerator-sized "electronics cabinet" (pictured to the left of Clark in figure 3.2).[97] Ideally, this box would be tucked into a closet and connected to the four modules via 30-foot cables. Ornstein noted, "We pushed this part as far out of sight as we could, thereby suggesting that it would someday disappear altogether."[98]

Using the Linc was a radically different experience from that of using most computers of any size in 1962. Instead of entering data onto punch-cards or via

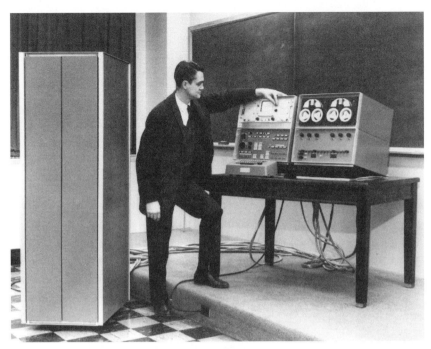

Fig. 3.2. Wesley Clark demonstrating the Linc prototype at Lincoln Lab in 1962. Photograph courtesy of Wesley Clark

a teletype and then receiving results on a paper tape, users interacted with the Linc by typing on a keyboard and watching the five- by five-inch display scopes for results. Knobs on the various components could be turned to manipulate, in real time, the data that was displayed on one or both of the scopes. When the machine was programmed, the numbers, symbols, and text that comprised the program's code were entered via keyboard and displayed on the scope. Despite the constraint of working with a 512-by-512-point black-and-white display, a wide variety of (either still or moving) text and images could be rendered.

The speed at which the Linc displayed what appeared on the scope was also adjustable. Robert W. Taylor later described to Mitchell Waldrop how using this feature allowed him to see that computers capable of no more than rear-ranging ones and zeros could build a "reality:"

> When I sat down at the LINC it had a little six-inch green and white display that looked like an oscilloscope, and a knob that let you adjust the speed of the machine. So you could turn up the speed, type an *A* on the keyboard, and the *A* would appear

on the screen very quickly—the *A* was made of dots, like a dot-matrix printout—or you could turn the speed down, and the *A* would build up very slowly. Also, you had a loudspeaker: the machine would click slow or fast according to what it was doing. So you had a sense of scale. You could see that this machine was building up a complicated reality through millions and millions of yes-no decisions.[99]

Linc's Triumph and LINC's Exile

Assembly of the Linc continued until just minutes before its first public demonstration in March 1962 at the NIH-sponsored Conference on Engineering and the Life Sciences. Clark and Molnar's presentation went smoothly and was well received.[100] Part of the credit went to Clark's stagecraft. As Samuel A. Rosenfeld reported in his twentieth-anniversary retrospective of Linc's debut, "Clark, with the flair of a showman, grabbed an ash tray overflowing with ashes and cigarette butts and poured the contents on the tape's read head. Even after several minutes of such abuse, the tape continued to operate with only two or three errors."[101]

In the course of the demonstration, several conference participants realized that the NIH itself had projects where the Linc could be used right away. That same afternoon, Robert Livingston, scientific director both of the National Institute of Neurological Diseases and Blindness (NINDS) and the National Institute of Mental Health, (NIMH) invited Clark and Molnar to try out the Linc in an actual laboratory environment. Livingston, who had been closely following Linc's development from afar, had found a task for which the Linc seemed to be custom-built. Arnold Starr, a neurophysiologist who had been working for Livingston in NINDS, had been for months struggling unsuccessfully to record the neuroelectric signals generated in cats' brains when they heard sounds. Despite much tinkering with the electrodes that were implanted in the brains of his cats, Starr could not distinguish neuroelectric signals from the electrical noise that the ear membranes created when a sound entered the auditory system. Compounding his frustration was the unreliability of his electronic components, not to mention the cats themselves, who only cooperated under certain conditions and even then not predictably.[102] He was, in short, stumped.

In the span of a single afternoon, Linc solved Starr's problem. After setting up the Linc in Starr's laboratory, Clark and Molnar connected one of the Linc's analog-to-digital input channels directly to a multiple-electrode array that Starr had implanted in the brain of his most reliable cat, Jasper. Then Molnar wrote a short program that commanded Linc to: (1) send a pulse to a device that would generate a click stimulus; (2) record the reaction to the click by the audio cortex; (3) repeat steps 1 and 2 as many times as desired; (4) display—in real time—the average neuroelectric response of the cat to the multiple stimuli.[103] Within hours of their attempt with the program, they isolated the neuroelectric response from the electrical noise and had gone on to command Linc to change the pitch and frequency of the stimuli, thereby gaining insight into how the brain reacted to particular patterns and intervals of noises. To Rosenfeld, Livingston recollected their wonderment at the new world the Linc opened for Starr to explore: "It was such a triumph that we danced a jig right there around the equipment. No human being had ever been able to see what we had just witnessed. It was as if we had an opportunity to ski down a virgin snow field of a previously undiscovered mountain."[104]

Linc's other early trials, however, did not produce such a sanguine reception. The following day, for instance, Clark and Molnar triumphantly wheeled Linc over to Mones Berman's laboratory to "see what [Linc] could do to isolate a very fast fluorescence transient produced in a particular biochemical reaction." After several hours of testing and adjusting, the Linc could not isolate the transient (and therefore the reaction) Berman sought.[105] Nevertheless, NIH's—and particularly Waxman's—interest had been piqued to the point where the ACCR promised Clark generous funding so that he could continue developing the Linc and then build several dozen replicas.[106]

Linc came together physically as the Lincoln Laboratory's support for its development fell apart. Already, Clark was already somewhat estranged from his colleagues over his recalcitrance concerning adapting the TX-2 for time-sharing. Further, his plans to devote his team's full time to developing the Linc were not shared by laboratory management beyond Papian. Particularly galling to Lincoln director Frederick C. Frick was a proposal by the CBL neurophysiological psychologist Thomas Sandel to set up a small "wet" laboratory adjacent to the TX-2 in order to use the large machine for real-time biological work. As Clark explained to Waldrop, Frick saw the proposal as an encroachment: "We were the only non-classified research group there. The lab director [Frick] didn't want non-military money and the shifts of power that would imply." Attempting to bring Clark back into line, Frick gave him an ultimatum: "I was told to knuckle under or leave."[107]

On the spot, Clark chose the Linc over the Lincoln Laboratory and announced to his stunned design team that they could switch projects or help him find a new home for the Linc. Most of the principals of the original Linc team chose to follow their computer wherever it went. For Severo Ornstein, who had long harbored misgivings about conducting research on behalf of the military, Clark's decision to leave Lincoln was heartening: "I was delighted to discover that, like me, Wes was hoping to find a way to do something with computers in a totally different, non-military arena."[108] But as Ornstein also recounts, he and the others were greatly motivated to pursue the Linc because they believed their project would be worthwhile: "Each of us had poured a lot of blood into the [Linc] development and we weren't inclined to let it go. Moreover, we had developed a conviction that we were on an exciting trail and that our futures lay ahead in biomedical computing."[109]

The disheartening search for an institution to support Linc consumed the second half of 1962.[110] Several members of the Linc team were almost immediately approached by Licklider, who offered them positions at Bolt Beranek and Newman, but that fell through in October when Licklider joined ARPA, where he distanced himself from Linc, lest he jeopardize the seemingly incredible support he had been offered to pursue time-sharing, which, of course, was the antithesis of Linc.[111] MIT, meanwhile, seemed to have no space to host a major development project that was not already fully funded. It was during that rootless time that Clark changed—or "backronymed"—Linc's name to the *Lab*-oratory *In*strument *C*omputer (LINC) to reflect the project's new orientation.

In the late fall of 1962, they found a savior in Walter Rosenblith, who had just successfully proposed that MIT host the Center for Computer Technology and Research in the Biomedical Sciences, an interdisciplinary institution that would house scientific and technical staff from several New England universities for the ostensible purpose of developing an effective, long-range biomedical computing program. To support the Center's first seven years of operation, the NIH had already committed to providing an astonishing $35 million. Within the Center was the vaguely-named Center Development Office (CDO), headed by Rosenblith and Papian which existed solely to garner multi-institutional support (namely from the NIH but also from major regional universities) for the LINC. As Clark recalls, the CDO's $1.5 million proposal to the NIH "was widely accepted almost at once," and funds to relocate the LINC team to a small building adjacent to MIT's main campus "magically appeared."[112]

Settling into their new home in January 1963, the LINC team rushed, over the next few months, to meet deadlines set by those who had secured them resources. The most pressing was that set by Bruce Waxman, who had secured funding from NIH and also NASA, via its Bioscience Program—in what Clark called a "dazzling display of civil service at its best."[113] Waxman had promised the two agencies that the center would be training dozens of teams of life scientists to use the LINC fruitfully by no later than the summer of that year. Further pressure mounted when the NIH publicized the $35 million grant for the center.[114]

In February, the NIH announced the LINC Evaluation Program, wherein researchers would get to take one of twelve LINCs back to their laboratories in exchange for spending six weeks in Cambridge learning how to use the machine.[115] The "LINC Summer," as the team called it, was structured as a hands-on experience, an approach they attributed to earlier disappointments with traditional teaching methods. As Rosenfeld explains, "Earlier, in 1961 and 1962, the LINC team had offered summer training courses on the basics of computer programming for laboratory applications. They were confident that in ten 8- to 10- hour days they could cover digital computer programming fundamentals." When, however, the classroom approach to training did not produce effective computer users, "the development team decided that no amount of purely academic discussion could prepare the scientists for the realities of computer maintenance and trouble shooting.[116] Beyond appreciating the pedagogical value of working directly with the computer, the LINC team wanted to prepare biologists to use a machine for which they alone would be responsible for operating and maintaining. Should trouble arise, there would be no maintenance organization to repair the LINCs. Though the LINCs were very simple compared to today's machines, their components were much less reliable, to the point where testing for bad wiring connections and replacing faulty pieces were unavoidable aspects of everyday use.

Then there was the matter of preparing the biologists to write software. As of the middle of 1963, the LINC's operating system, LAP, was not developed enough to be of much utility to the users, nor was there an extensive library of prewritten programs. Given that each user would have unique needs, as Ornstein points out, "Virtually all of the software that a user would employ would have to be developed and written directly by that user, who would thus be intimately familiar with its purposes and implementation."[117]

For the dozen machines, NIH received a "surprisingly large number of proposals submitted (72)," many from top research groups. As Rosenfeld put it, "Even with little knowledge of LINC's capabilities, it was obvious to many researchers that a small, on-line computer in their own labs was a potential boon worth the investment of a summer of tinkering in the suburbs of Boston."[118] With the exceptions of geneticist Joshua Lederberg, the dozen winners all conducted research in physiology or psychology. Partly this can be attributed to the ACCR's agenda of promoting work that directly advanced the NIH's mission of improving medicine, and partly it is because the physiologists' and psychologists' proposals most closely matched LINC's specific capabilities. (Chapter 4 explores how several groups of researchers put LINC to use, while Chapter 5 examines Lederberg's use of LINC—and many other systems—in his effort to find and determine the structure of "Martian amino acids.")

Although Clark and Molnar had demonstrated a functional prototype of the Linc at NIH in early 1962, that machine was only superficially met the objectives of the plan Clark had pitched to NIH. This precipitated a scramble. Between January and June 1963, the LINC team had to finish the control logic circuitry, expand the memory to 2K, render the LAP functional for users other than experts like Clark and Molnar, get the tape unit to read and write consistently, and wire the thousands of circuits in each of the sixteen machines' electronics cabinets. Severo Ornstein described the effort as "the most intense thing any of us ever did," noting that for months on end the core team (now Clark, Molnar, Ornstein, Wilkes, Bill Simon, Norm Kinch, and Don Maltor) "worked without regard for the clock until we were ready to drop."[119] Much of the work was improvised as well, as Ornstein colorfully illustrates: "One of the crew (Don O'Brien) reported a vivid dream in which Wes [Clark] was driving a steamroller directly towards the edge of a precipice while Charlie [Molnar] was furiously attempting to attach wings. Bill Simon sat in the rear, speed-reading a book on aerodynamics!"[120] The only area where they had any significant leeway was, thanks to the NIH's largesse, that of price. Though Clark had set a goal of $25,000, the assembled LINCs cost roughly twice that, with most of the money going to the memory and logic circuitry.[121]

On July 1, 1963, the first cohort of biologists arrived at the center to begin their month of LINC training. The LINCs, however, were still not ready. To buy time, and also to get a sense of what the biologists knew about computers and programming, the LINC team provided—against their better judgment—the biologists with two weeks of classroom instruction on the use of computers. Immediately it became clear that the biologists knew almost nothing about computers. In just two weeks the course could not offer the comprehensive mathematical and engineering education Robert Ledley had suggested in 1959 would be necessary to bridge the gap between biologists' current knowledge and what they needed to know to use computers.[122] It could, however, as Clark put it, enable the biologists to "learn enough computerology to give them the confidence needed to take their machines home to their own laboratories."[123]

For the biologists, the course made clear the scale of the task of incorporating a computer into their research. Several of the campers, Clark recalls, had shown up in Cambridge with golf clubs, so unfamiliar with computers that they were unaware of how much work learning to use them entailed.[124] The biggest challenge was teaching the biologists to program on the machine level—that is, without higher level languages or compilers. The few biologists who were familiar with computers, such as Lederberg, remembered being indignant that the LAP had not been developed to the point where excursions into machine code were unnecessary. But Clark recalls that "the general acceptance of machine-level programming as the price of dealing with such a small memory had been cheerful enough."[125] One researcher who was willing to pay that price was C. Alan Boneau, a Duke University psychologist, who in 1965 summarized what he believed were his accomplishments during the LINC Summer as well as the consequences of his computer training. In his evaluation of that program, he reported, "I feel that the month at Cambridge, while hectic, was a very worthwhile experience, which netted a tremendous amount of theoretical and practical skills which have stuck with me." He explained that after his initial training his computer skills had grown considerable, and that he was able to do work that had seemed beyond his ability just months before. For instance, he noted, "At present I experience no qualms about running down some malfunction in the machine (which usually turns out to be something else) and have uncovered defective diodes and transistors with no trouble. [Since the 1963 LINC Summer] I have designed and built supplementary circuitry following the DEC logic requirements for running ancillary equipment and feel that I know enough that if I pushed I could design my own computer (at least the logic) at this point." Such capability, while impressive, did not come easily. "Admittedly," he wrote, "most of these skills came about the hard way, the Cambridge stint furnishing guidelines, but no details, and many the long hour I sweated over difficulties that came up when I was trying to get it to do things that weren't in the original plans."[126]

Ten days into the course, the LINC construction was still not on pace to provide any of the campers with hands-on experience before their month was up. The biologists, meanwhile, were growing restless in the classroom. When

Molnar joked that the process could only be sped up if the biologists assembled the LINCs themselves, Clark jumped at the suggestion and put the biologists to work. The decision turned out to be fortuitous. Few of the biologists had much experience in building electronic devices, most having not even dabbled with the radio assembly kits (such as Heathkits) that were popular in the early 1960s.[127]

Once the LINCs were assembled, each of the groups had to write a program for the LINC for a problem from their own laboratories. Within two weeks all of the groups had written and run their programs, with Clark noting, "For the most part the participants had all taken to the unfamiliarity rather well."[128] By month's end, the biologists had packed their LINCs into moving vans, whereupon the machines, in Molnar's words, "dissolved in the laboratories around the country." With the second cohort (August 1963), things went much more smoothly. Better still, the experience of building the LINCs prepared them for task of reassembling machines. Molnar proudly pointed out that the record time from arrival to "reassembled and running" was about thirty minutes.[129] By the end of the summer 1963, about a dozen LINCs were installed in biologists' laboratories.

While the LINC team was busy training biologists to use their new computers, their host, the Center for Computer Technology and Research in the Biomedical Sciences, was falling victim to its own success in generating interest and excitement. The center's large budget and heavy presence in the press had caught the MIT faculty by surprise. By the late summer, many had concluded that the center would soon become a major MIT institution and began to more closely scrutinize its structure and rapid growth. Other than Rosenblith, no prominent MIT faculty were involved in the center; none of the principals of the center's flagship LINC project had "serious faculty positions."[130] It also appeared to the faculty that the MIT community had little say in the center's direction, given that it was supported almost entirely by federal grants. Furthermore, the center's interdisciplinary nature put it into direct competition with a wide array of more established MIT departments and projects.

In the fall of 1963, a faculty group headed by Provost Charles H. Townes offered the LINC group regular faculty positions—Clark would be fully tenured upon entry—provided they integrated the center into the mainstream MIT administration. Otherwise, Townes informed them, MIT would not affiliate with the center, nor would it provide it any institutional support. The LINC team, which had thrived in the relative autonomy of NIH oversight, balked at

Townes's proposal, ultimately deciding that as long as they had access to the NIH money, they had no major reason to continue developing biomedical computers at MIT.[131]

MIT cut its institutional affiliations to the center swiftly, and the LINC group had to start looking for a new home at "a university with good engineering and medical schools in which the top management would look favorably on our enterprise of interbreeding the two disciplines."[132] Such universities were few and far between, even though developing biomedical electronics was high on the NIH's agenda. In early 1964, after looking at Yale University and the University of Rochester, Clark entered serious discussions with the administration of Washington University in St. Louis on the possibility of establishing a thirty-person, multimillion-dollar center for developing computers like LINC.

Washington University had several qualities that made it attractive to Clark. First, its Provost, George Pake was not only enthusiastic about computing but also LINC's particular ideals, both in biomedicine and computer architecture.[133] Indeed, his commitment to biomedical computing was so strong that, according to Ornstein, "Pake confidently told the NIH people that he intended to take us all on as faculty whether or not NIH decided to continue their support of our activities."[134]

Washington University was also home to Jerome Cox's Biomedical Computer Laboratory (BCL). Cox was an electrical engineer who had served as a valuable consultant to the LINC team during its construction, working out several key problems pertaining to the interface of the core memory and the logic circuitry. In 1960, Cox had developed his own digital computer, the Histogram Average Ogive Computer (HAVOC), which he used to record evoked average responses from hearing-impaired infants to ascertain the degree of their hearing loss.[135] Unlike LINC, HAVOC was a special-purpose computer and therefore could not readily be reprogrammed.[136] Following HAVOC's success, Cox had seriously considered building a general-purpose digital computer, but he abandoned that plan when he saw the LINC prototype and joined the LINC effort.[137]

Cox was also heavily involved in the NIH-ACCR, serving on that committee as well as the LINC Evaluation Board. With the ACCR's support, Cox established the BCL at the Washington University School of Medicine in 1962 for the purpose of developing and promoting the use of machines like HAVOC among research physicians. When he saw that LINC needed a home, Cox jumped at the opportunity, first by stoking Pake's enthusiasm for LINC, then by flying out to Cambridge in the early spring of 1964 to ensure that the grant paperwork for a possible move to St. Louis was proceeding apace. Cox's aggressive courtship of the LINC group very likely kept the project from dissolving. When he showed up in Cambridge, he found the LINC group adrift and its leader depressed.[138] Unmotivated to write more grant proposals for establishing a home, Clark had retreated to what he enjoyed, working on the LINC and playfully arguing about ideas. In order to set up shop at Washington University, though, the LINC group needed to formally explain to the NIH what they would do in the long term.

After a great deal of cajoling from Cox, Clark settled on proposing to the NIH an expansion of his vision of interactive computing. It was still quite vague, and amounted to giving nonspecialists the tools to design their own computers. While describing this vision, Ornstein recalled, "We felt that it was important to be able to design computers, and related pieces of special purpose digital hardware, far more easily than was then possible. It should be feasible, Wes felt, to come up with a limited set of building blocks that were truly logical elements of significant power, in which the rules for interconnection should be extremely simple." As Clark imagined it, "The builder should not be required to have any electrical engineering background whatsoever, so all questions of electrical loading, timing, etc, would somehow have to be pre-solved. One should furthermore be able to build systems of arbitrary size and complexity; the units would need to be extensible."[139] They called their building blocks "macromodules," though Ornstein concedes that giving these tentative musings such a concise name was tantamount to "lending them a reality which, at that stage, they didn't possess at all."[140] Regardless of the proposal's plausibility, the NIH was sufficiently impressed that it renewed its long-term commitment to the LINC group.

Between Pake and Cox's promises and goading, both the NIH and Clark were persuaded to move the LINC effort to Washington University. There, the LINC team was housed in its own facility, the Computer Systems Laboratory (CSL), a "twin sister" of Cox's BCL. The move to St. Louis, of course, precipitated several departures; most notably, Mary Allen Wilkes left the group to take a trip around the world. Molnar, too, was unable to move to Missouri immediately because he needed to stay another year in Massachusetts to complete his Ph.D. and military assignment. Ornstein, meanwhile, harbored doubts that he would be happy in St. Louis and committed hesitantly for a maximum of three years there. Nonetheless, the bulk of the group, including Molnar, had made the migration by late 1965. Once settled in St. Louis, they began to study the effect of their machine on the life sciences.

LINC, the First Personal Computer

LINC was highly influential in computer design in the 1960s and beyond. Unlike most computer systems then or now, the LINC's design specifications were was made entirely accessible to the public and were not protected by patents or other restrictions—its development, had after all, been publicly funded. Thus, anyone was free to duplicate the LINC and, if he or she so chose, sell it. Seeing a potentially lucrative market in laboratory computers, Digital Equipment Corporation began to offer clones of Clark's 'classic' LINC as well as the LINC-8—a PDP-8/LINC hybrid—to biomedical researchers starting in the mid-1960s. Figure 3.3 shows an advertisement for one of these machines that appeared in the May 1966 issue of *Scientific American*. The LINC-8 offered several substantial improvements over the original LINC, including more support for general-purpose computing subroutines and a larger memory. Although DEC only managed to sell about 50 LINC classics and 150 LINC-8s, its later minicomputer models incorporated many aspects of the design of the original LINC. For instance, the popular PDP-12 (initially called the LINC-8/I) enabled users to emulate most of the functions of the original LINC on a platform that also provided a general-purpose computer much more powerful than the original LINC.[141] Almost thirty-seven hundred PDP-12s were sold before DEC discontinued the model in 1971. The LINC's magnetic tape, called LINCtape, was reincarnated as DECtape, which, along with a LINC-inspired tape drive, was used with most DEC machines during the mid-1970s.

DEC was not alone in building LINC variants. Stating in 1964, another Massachusetts company, Spear Electronics, began to sell its "micro-LINC," which was a standard LINC modified to be more "friendly" to neophyte computer users. "In spite of its extremely sophisticated approach to laboratory data acquisition and processing," Spear boasted, "you will find that a Spear micro-LINC remains affable and unassuming—as a computer should that costs less than $50,000."[142] Unlike the original and DEC LINCs, Spear's LINC provided an operating environment that could with "only a few hours of training" be used "with no need for a basic computer background." Instead of writing programs, users chose the programs they wished to run from among a large library of pre-

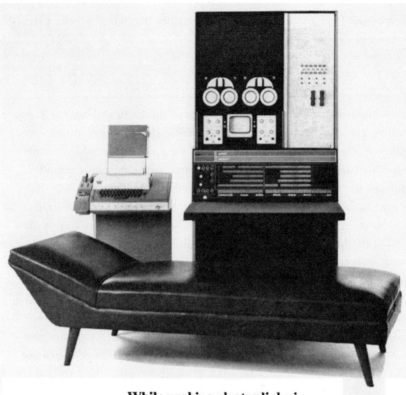

While probing electrodialysis,
a man suffered mental paralysis.
His friend, the LINC-8
alarmed by his state,
revived him with real-time analysis.

When LINC-8 goes on-line with your experiment, a dialogue begins. True dialogue. What you say to your friend depends upon what your friend is saying to you.

LINC-8 is a full laboratory computing facility for life, physical, and earth sciences. It has inputs, outputs, and a high speed digital computer in-between. It listens to your problem, collects analog or digital data directly from your experiment, analyzes it, then displays the analysis in a form to give you new insights,

and at a speed that lets you do something about it. Like change the parameters.

The original LINC was conceived at M.I.T. to be the most creatively approachable computing system ever designed for the laboratory. LINC-8 is all the LINC was, except it is about 5 times faster, 50% larger in memory, in a single cabinet, with teletype output in addition to the scope, all for less money. Two voluminous software packages help you to freely associate.

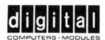

COMPUTERS · MODULES

DIGITAL EQUIPMENT CORPORATION, Maynard, Massachusetts 01754. Telephone: (617) 897-8821 • Cambridge, Mass. • Washington, D. C. • Parsippany, N. J. • Rochester, N.Y. • Philadelphia • Huntsville • Orlando • Pittsburgh • Chicago • Denver • Ann Arbor • Los Angeles • Palo Alto • Seattle • Carleton Place and Toronto, Ont. • Reading, England • Paris, France • Munich and Cologne, Germany • Sydney and West Perth, Australia • Modules distributed also through Allied Radio pared "biomedical and statistical analysis routines."[143] By the late 1960s, however, the micro-LINC was discontinued because most researchers who wanted an interactive computer wanted one with the capabilities of the LINC-8.

LINC and its variants were commonplace in laboratories until they were replaced by microcomputers, typically Apple Macintoshes, in the early 1980s. That a personal computer could serve a lab in the LINC's stead was hardly coincidental, and indeed several prominent computing figures have hailed the LINC as the progenitor of personal computing. C. Gordon Bell, the developer of DEC's VAX minicomputers and later a prominent researcher at Microsoft, accorded the LINC the status as the "first PC." As Bell put it, "the microprocessor, memory, and mass-storage technology appearing in 1975 [led] directly to the personal computer industry . . . nevertheless, the first personal computer, the LINC, was built in 1962, long before its predicted technological time."[144] Alan C. Kay, "the grandfather of the Macintosh," whose Xerox PARC computer interfaces inspired those of Apple and Microsoft, was in turn inspired by the LINC. In 1985, while addressing his colleagues at Apple, Kay declared the LINC "the first personal computer ever invented by man" and noted that "what didn't find its way into the DEC minicomputers is what it [LINC] was all about, which was a personal interactive computer."[145] He reiterated this claim in 1996, labeling the LINC "the first PC."[146]

Dynabook, Kay's 1972 design for a laptop-like "personal computer for children of all ages," embodies ideals that resonate strongly with those found in the LINC. "Imagine," Kay and Adele Goldberg wrote in their description of the Dynabook, "having your own self-contained knowledge manipulator in a portable package the size and shape of an ordinary notebook. Suppose it had enough power to outrace your senses of sight and hearing, enough capacity to store for later retrieval thousands of page-equivalents of reference materials, poems, letters, recipes, records, drawings, animations, musical scores, waveforms, dynamic simulations, and anything else you would like to remember and change." What made Dynabook special, Kay argued, was not just its capacity to store many kinds of information but that it could be used in real time. "There should be no discernible pause between cause and effect," he wrote, and explained that "one of the metaphors we used when designing such as a system,

Fig. 3.3. (opposite) Advertisement for the LINC in *Scientific American*, May 1966. Digital Equipment Corporation hoped its LINC variants would appeal to biomedical workers frustrated with sharing centralized computers.

was that of a musical instrument, such as a flute, which is owned by its user and responds instantly and consistently to its owner's wishes. Imagine the absurdity of a one-second delay between blowing a note and hearing it!" As Kay saw it the "desires for flexibility, resolution, and response lead to the conclusion that a user of a dynamic personal medium needs several hundred times as much power as the average adult now typically enjoys from a timeshared computing." Thus, he (and other computer developers) faced a choice: "This means that we should either build a new resource several hundred times the capacity of current machines and share it (very difficult and expensive) or we should investigate the possibility of giving each person his own powerful machine. We chose the second approach."[147] The exemplar of that second, individualistic approach, and apparently Kay's inspiration, was the LINC.

LINC also influenced Kay's concept of the computer as a "metamedium"—that is, that the digital computer "can be all other media if the embedding and viewing methods are sufficiently well provided." In a 1977 essay coauthored with Adele Goldberg, Kay explained that "this new 'metamedium' is active—it can respond to queries and experiments—so that the messages may involve the learning in a two-way conversation." Thus, a real-time digital computer would not be treated like a device explicitly designed—as computers originally had been—to perform arithmetic and logical tasks but was rather a medium resembling that of "an individual teacher." Here too the precedent had been set by LINC, which was a digital computer that could be used to perform tasks of laboratory instruments, and could, once programs were written for it, be treated by users in the same way they had treated those instruments. On this new role of the computer, Kay and Goldberg wrote, "We think the implications are vast and compelling."[148]

At Xerox PARC, in Palo Alto, California, where Kay worked in the 1970s, the LINC also left a legacy. Xerox's 1972 Alto computer—initially called "the interim Dynabook"—which arguably served as the basis for many of the projects later pursued by Apple and Microsoft, embodied many of the LINC's ideals. Like the LINC, the Alto was small, completely controlled by the user, graphically oriented, and could be used in real time. Instead of twisting knobs, the user interacted with Alto via a device that gave them much more precise control, Douglas Engelbart's "mouse." The Alto's developers did not draw directly from the LINC to design their system—they were a generation too young to have been involved in the LINC's construction—but their mentors and managers at Xerox PARC were quite familiar with the LINC and sympathetic to Clark's approach to computing. George Pake, the Washington University provost who had fostered LINC's development in St. Louis starting in 1964, was Xerox PARC's founding director. Robert W. Taylor, who regarded his ARPA-related visits to the St. Louis LINC group as a formative experience, was the manager of Xerox PARC's Computer Science Laboratory from 1970 to 1983. Beyond creating an environment that was hospitable to LINC's ideals, Xerox PARC management hired several participants in LINC's development. Most notably, Severo Ornstein, part of the original LINC team, joined Xerox PARC in 1976, working there for several years on an interface for laser printers and on Mockingbird, a musical score editor.

Though Xerox was only a marginal player in the computer market when it boomed in the 1980s, developments at Xerox PARC, some of which had roots in the LINC, profoundly shaped the design of the personal computer. In 1979, Steve Jobs, the cofounder of Apple Computer, visited Xerox PARC and was inspired by the Alto to build a small computer with a graphical user interface (GUI), which he called the Lisa. The Lisa evolved into the Apple Macintosh, which debuted in 1984; a similar system, Windows, was developed by Microsoft for IBM PC–compatible computers in the early 1980s. The personal computers that were inspired by the machines at Xerox PARC were built around microprocessors, and they were cheap enough for millions of Americans to afford, two qualities not shared by the LINC. Nevertheless, LINC stands out among these machines' ancestors not just because of its priority but also due to the explicit way in which LINC introduced the particular—and at the time of its development, highly unconventional—set of ideals around which personal computers have been built. Most importantly, LINC was a successful revolt from centralized, time-sharing computing. It demonstrated that a real-time interactive computer could be built for individuals and small groups, and that the computer's use did not necessarily need to be institutionally governed. LINC was, as Clark concluded in 2007, "a real beginning." He remembered, "What excited us was not just the idea of a personal computer. It was the promise of a new departure from what everyone else seemed to think computers were all about, a corrective point of departure from an otherwise overwhelming mainstream." From his perspective, "The need [for a machine like LINC] was entirely real, the opportunity was there, the resources superb. Just build and demonstrate a sound counterexample [to the centralized norm] and see to it that it was used

humanely, a complete if small computer that did interactive real-time work efficiently, one that could simply be turned off at night with a clear conscience, just
taken for granted, no administrators. For us, it was the point of departure."[149]

Those who were seduced by the LINC paid dearly for their passion. Not only
were they cut off from the major patron of computer research, the military, but
they were also cast out of the geographical center of the computer development
world circa 1960, MIT. Few of them, however, would have had it any other
way. In the early 1960s, when Clark conceived of LINC, the very notion of an
interactive general-purpose digital electronic computer was embraced by only a
handful of people, mostly his colleagues at the Lincoln Laboratory. When Clark
went a step further and declared that such computers could only achieve their
full potential if each individual user had complete control over all aspects of
the machine's operation, he alienated most of those sympathetic to alternatives
to batch-processing computing. While his colleagues devoted their energy to
developing time-sharing architecture for real-time interactive computers, Clark
was spurred by the unique needs of biologists to develop a smaller, interactive
computer over which the user had total command. Only computing in real time
could let biologists modify experiments as they progressed, a near necessity to
anyone working with volatile, capricious living subject matter.

4

A New Way of Life

Computing in the Lab, in the Clinic, and at the Foundation

B y 1965, dozens of laboratories and clinics across the United States were operating electronic digital computers. For the users, installing and beginning to make regular use of these computers was an exciting process. They had at their disposal machines that could perform calculations many times faster than human beings, and many had generous federal support—especially from the NIH—to acquire the skills they needed to make productive use of the equipment. Whether their computers were room-sized IBM 7090s or refrigerator-sized LINCs, those who had access to computers found that using them profoundly shaped the way they thought about their research or patients and the way they worked on a day-to-day basis. They also learned through direct experience that adopting computer technology, while generally rewarding, required much more effort, dedication, and patience than they had anticipated. In the words of two physician–computer experts working in the 1960s, "The discrepancies between the visions and the realities are startling."[1]

Amid the hype and hope surrounding computers in the 1960s, candid assessments of their use were rare and not widely distributed. At stake were multimillion-dollar federal grants and corporate contracts, not to mention the users' prestige and egos. Observing American biomedical computer use from Britain, David E. Clark wrote, "People don't like washing their dirty linen in public, and so many reports are difficult to seek out."[2] However, anyone who went through the trouble to extract one of the progress reports submitted to the NIH's Computer Research Study Section would have found frank, technically competent, and sometimes even humorous evaluations of computer use in research and care. Though written over forty years ago about decades-outmoded computer systems these reports make strikingly clear that many of today's challenges related to computer use in biology and medicine have been encountered before.

For the NIH and other major sponsors of biomedical computing, such as the USAF and the NSF, the "impact" of the computer on research and care was a major concern and was monitored closely.[3] On the one hand, computers had been a large and risky investment for these agencies. The mathematics and engineering training equired to program a computer was simply not part of a biologist's or a physician's traditional education. Worse, living systems, because they were so enormously complex and dynamic, were difficult to quantify or otherwise reduce so that they could be examined using a digital computer. On the other hand, computers offered great hope that vast amounts of information could be managed and from that information wisdom could be extracted to allow enormous strides in basic research and patient care.

Even in the early 1960s, when the NIH's early efforts to computerize biology and medicine were just getting under way, some general patterns of computer use had become apparent. One particularly keen early observer was NIH-ACCR member Max A. Woodbury, a mathematician who had worked on UNIVAC with J. Presper Eckert and John Mauchly, most famously to devise the algorithms that predicted Eisenhower's landslide victory over Stevenson in the 1952 election, before gravitating toward the life sciences and becoming Professor of Experimental Biology at the New York University's Medical School. Woodbury took an anthropological—and also rather sardonic—approach to describing the experiences of biomedical computer users. In 1963, after several frustrating site visits for the ACCR, he wrote that "hopes and fears alike show up only too clearly in attitudes toward computers and very secondarily, with the persons who—well—interact with them. The range from 'blind trust,' to ostrich-like behavior, to suspicious dislike or even hate, reflects the belief in magic, black and white, still prevalent in this day and age."[4]

Though Woodbury's analysis was tongue-in-cheek, it pointed to a serious problem, a "tendency to place a magical interpretation on computing activities—leading us to say, for example, 'let's feed the data into a computer and see what comes out' or the reverse side of this same man-made coin 'computers can do nothing they are not told to.'" As a consequence of these "polar attitudes," efforts to use computers were generally guided into two counterproductive channels. First, "an effort on the part of programmers to package programs in a closed form with little flexibility and such that the user specifies only a few knob settings on the 'idiot proof' magic black box at hand." And second, "the user specifying to a programmer those aspects which he understands and the programmer codes it for him." In both cases, "the final result is a program written by one person to the perceived specifications of the other," a situation that Woodbury believed ultimately pointed to "a separation between man and his tools."[5]

In laboratory research settings the "separation" Woodbury perceived was largely overcome when scientists gained access to small, real-time computers like the LINC, which allowed them to do much of the programming work themselves as experiments progressed. In efforts to computerize medicine, however, the gap that existed between the user and the computer became a major—and sometimes insurmountable—obstacle. When the intellectual and institutional requirements of running a computer collided with the day-to-day requirements of running a hospital, even the best-led and best-funded efforts to computerize healthcare centers came up far short of their initial goals.

The great difference between biological and medical computing had not been anticipated. In the late 1950s and early 1960s, the vast majority of the computer work being done in biology and medicine fell under the aegis of "bio-medical computing." Early visionaries, like Ledley, Lusted, and Waxman, saw little distinction between the "bio" and the "medical" applications of computing and used the terms interchangeably. Indeed, most American laboratories and hospitals that received significant federal funding in the early 1960s were evaluated by NIH-ACCR and its successors, the CRSS and DRFR. However, when biologists and physicians began to report back to the NIH in the mid-1960s, it became apparent that biology and medicine each bore their own set of distinct challenges when it came to computerization. Consequently, separate communities and later professional societies and journals formed in bio-computing and medical computing. These groups, which were heavily intermingled from the start, share many of the same broad goals—such as battling disease—but were also shaped by quite different experiences using computers.

Computers as a Way of Life in the Lab

For the biologists, utilizing computers for research was an extraordinary challenge. The most thorough and forthright accounts of the process of computerizing laboratory work can be found in mid-1960s reports to the NIH on the use of the LINC. Examining them reveals how using computers shaped how scientists thought, worked, and lived. These cases are mostly confined to physiology and psychology but can be viewed as representative of the problems faced by researchers working outside those fields. Though biologists employed a wide variety of digital computers and programming languages, they all had to learn the basics of computing. A particular advantage of looking at the use of the LINC is that small-scale real-time computing, while certainly not the norm in the 1960s among the general population of scientific computer users, has been the dominant mode of computing in biology since the late 1970s, when biologists began using microprocessor-based personal computers in large numbers. With the crucial difference that prepackaged software suitable for biology research was almost completely nonexistent in the early to mid-1960s, the experience of the dozens of the early LINC users resonates—in a way that experiences using large, centralized machines does not—with those of thousands of researchers who adopted personal computers in later decades.

One reckoning came on March 18, 1965. That day and the next at Washington University's Computer Research Laboratory (CRL) were devoted to the "Convocation on the Mississippi," the final meeting of the NIH's LINC Evaluation Program. There, the dozen groups of biologists who had used the LINC since the early fall of 1963 would report (1) what, if anything, they had accomplished with the LINC; (2) whether or not they had found the effort to use the computer worthwhile; and (3), their future plans for computer use. They would also inform the NIH if they wished to continue using the computers, but it would then be up to the NIH to judge whether or not the researchers could keep the machines.[6] From the results of this field test of computers, the NIH would then make a decision on continuing support for small-scale computers like the LINC.

For the LINC team in St. Louis, the stakes could not have been higher. In the years since its members had departed MIT, they had all but lost the debate over time-sharing. While J. C. R. Licklider's ARPA poured millions of dollars into developing time-sharing systems for military and civilian researchers, Clark's group could count on only the NIH to support their development of small computers over which the individual user had complete control at all times. Granted, Licklider still took a strong interest in Clark's work at Washington, to the point where he dispatched his protégé, Robert Taylor, to St. Louis to examine the LINC. Taylor was impressed, noting to Mitchell Waldrop, "A Teletype was one kind of interaction, Spacewar [a 1962 game for the PDP-1 in which two spaceships, each controlled by human player, shoot at each other] was another. E-mail was still another, but the LINC was somehow more dynamic than any of them."[7] Nevertheless, when Jerome Cox petitioned Licklider to support greater production of small, personalized computers like the LINC, Licklider declined on the grounds that a machine like the LINC would still be far too expensive for regular people to afford.[8] Thus, the LINC's future rested in the hands of the biologists.

The LINC team need not have worried. Not only were the biologists pleased with the LINC but, having used it, they could not for the most part imagine returning to laboratory life without such a machine. Their reports to the LINC Evaluation Program show that they incorporated the LINC into their existing work and that they were propelled into new research agendas by using the machine. Twenty-seven of the biologists who used the LINC—"LINC-lunks" as they called themselves—were so moved by the experience that they dedicated a resolution to LINC's developers thanking them "for supplying the undersigned with one of the most challenging, interesting, and educational experiences of their lives by introducing them to an exciting and powerful new experimental tool and technique and opening up a new world of ideas, possibilities and expectations."[9]

The atmosphere at the conference may have been genial, but the discussion was frank, with biologists praising the LINC and also not hesitating to communicate what they believed to be its shortcomings. Twelve groups who were granted a LINC by the NIH gave thorough accounts of their work with the machine, but three of these testimonies are particularly effective in illuminating how the LINC—and indeed computers in general—transformed research.[10] First to be examined is LINC's use by George S. Malindzak Jr. and Frederick L. Thurstone, both heart physiologists based at the Bowman Gray School of Medicine at Wake Forest University. Their experience highlights how the LINC broadened their research agenda by vastly speeding up the process of data acquisition. It also demonstrates that using the LINC brought unwelcome changes to the lab, leading to resistance among graduate students and technicians to working with computers. As physiologists working in a small laboratory setting, Malindzak and Thurstone were representative of the majority of LINC's users. Furthermore, their account was regarded by the LINC development team as paradigmatic. Also presented are the cases of two groups of psychologists, led by Donald S. Blough and C. Alan Boneau, of Brown University and Duke University respectively, both of which used LINC in studies of operant conditioning in pigeons. In a loose sense, the LINC work with pigeons is a twin study, and by examining each of these groups in its own right, many of the epistemological and institutional changes wrought by LINC become apparent. Though the two groups of psychologists were employing LINC in similar studies, their approaches to using it were distinct. Thus, by comparing the two groups of psychologists (and by comparing both to the physiologists), one can get a sense of the degree to which local conditions shaped computer use and of the computer's capacity as an agent of change.

In the end, George Malindzak and Frederick Thurstone were "thrilled" with the LINC's performance and reliability, but they were considerably less pleased by the difficulty of integrating the little computer into their working laboratory at the Bowman Gray School of Medicine. Before acquiring the LINC, they had extensively used analog equipment to study how blood flowed through arteries, especially the aorta. Typically, they collected data from live mice implanted—"instrumented" in their terminology—with recording devices called flowprobes, which measured the velocity of the blood as it traveled through an artery. The flowprobes were attached via wire to analog amplifying and recording devices. Prior to their acquisition of LINC, analog-to-digital conversion was performed by hand and processing was accomplished on the university's IBM 1620 computer, for which Malindzak and Thurstone had written several small FORTRAN programs.

By using the LINC, the two researchers were able to quickly determine if their flowprobes were working correctly and then display and analyze their data. Once the equipment was demonstrably working, the LINC allowed them to compute and display graphs of harmonic amplitudes and phase angles for each of four simultaneously measured aortal pressure functions. Here the LINC proved very helpful by allowing them instant access to results, which, in turn, let them isolate useful data. As they explained, many of their experiments produced " 'bizarre' results," namely they "showed a non-linear (almost random) distribution of mean arterial pressure and harmonic phase angle with distance along the aorta." While they believed that "this [phenomenon] could be real," they found it "difficult to justify on the basis of arterial dynamics." The problem was that the causes of the phenomenon, such as clot formation within the tubes—called cannulae—they inserted into the aorta to deliver or remove fluids were "difficult to detect with conventional monitor equipment."[11]

Before using the LINC, the "bizarre" data only became apparent after extensive processing on the offsite IBM 1620. They reported, "One could run through a complete experiment without knowing until final processing is done that the data does not meet the criteria for successful numerical analysis." That is, they did not learn until long after the experiment was over if their data had been corrupted by clogged cannulae. With the LINC, however, they were able to monitor—in real time as the data was being gathered from the subject—spatial distribution of mean pressures, as well as harmonic amplitudes and phase angles for each pressure function. Consequently, they were "able to detect prior to actual processing whether or not the data collected during the experimental phase meet the criteria for the numerical analytical scheme." If the LINC detected anomalous data, they reported, then "corrective measures are taken and subsequent data is earmarked as 'good.'"

Having accomplished their initial mission of reliably measuring pulsatile flow, thanks to the LINC, Malindzak and Thurstone began to investigate hitherto inaccessible phenomena. As they reported to the LINC Evaluation Program they had studied the "hydrodynamics and transmission characteristics of the mammalian arterial system" in three completely new ways. First, they had used the LINC to investigate "the degree to which reflections of the arterial pressure pulse are present in the aorta and the extent to which the reflections distort and modify the pressure pulse contours"—recording the pulsatile reflections necessitated a degree of precision that their old instruments had not afforded them but that the LINC could. Second, they used the computer to explore "the physical nature of the temporal and spatial variance of reflected energy in the aorta trunk and the establishment of a quantitative basis for its prediction." Third, they wrote programs to measure "the effect that varying amounts of reflections have on overall cardiac performance in particular, the total work of the heart." To access the second and third points on their agenda, they developed a "method of numerical analysis based on Fourier analysis of complex pressure pulses . . . that describes the transmission of the pressure pulses within the circulatory system."[12]

Within months, however, the LINC was producing so much useful data that Malindzak's and Thurstone's time on the 1620 was not sufficient to run all the transforms they wanted to. Rather than pay for extra sessions on the 1620,

Malindzak and Thurstone decided to develop the 1620's FORTRAN Fourier analysis routines for the LINC. Making an effort to "utilize the LINC as
extensively as possible without jeopardy to the on-line research program," they
used the LINC while it was "offline"—that is, not connected to any live subjects—at night and on weekends to perform Fourier analysis of arterial pressure
pulse data. This enabled them to produce—usually overnight—an amplitude
and phase for each desired harmonic for each of four channels of information.
They reported that the results of these analyses were then transferred to punch
cards and "fed to an IBM 1620 for further processing in terms of incident and
reflected vectors."[13]

Implementing the Fourier analysis routines on the LINC proved to be a
considerable challenge. Writing the necessary arithmetic subroutines (such as
floating point, add, subtract, multiply and divide, sine, cosine, arctangent, and
log) needed to carry out Fourier analysis required the efforts of several programmers over the course of a year.[14] Once the subroutines were complete,
Malindzak and Thurstone began to use LINC in a new capacity, noting, "It has
been only since our arithmetic routines have been working properly that we
have come to realize the full potential of the LINC in regard to our research
program. What we have viewed as a sophisticated A-D convertor prior to this
time has now become a useful laboratory tool."[15]

The LINC may have given Malindzak and Thurstone access to areas of
research that had been hitherto beyond the means of their small laboratory, but
pursuing the new agenda that the LINC made possible proved disruptive. In
several important ways, their experience belied Molnar's claim that "one consequence of the LINC style was that the LINC could enter the existing laboratory
of an investigator without a need to create new organizations and new staffs to
put the tool into use."[16] Hardest hit were the lab's graduate students, who were
now required to master the LINC in order to conduct research. As Malindzak
and Thurstone reported, their students responded negatively to the LINC for
"three very good reasons." First, "Most of the students are not to the point in
their program where processing experimental data is an important consideration." Second, "[students] who are aware of this need have been discouraged
by the amount of programming required to supply simple basic routines which
are easily available on any machine using FORTRAN." And third, "There is no
reference programming manual from which they could learn LINC symbolic
programming techniques."[17] Taken together, these three reasons show that the

learning curve to using the LINC was too steep for the purpose of most graduate students' work, so they avoided the machine.

At the same time graduate students refrained from using the LINC, Malindzak and Thurstone's use of it intensified. Consequently, the presence of the
computer deepened the divide between the graduate students' experiments and
those conducted by Malindzak and Thurstone, whereas before the computer's
arrival the work of faculty and students had been tightly integrated. Its presence had therefore cleaved training and research by rendering the laboratory's
research, now wholly dependent on LINC, too esoteric to be used for training. This circumstance, in turn, increased the faculty workload dramatically,
because they had to conduct an increasing amount of the experimental labor
themselves and because large parts of the graduate training regimen could no
longer be carried out on the job, so to speak.[18]

To alleviate their new workload, Malindzak and Thurstone brought professional computer programmers into their lab, another entirely new development,
and one that contradicted Clark's calls for scientists to treat the LINC just like
any other laboratory instrument. Treating the LINC as a computer rather than
an instrument, however, turned out to be disastrous, due mostly to the vast differences between operating the LINC and operating virtually any other computer on the market. The lab chiefs reported, "We have tried to train three
programmers . . . on the LINC thus far. The first had a nervous breakdown, the
second simply didn't want to learn and the third quit to take a better job. In all
three cases it required no less than two months before these programmers could
write a new program with confidence."[19]

Being early adopters of and becoming dependent on the LINC, Malindzak
and Thurstone discovered, had also isolated them from their colleagues in the
broader physiology community. With LINC as their primary research instrument, they found they had increasingly less in common with colleagues who
were still using analog devices. Preoccupied with the LINC, their discourse
diverged sharply from that of their colleagues. Even those who used digital
computers for analysis had little to offer someone seeking advice about specific
problems on the LINC. Such social isolation, Malindzak and Thurstone concluded, greatly undermined their productivity, and indeed many of the institutional goals of the NIH effort to promote computers in the first place.

What Malindzak and Thurstone believed most harmful was their lack of
access to a community of computer users, which they argued was just as impor-

tant as access to the machine itself. Without a community of computing biologists, they maintained, it would be very difficult to develop the software necessary to make the LINC a versatile research tool. They noted, "This limitation is exhibited most clearly in the lack of available basic computer programs and in the insufficient communication among those who are using the LINC computer and attempting to increase its effectiveness in their research." They also feared that poor communication between LINC users would lead to expensive but redundant work at multiple institutions. "With the present investment in programming and trained personnel," they warned, "duplication of this effort would be impractical if not foolhardy."

To overcome the problems posed by the dearth of circulated programs and the lack of communication among biologists, Malindzak and Thurstone called on Washington University to "establish at the earliest possible date a centralized programming staff and office which would be charged with the function of alleviating these difficulties." Until a reliable system for distributing programs was established, they felt it necessary to report that "it is probable that many investigators can best apply their programming and research efforts to machines for which greater support information is available." This remark they qualified with a stinging conclusion that "this may be true even though the most significant features of on-line operation and rapid analysis which the LINC possesses may not be available [on any other computers]."[20]

While physiologists scrambled to accommodate the volumes of new data produced by using the LINC, psychologists found that their little computers allowed them to design experiments that were radical departures from the scope and aim of their previous work. Moreover, the LINC allowed them to access "subtleties" that, in turn, opened major new paths of inquiry. Two groups of psychologists reporting to the Washington University Convocation, led respectively by Donald S. Blough of Brown University and C. Alan Boneau of Duke University, used the LINC in their investigations of the same phenomenon, operant conditioning in pigeons. By examining the commonalities and major differences between each group's LINC experiences, many of the changes the computers were bringing to the study of the mind become clear.

In order to appreciate how using LINC affected laboratory psychology work at Brown and Duke, one must be familiar with the fundamentals of operant conditioning. Like classical (Pavlovian) conditioning, operant conditioning (also known as instrumental conditioning or instrumental learning) involves the subject's response to a stimulus. Unlike classical conditioning, however, the response in operant conditioning is *voluntary*. The best known example of an experiment based on operant conditioning is the "Skinner box." Psychologist George Boeree colorfully describes one of the phenomena B. F. Skinner observed in 1940. Setting the stage, Boeree writes: "Imagine a rat in a cage. This is a special cage (called, in fact, a 'Skinner box') that has a bar or pedal on one wall that, when pressed, causes a little mechanism to release a food pellet into the cage." Then, something important happens: "The rat is bouncing around the cage, doing whatever it is rats do, when he accidentally presses the bar and—hey, presto!—a food pellet falls into the cage! The operant is the behavior just prior to the reinforcer, which is the food pellet, of course. In no time at all, the rat is furiously peddling away at the bar, hoarding his pile of pellets in the corner of the cage." In the case of this rat, "A behavior [the operant, or pushing of the bar] followed by a reinforcing stimulus [the conditioning, or receiving of the food pellet] results in an increased probability of that behavior occurring in the future."[21] Besides "positive reinforcement" (described above), operant conditioning provides a framework to understand the phenomena of "negative reinforcement," in which a subject learns to avoid a particular voluntary behavior when that behavior is followed by experiencing a negative or unpleasant stimulus. Lastly, "extinction" of the operant behavior is the phenomenon whereby the subject ceases a particular behavior after a period during which the reinforcing stimulus is absent; for instance, if there is a long period during which no food drops into the cage after the rat pushes the bar—even many times—the rat will eventually stop pressing the bar.

Like Skinner's rats, the pigeons at Donald Blough's laboratory at Brown University had been conditioned to exhibit particular behaviors, namely to peck at keys illuminated from behind by small lights of fixed wavelength and intensity. If a pigeon pecked a lit key, it would receive food reinforcement. What Blough wanted to investigate were the mechanics of extinction. His methodology: "Following a number of sessions . . . food reinforcement ceased and the light on the key varied randomly in either wavelength or intensity. Responses emitted during these changes were categorized by both stimulus and inter-response time." By accurately measuring the responses over the period of extinction, Blough hoped to observe precisely how responses changed in the absence of stimuli.[22] All of the stimuli were controlled by the LINC, which also recorded all of the responses—in the course of a workday, the pigeons often pecked keys more than ten thousand times.

In order to pursue this inquiry Blough employed the LINC to clear several major hurdles, some behavioral (on the part of the pigeons—as opposed to the researchers), others technical. In the former category was the problem of inter-response dependencies. In a primer to other LINC users, Blough illustrated why this phenomenon had frustrated his work. Normally, he explained, an effective way to measure the influence of a stimulus (and other variables) is to measure the rate at which an animal responds to that stimulus. However, in situations where there has been operant conditioning, the animal's response rate is governed by "inter-response dependencies"; that is, "when behavior is maintained for many hours by intermittent reinforcement, behavior patterns emerge and responses become 'chained' together." These dependencies can be very strong, to the point where even greatly changing other variables seems to have little effect on the animals being tested. For instance, once pigeons became trained to expect food only at particular intervals—say once per hour—they settled into "superstitious" behavior patterns and would only peck food-producing keys at those intervals, even if many other conditions in their environments had changed. Pigeons that had developed inter-response dependencies therefore ruined studies of response times because they were stuck in a pattern. Sometimes the inter-response dependencies were easy to spot, but in other cases, such as when the inter-response times the pigeons had become accustomed to were very short, their influence could escape the researcher's notice. Even with the best equipment, Blough noted, "this influence is hard to evaluate and to control."[23]

Using the LINC, Blough's group was able to overcome this vexing problem. The team programmed the LINC to "reinforce . . . only those responses that terminated inter-response times which had occurred least frequently in the immediate past." According to Blough, this "schedule," which would have been extremely difficult for a human technician to consistently maintain, "discouraged response-to-response dependency, while generating stable response rates and uniform behavior among subjects."[24] This technique was used to provide data for several published microbehavioral studies. For instance, Charles P. Shimp, one of Blough's graduate students in 1965, authored a 1974 *Journal of the Experimental Analysis of Behavior* article, demonstrating that there was a linear relationship between inter-response times per feeding opportunity and the number of feeding opportunities.[25]

While offline, the LINC was used extensively to process the data it recorded. As Blough explained, "The LINC computed condition probabilities that a response would occur, given that a particular stimulus was present and that a particular interval had elapsed since the previous response."[26] The results of these analyses—usually available the day the data were acquired—were extensively used to plan future experiments. Experimental planning was also catalyzed by the histograms LINC generated in real time.

The LINC also allowed Blough's group to gather and organize much greater volumes of accurate data than previously possible. The LINC could control the stimuli and measure responses in six separate pigeon boxes (each containing one bird). To do so, the LINC was programmed to display a light (or a pattern of lights) of a particular wavelength for a certain amount of time and at certain intervals. Humans could conduct this work on a coarse level, but the LINC made it possible to implement stimulus regimens where the interval between the time a bird tapped a lit key and the time the bird was exposed to the next stimuli was decreased or increased by increments as short as fifty milliseconds.

Like the physiologists Malindzak and Thurstone, Blough found that his LINC allowed him to envision a much more ambitious agenda. In his words, LINC "not only enables us to do more easily what we formerly did with relay and solid-state programming equipment, but it has opened up entirely new possibilities." Having used the LINC to create and monitor a complex stimulus-reaction environment for pigeons, Blough hoped to use the machine to find a way to "drastically reduce individual differences [among pigeons] and make possible a rational quantitative treatment of the rate measure." Moreover, he planned to use the LINC's interactive environment to study such responses in humans. Noting that "the display capacities of the LINC encourage us to add some human perceptual studies to our program," Blough sought to monitor human subjects as they performed conditional tasks on the LINC.[27] This new agenda, however, made his team wholly reliant on their computer. By 1965, he would report sincerely, "Our research now depends entirely on the LINC. . . . Most of the research we are doing now and plan to do would be impossible without the machine."[28]

For Blough, integrating the LINC into the laboratory proved far less disruptive than the experiences of Malindzak and Thurstone. Ignoring boasts that the LINC could be quickly and easily programmed by biologists unfamiliar with computers, Blough imported an engineer who had a strong interest in psychology, Lloyd Marlowe, to write software and manage hardware for the computer on a part-time basis. Marlowe wrote over fifty programs and created a "meta-system" to let users call up those programs and to let them set parameters for graphic displays.[29] Blough's three graduate students all conducted experiments that relied on the LINC, but the amount of time they spent pro-gramming—as opposed to operating—the LINC was strictly limited. Once his group had the programs and hardware integration they needed, Blough was satisfied with LINC's operation and approachability: "Though I started with no special knowledge of any computer, I have been able to make effective use of the LINC, and to keep it going with relatively little outside help." He was con-cerned, however, that "those of us with no programming background" lacked access to teaching materials about programming. To remedy this, he called on Clark's group to "mak[e] available a graded series of pre-written, annotated pro-grams for newcomers" and to publish "detailed handbooks on the nature of the machine and its programming."[30]

Meanwhile, in C. Alan Boneau's laboratory at Duke University's Department of Psychology, a LINC was being employed in another investigation of operant conditioning of pigeons. Instead of using the LINC to examine the minutiae of behavioral extinction, Boneau hoped the little computer would enable his labo-ratory to reap insight into the color discrimination problem, or color-blindness. The setup of Boneau's experiment was as follows. First, a pigeon was placed into a box with a volume of about one cubic foot. On one side of the box were two holes, a small round hole at head level and a larger (two by two inches) hole at ground level. Behind the smaller hole was a piece of translucent plastic hinged so that it moved when the pigeon pecked into the hole. The larger (bottom) hole contained a trapdoor that, when opened, allowed pigeons to access food. To run the experiment, researchers would project monochromatic light from the rear onto a plastic key—the light source was a variable monochromator controlled by the LINC. Researchers could instruct the LINC to vary the intensity and color of the light. Furthermore, a shutter, also controlled by the LINC, inter-rupted the projected light at specified times and intervals.[31] As Boneau explained, "The basic procedure consisted of a series of short presentations of the various stimuli, food being made available for a short period if several conditions were met."[32] For instance, the shutter would be opened, letting a particular color of light through to shine on the key; then, if the pigeon pecked that key, the shut-ter would be closed and the hole containing the food would become accessible for a few seconds. If the pigeon continued to peck the "correct" color, the food hole would be open for longer and longer periods, but if the pigeon pecked the "wrong" color, access to the food was denied, either outright or by decreasing the amount of time the food hole remained open. Typically, the total elapsed time of a trial was about five seconds, and thousands of trials were conducted in the course of a day.[33]

As with the pigeon experiments at Brown, the LINC controlled all of the mechanical components of the study and recorded the trial data produced by the birds. Before the LINC arrived, all of these functions were carried out by technicians using specialized electronic equipment. Boneau reported that replacing them with the LINC did not disrupt the process of his experiments, noting that "there have been absolutely no procedural changes in the research program *necessitated* by LINC." There were, however, "a few (and undoubtedly will be more) [procedural changes] which were inspired by the presence of the LINC."

Evoking "LINC's capabilities to squeeze more information out of the experimental situation," Boneau presented to the LINC Evaluation Program a portrait of a laboratory that had its agenda and practices irrevocably transformed by the little computer. First, using the LINC allowed Boneau to consider many more variables in his studies. For instance, prior to installing the LINC, Boneau measured only the number of pecks occurring in an extended number of trials, but with access to the LINC "we were soon measuring the latency of the peck and storing the complete sequence of latencies together with the stimuli and reinforcement information." More important, having the programmable LINC on hand also allowed Boneau and his colleagues to craft their experiment as it proceeded. They reported, "It occurred to us that the lumping of the data was probably observing short range temporal effects contingent upon individual reinforces and long range effects like changing drive level over time as the bird gradually ate enough to near satiation." They continued, "Consequently, we decided to record the latency on every trial, keeping an ordered list of stimuli and the latency of the response of any to them. We would then be able to go back over the data, pulling out various interesting aspects of them as we saw fit."[34]

By incorporating these new parameters into their ongoing study, Boneau's group began to see in the data accumulated by the LINC trends that had until then not been apparent. This, in turn, enabled them to conceive new questions to pursue. The strongest instance of computer use raising new inquiries in Boneau's lab involved a trend his group spotted in the LINC data. Boneau described it: "There gradually emerged out of these data a relationship between latency on the one hand and accuracy on the other. The longer we waited before responding, the more likely was the bird to give a response to a reinforced value." Curiously, as Boneau noted, "From all we can tell at present, the performance for a given latency is invariable, no matter the circumstances from which the latency came."[35]

In their attempt to elucidate a cognitive mechanism to account for the pigeons' behavior, Boneau's group turned to the LINC once more. Specifically, they wanted to determine if "some sampling process is taking place over time and that the increase in accuracy is simply a function of the fact that a larger sample was taken." To create an experiment to illuminate this phenomenon, they employed the LINC. At the 1965 Washington University meeting, Boneau said that the LINC would be programmed to display a stimulus light of a particular wavelength for a variable length of time—between one-quarter and one and a half seconds—and then replace it for the remainder of the two-second trial period with a white light. Once the LINC was programmed, Boneau explained, "we will then be able to compare the latency distribution across stimulus values for the various exposure times. We expect that this procedure will interfere with the performance at the shorter exposures, but if it doesn't it will rule out the sampling hypothesis."[36]

In his testimony to Clark's group, Boneau was adamant that only the LINC made possible the conception and pursuit of his new agenda, claiming, "It is quite likely that we would never have become involved in these problems without LINC." The basis of this assertion, he explained, was that "there is entailed an extremely large amount of data, at one time we were sorting through some one million relevant trials. The analyses tended to be somewhat complex, and only because of LINC were we tempted to do them at all."[37] From Boneau's perspective, the LINC had opened new pathways not because it was a computer per se but because it was interactive in real time. He conceded, "It is possible that some of the data sorts could have been handled by a big computer if we knew what we were looking for." But he continued, "With the LINC, however, we were in a position to change the analysis slightly when something seemed to be coming out, and we spent a few hundred hours at this task zeroing in on hidden meaning, a venture which would have been prohibitive on the big computer, to say nothing of inconvenient."[38]

LINC's prominence in shaping the intellectual contours of Boneau's work was reflected in the time and effort he devoted to using the computer. Tellingly, in the year following the 1963 LINC summer training program, Boneau dedicated his entire sabbatical to computerizing his laboratory. He recalled that this work was consuming and often dismaying: "There were times when I thought

the machine was a monkey on my back and resented the uncompromising demands for time. After spending into the wee hours several nights in a row trying
to get something to work one develops a perspective verging on despondency
which fortunately usually vanishes with a couple of nights' sleep." Essentially,
Boneau was working with the LINC full time. To "capitalize on the machine,"
Boneau found, he had to make sacrifices elsewhere, resulting in his becoming
"pressed, harried, and stressed," though he added that "I wouldn't trade the
experience for anything."[39] By early 1965, Boneau had invested so much in getting his LINC to work that he could not bring himself to stop spending time on
it even in the face of the possibility that the NIH would not allow him to keep
the computer: "Many times I felt that the time and energy devoted to the LINC
(which had to be pried loose from other activities) would go up in smoke if the
stewardship were only temporary, but LINC demands and gets."[40]

Looking beyond the cases described in the preceding pages, several general
claims can be made about the LINC's presence in the laboratory. With a real-
time interactive computer in the lab, experiments became more quantitative but
also less rigidly structured than work that had to be prepared for a mainframe
at an offsite computing center. Though the NIH had hoped the LINC would
serve as an effective link between biologists and larger computing facilities, most
labs restricted their computer use to the LINC itself. When these labs wanted
more computing power, they generally augmented their original LINC with
similar lab-based computers. The irony here is that instead of helping biologists
adapt to the requirements of the computing center, the LINC undermined the
centralized mode of computing. Small and versatile, the LINC was, however,
not the "ordinary instrument" its architect, Wesley Clark, had hoped it would
be. Instead, it was a device that required considerable dedication among its users
and often the presence of a new person in the lab, the computer expert, usually
someone with a background in mathematics and engineering rather than biology. Once labs made the investment in training and personnel, they became
locked into agendas that could not be pursued without a cascade of evermore
powerful computers.

Despite Wesley Clark's fervent wish that the LINC would come to be regarded as no different from any other laboratory instrument, biologists made
many remarks that indicated that they saw clear distinctions between the LINC
and instruments like microscopes, centrifuges, or oscilloscopes. What made the
LINC special in the minds of its users was primarily that writing computer
programs to solve a problem helped them to restructure their thinking about

that problem. As Ernst O. Attinger, research director of a cardiology laboratory at Research Institute, Presbyterian Hospital, Philadelphia, reported, "The extensive use of LINC has impressed upon each member of the staff the importance of clear and careful formulation of a problem."[41] Meanwhile, for Stanford University's Joshua Lederberg and Lee Hundley, thinking about biochemistry problems in terms that could be programmed on the LINC altered their conception of them: "LINC has been a most demanding teacher in its own right. It has changed and simplified our approach to many problems. It has also made possible experiments which would otherwise have been too time consuming to perform."[42]

Interacting with LINC was also cast as the means to the end of becoming an effective computer programmer. After expressing his dissatisfaction with LINC manuals and training courses, Bernard Weiss, who used LINC in the course of neurophysiology and psychology research on monkeys at the Johns Hopkins University Medical School, declared that "the LINC itself is an excellent teacher." Though Weiss had tremendous difficulty surmounting the engineering (hardware) challenges posed by incorporating LINC into his experiments, he found that his development as a programmer surprised him: "Programming skills, I found, once a computer was available to use as a teaching machine, were more readily acquired than I anticipated."[43]

Once biologists started using the LINC, they became locked into agendas that required constant, reliable access to computers. For Fred S. Grodins, a Northwestern University physiologist, there was no turning back from using the LINC. At the 1965 meeting of the LINC Evaluation Program he proclaimed that "the LINC has become a way of life in this laboratory and its loss would be considered a near-catastrophe."[44] In his studies of variance spectra of finger and hand tremors, Grodins had come to rely on the LINC not only to isolate data but also to conceive more complex models of tremors. Similarly, Joseph Edward Hind, a neurophysiologist based at the University of Wisconsin's Medical School, found that using the LINC "revolutionized the analysis of neuronal responses. Not only did it speed up data analysis by more than two orders of magnitude, but it also provided rapid, 'on-line,' feedback of processed output that enabled hitherto impossible experiments to be carried out."[45] Hind and his colleague, Chris D. Geisler, an electrical engineer jointly appointed to the Department of Physiology, noted in 1965 that using the LINC helped their group to plan larger, long-range computerized projects. They also explained that while planning for the future it was difficult to resist the temptation to spend enormous amounts of time creating novel programs for the LINC. Giving in to such temptations, they invested much time developing programs and standardizing their LINC for an anticipated larger group of users, rather than operating it as "essentially a personalized instrument for use by an individual."[46]

Using the LINC turned out not to be a casual endeavor but rather an all-encompassing one. In essence, they had to become full-time computer operators and programmers. All told, programming and operating the LINC in 1964 consumed Hind's entire time and half of Geisler's. As noted, they were hardly alone: whole sabbaticals were devoted to integrating LINC into the laboratory, and investigating questions that emerged via its use tended to require even more programming. Hind and Geisler's solution was to "recommend that participating laboratories be advised to hire a programmer and perhaps an engineer. It is unreasonable to expect a scientist with a full-time research program to handle all the responsibility for LINC in dynamic-evolving situations."[47]

Many laboratories did just this. In Philadelphia, for instance, Attinger took the step of importing into his cardiology research laboratory an electrical engineer, Antharvedi Anne, who became the machine's primary user. LINC, Attinger found, was "relatively simple to operate," but he concluded, "I am not convinced at all that a biologist without either mathematical and computer experience or the assistance of a good engineer will be able to make use of the LINC and its particular features."[48] Fortunately, as he continued, his lab had Anne, "who has made "maximal use of the special features on the LINC for our purposes." The biologists could use the LINC for minor tasks without Anne's assistance, but whenever a program needed to be written or equipment needed to be connected, the task fell exclusively to him. Moreover, as Attinger explained, with Anne as an intermediary, the biologists became dependent on LINC but also on Anne because they never learned how to program it. He reported that [Anne "has given a number of courses on computers to our staff, so that most of them are able to use the LINC, although they would be somewhat at a loss if they had to write their own programs for their rather complicated analyses."[49] Consequently, of the twelve papers and professional talks that Attinger's laboratory produced between 1964 and 1965, Anne was listed as an author of six.[50]

Also hiring engineers was Nelson Y. S. Kiang, of the Eaton-Peabody Laboratory of Auditory Physiology (EPL), a spinoff of MIT's Communications Biophysics Group, founded in 1956 and based in Boston in the Massachusetts Eye and Ear Infirmary. Wholeheartedly, Kiang agreed with Clark's call not to accord the computer any special status; "Our philosophy was to use the LINC as a tool just like everything else," he explained.[51] Programming the LINC and connecting it to the analog auditory recording equipment in his laboratory, however, proved too time-consuming and complicated for the physiologists to undertake alone. Kiang's solution was to recruit young engineers, often still in graduate school and then "train them to be biologists." Much of the engineers' value, Kiang recalled, was their mastery of tacit knowledge required to reconfigure the LINC. Given that "LINC's wiring was not thoroughly documented," being systematic about rewiring LINC was difficult for biologists inexperienced with electronics, and Kiang said that in the long run he found that "it was easier for me to train engineers as biologists than it was to train biologists as engineers." For their part, two of the engineers, Ishmael Stefanov-Wagner and David Steffens, found the EPL work sufficiently rewarding that they made careers of it, helping run LINC-based experiments for twenty-eight years, or until 1993, and staying on at the laboratory after the LINC was replaced with an Apple Macintosh.[52] Though most labs went the route of importing engineers, in some cases one of the researchers would become a full-time computer specialist. For instance, William Talbot, who operated the LINC while pursuing a Ph.D. at the Johns Hopkins University Department of Physiology under Vernon Mountcastle, became so proficient at programming and rewiring the LINC that he eventually pursued a career in computing rather than as a physiologist.[53]

Beyond opening new research agendas and introducing new personnel to the lab, using the LINC perpetuated more computer use. In essence, research conducted on the LINC had raised questions that the LINC itself was incapable of providing the means to investigate. Charles Molnar saw this too and later cast it as an irony of meeting LINC's initial design goals. As he characterized it, "The primary objective of the LINC design had been to create a tool that would address issues of data collection and management and provide interactiveness with the user and the laboratory environment." However, he found that in the years since LINC's introduction, "It was surprising to see how rapidly the removal of these bottlenecks led to pressure to improve the arithmetic and computational capabilities of the LINC."[54] Indeed, many of the life scientists who reported their experiences at the 1965 meeting of the LINC Evaluation Program expressed a desire for more powerful and much more expensive computers. Stanford-based users Joshua Lederberg and Lee Hundley made it clear that "this desire for a larger capability has certainly been the result of the use of LINC itself," adding that "we feel that future developments must proceed in this direction if full advantage is to be taken of the LINC program."[55] As in the case of Malindzak and Thurstone, Lederberg and Hundley's LINC produced too much interesting data for the LINC itself to process in a reasonable amount of time. Consequently, they made plans to acquire a much more powerful computer, an IBM 360 (see chapter 5).

"What Would I Want with a Computer in My Laboratory?": Selling the LINC Vision

Demand for computers was not necessarily innate to the biology lab. Rather, much of the demand was generated by outsiders, first by the NIH and then, to a larger extent, by computer manufacturers. After the 1963–65 LINC Evaluation Program was deemed a success by the NIH, private companies like Digital Equipment Corporation and Spear Electronics attempted to use the findings of that program to help them market the variants of the LINC they were beginning to build. To convince potential customers of the merits of a computer, these companies trained their sales forces to craft feasibility studies for the labs they visited. Often, biologists needed to be convinced not only that the computer would help them conduct their research but also that investing in a computer would not disrupt day-to-day operations.

When it came to spreading the gospel of computing, commission-driven salesmen were by far the most zealous missionaries. Those working for DEC were particularly aggressive. The company saw a market for its LINC variant, the LINC-8, in the thousands of biology labs that did not use computers—and did not express interest in using computers—as of the mid-1960s. To train its sales force to become more effective in convincing researchers to purchase the LINC-8, DEC developed a role-playing exercise called "Now, what would I want with a computer in my laboratory?" A close look at this exercise in persuasion, which DEC circulated internally in the form of a skit, reveals how the company sought to create demand for its product. It also sheds much light on what DEC saw as biologists' intellectual and institutional anxieties regarding computer use, as well as on how the company believed it could use such qualms to its advantage.

The play's setting and cast are simple; it is merely a conversation "overhead during a long cup of coffee with John Q. Scientist and DEC." It begins with the hesitant scientist asking the DEC salesman, "Now, what would I want with a computer in my laboratory?" The salesman replies by stating that "several people in your field have been getting a lot of help from them in the last few years," and asks the scientist if he is presently using a computer at all. With a tinge of hostility, the scientist explains that he is not, "but two of my grad students have been running problems at the computing center, and judging from their gripes, I want nothing to do with it."[56]

The scientist then launches into a polemic against the shortcomings of off-site, batch-processing computing. "Apparently it takes weeks to get anything to work. They spend a couple of days writing a program, then they find out about their mistakes, at about one mistake day." Exasperated, the scientist continues, "When they finally get a working program, they get back long lists of numbers which they pore over and sometimes plot on graph paper. Half the time, the program doesn't do the job they wanted, and they start all over. I haven't that kind of time or that much patience. They say that this 'time-sharing' will speed it up, though." Upon hearing the term *time-sharing*, the DEC salesman interjects, "Whoa there!" and then attempts to steer the scientist away from thinking about using a centralized, time-shared computer. The better alternative, the salesman explains, is "a computer right in your laboratory that will show you the results as things are happening. You have immediate access to both the program and the data. It could do a lot more for you than the computing center could."

At this point, the scientist becomes excited about the potential of such a system but then checks his enthusiasm by contemplating its cost. This, according to the script, prompts the salesman to begin his pitch, "Digital and other companies have brought that investment down to a very reasonable figure, especially when you consider the performance you are buying." Instead of just reciting the LINC's capabilities, the salesman is instructed to ask the scientist about his particular research goals and instrumentation needs in order to ferret out specific potential applications for a small, general-purpose digital computer. His foot in the door, the salesman tells the scientist, "I'd like to go over your operation with you to see if you aren't missing some pretty good bets on computing" (2).

Again the researcher hesitates, because he apparently does not see what computers have to do with the daily operations of his lab. Here the salesman must persuade the scientist that the computer is not just "a desk calculator" but can be useful in many aspects of research, and he attempts again to draw out the scientist on what exactly happens in the lab. The scientist in the skit, it turns out, is researching the effects of various drugs on the vagus nerve. After each dose of drugs is injected, a lab technician using a polygraph measures the changes in heart rate and blood pressure, and plots it on a curve. Generating a meaningful curve takes about forty-five minutes, and there is little variation in terms of readings and calculation. Day after day, much plotting and arithmetic work is repeated.

When the salesman asks why the scientist did not consider automating the work, the latter replies: "We thought of sending the raw readings to the computing center for punching and calculation, but the time and effort weren't worth it. This whole experiment would be over before we got a good working set-up there." With the scientist's unfulfilled desire for computing capabilities now established, the salesman pounces, explaining that having a LINC would allow the lab to write its own program, to "debug it on the spot," as well as perform the calculations required to generate curves. The intrigued scientist then exclaims, "You've just moved the computing center into my lab!" (2).

To tantalize the scientist further, the salesman is instructed to remain blasé about the mere *presence* of computational power in the laboratory; rather, he emphasizes that with a LINC, the researchers will all but eliminate the necessity of manually recording and processing data. The whole quantitative aspect of the experiment, the salesman explains, could be automated: "Why not have the computer read heart rate, blood pressure, and timing events right from the polygraph, perform the computations, and display the curves while the experiment proceeds?" (3) Furthermore, he says, the LINC would not just take a "passive role . . . as a data-gatherer and analyzer," but "can work with you to *run* the experiment too" by controlling stimuli, be they noises, heat, or even injections via a motor-driven syringe pump. Best of all, though, the results would be available immediately, whereupon they can be placed in a permanent record on LINCtape at the researcher's discretion. Paper records would be almost eliminated, and the scientist could see for himself "the saving of the time and errors involved in reading those paper records" (4, emphasis in original).

The scientist, listening to the sales pitch and impressed by the LINC's convenience, is still unsure that such a capable computer would be easy to set up and use, especially considering that he is unfamiliar with computers. Noting that the LINC will replace much of his analog recording equipment, the scientist anxiously predicts, "I can see us spending a few months just getting a system like that put together, not to speak of making it run." Again the salesman assuages the customer's doubts, claiming, "When we say our computers are approachable, we mean it," and adding that setting up the computer and writing programs should not amount to more than a few days' labor.[57]

To seal the deal, the salesman explains to the scientist that the LINC could empower him by accommodating a wide variety of experiments, including ones that he hitherto lacked the instruments to conduct. "When you need changes," said the salesman, "you change programs, not equipment. Your computer can be an averager, a correlator, a histogrammer, a controller, a calculator, a display device. . . . It can be anything you program it to be" (4). Finally, the salesman would leave the scientist with the notion that the LINC had enormous peda-gogical value in a field that was inexorably computerizing. After continuing to raise the specter of biology's inevitable computerization by bombarding the biologist with computer-driven success stories, the salesman points to the labo-ratory's graduate students and concludes that they "would gain the education of working with a computer, for in the life sciences they will do that after they leave school, certainly" (5).

DEC was not alone in trying to foster demand for LINC variants among biologists. Stating in 1964, another Massachusetts company, Spear Electron-ics, began to advertise its micro-LINC, which was a standard LINC modified to be more "friendly" to neophyte computer users. "In spite of its extremely sophisticated approach to laboratory data acquisition and processing," Spear boasted, "you will find that a Spear micro-LINC remains affable and unassum-ing—as a computer should that costs less than $50,000."[58] Unlike the original and DEC LINCs, Spear's provided an operating environment that could with "only a few hours of training" be used "with no need for a basic computer back-ground." Instead of writing programs, users chose the programs they wished to run from among a large library of prepared "biomedical and statistical analy-sis routines."[59] By the late 1960s, however, the micro-LINC was discontinued because most researchers who wanted an interactive computer wanted one with the capabilities of the LINC-8.

Computers in the Clinic: The Big Picture

As was the case in biology, a large portion of the introduction of computers to medicine in the United States was overseen by the NIH. Though hospi-tals received money and reported to the same NIH entities that supported the research laboratories, drawing from the same small body of literature, there was a large difference between the experience of biologists and physicians when it came to adopting computer technology. While all computer projects sponsored by the NIH ostensibly supported the HHS's ultimate mission of improving Americans' health, those with an immediate clinical component faced several challenges not found in laboratory environments. First, there was the need to handle much greater amounts of information much more reliably than could lab-based researchers. (The consequences of an error in, say, a medical record could be lethal.) There was also the matter of computerizing a much larger operation than a laboratory. Biologists typically worked in groups of under a dozen total people (including students and technicians), whereas hospital staffs numbered in the hundreds or thousands. Finally, hospitals were intensely scrutinized by the public. Though the public was not necessarily alarmed by the specter of computers making life-and-death decisions, there was great concern about the potential effect of computers on the cost of medical care.

Computers were first used in medical settings in the early 1960s, in many cases inspired by Ledley and Lusted's late-1950s advocacy work and supported by the NIH. Hospital computing pioneer Morris F. Collen (b. 1913), who surveys these early systems in his book, *A History of Medical Informatics*, shows that before the mid-1960s they tended to be limited in scope, aiming to computerize only small parts of a hospital's operations—often only provisionally—and they tended to be research- rather than clinically oriented.[60] Most of these first-generation systems were the first computers a hospital had, and most therefore were used for training and experimental purposes, rather than with actual patients. For instance, the NIH-sponsored Johns Hopkins Hospital computer facility, pointed to by Collen as a great success, spent almost a decade (1961 to 1970) developing prototype systems for clinical use. Though the hospital did not fully computerize its records system until the early 1980s, by acquiring a computer early it became a central training point for leading personnel in hospital computing.[61]

Other early medical systems saw limited distribution because they were geared much more toward research than patient treatment. One system in this category was Lee Lusted's Primate Information Management Experiment (PRIME), which tracked many variables, over several years, related to the health of chimpanzees that were the subjects of medical testing. With PRIME, Lusted gathered data much in the same way as he and Ledley had proposed in 1959, thus enabling statistical analysis of data gathered for one, several, or all of the chimpanzees being tracked. Lusted cast PRIME as "an operational model for a hospital automated information system," but its orientation toward producing data for statistical analysis rather than easing patient management limited its spread to research facilities rather than hospitals.[62] On the NIH campus itself, meanwhile, Arnold Pratt's DCRT initiated several one-off projects on the agency's IBM 650 and (starting in 1963) IBM 1620 to automate data-gathering operations at the NIH's Clinical Center, a major research hospital. Though the DCRT would expand dramatically after acquiring an IBM 360 in 1966 and continue that expansion well into the 1970s, when it enjoyed a golden age of sorts, its early projects had few direct descendents.

One pre-1965 system that was exceptional, both in the sense that it generated a lasting legacy in terms of direct patient care and that its development was not majority-sponsored by the NIH, was Morris Collen's own multiphasic screening system, which he developed for Kaiser Permanente (KP).[63] Collen, who had been recruited to the Kaiser Company in 1942 fresh from completing his residency in internal medicine by Sidney Garfield (the surgeon who cofounded KP with industrialist Henry Kaiser in 1945), had from the beginning of his career been interested in developing holistic, systematic approaches to treating serious medical conditions in large populations. Following his successful quantitative-oriented and protocol-driven effort to treat and limit the spread of pneumococcal lobar pneumonia—an extremely dangerous illness before the development of penicillin—among workers in Kaiser's shipyards during the war, Collen quickly rose through the ranks of the Kaiser Company's and later KP's healthcare systems.[64] By the mid-1960s he was a powerful figure within KP's rapidly growing medical system, and used his position to steer company resources toward computerizing patient screening. A *Newsweek* article titled "Enter the Robot M.D." describes Collen's vision and the operations of a completed system that would help to fulfill his desire to make many aspects of maintaining a person's (and arguably a whole population's) general health much more systematic. The major bottleneck in healthcare, as Collen saw it, was that there was "no adequate means for screening large numbers of healthy people for disease. It's expensive; doctors and patients don't have time. There just aren't the resources to give everyone a physical exam every year—acutely ill get priority." By way of example, Collen pointed to cervical cancer, where thirty-nine of forty cases went undetected before the disease became potentially lethal, and diabetes, where forty-nine of fifty cases went undetected before the condition made someone acutely ill.[65]

Collen's solution was what he called "multiphasic screening"; that is, "the use of automated equipment to carry out disease detection on a massive scale." In KP's prototype system, computers tracked a "comprehensive battery of tests" administered by physicians, nurses, and the patients themselves. The thirty-one screening tests, which involved patients going "from station to station" within the screening center, included, "physical examinations, comprehensive laboratory tests, electrophysiology tests, radiographs, and an automated self-administered medical history."[66] *Newsweek* reported that it took the average patient about 2.5 hours to complete the tests, and that "if abnormalities are detected, additional tests may be applied."[67]

By the late 1960s, many of KP's 2 million patients had been screened using Collen's system. Jochen R. Moehr, today one of the leading figures in medical informatics, recalled that "within a decade, Dr. Collen accumulated several millions of health checkup data sets on more than a million subjects, creating in the process not only a prototype electronic health record, but also a phenomenal and unique basis for research, and this despite the immaturity of the technology available in the fifties and sixties."[68] Though the KP computerized multiphasic screening system was massively used and exemplary, and though Collen predicted in 1966 that "in ten years, every large medical center will have a major automated multiphasic-screening facility," the general concept of multiphasic screening did not fare well in the following years. Even from the outset, as is apparent in *Newsweek*'s otherwise laudatory coverage of the system it was clear that many physicians objected on the grounds "that the read-out from a computer is no substitute for sound medical judgment." During the 1970s, multiphasic screening's popularity diminished due to widespread physician and public objections. Among physicians, doubts grew about the major premise of the multiphasic screening: that dedicating massive amounts of resources to building computerized screening systems would indeed be less expensive than treating diseases once patients presented acute symptoms. The general public, meanwhile, objected to the impersonal nature of the screening and the notion that a data-entry or computer programming error could have serious consequences for one's well-being.[69] By contrast, within the community of medical computing enthusiasts Collen's system was warmly and continuously embraced. In 1993, the American College of Medical Informatics would establish the annual Morris F. Collen Award, which in Moehr's words, "is considered the 'Nobel Prize of Medical Informatics.'"[70] Among subjects of this book, the award has been bestowed upon Robert Ledley, Homer Warner, Donald Lindberg, Octo Barnett, Joshua Lederberg, and Collen himself.

The closest to a comprehensive and independent contemporary account of the immediate effects of the NIH's computing policy on medicine can be found in David E. Clark's 1967 report, "Computer Requirements of the Hospital and Medical School." Clark, the director of the Medical Computing Unit of the University of Manchester (and of no relation to LINC architect Wesley Clark), was dispatched by the UK's Medical Research Council (MRC) in 1966 to survey computer use by American biomedical researchers.[71] Clark's mission was to take stock of the situation in the United States and make recommendations for how computers could be employed in British laboratories and hospitals. In the second half of 1966, Clark visited seventy medical computing installations in twenty-two cities in the United States and consulted experts like Robert Ledley and Ralph Stacy.

Clark was particularly impressed with the growth of American biomedical computing and the NIH's role in fostering that growth. To spur his compatriots to overcome an "American lead in excess of five years," he cast what he saw in America as a national mobilization toward computing, driven by President Lyndon B. Johnson's Medicare and Medicaid programs. He reported that there were so many—forty thousand by his count—computers in the United States and they had so proliferated in so many aspects of life that it would be fair to claim that "the computer is no longer regarded as a special piece of apparatus— a symbol of prestige like the automobile—life could not go on without one, they are just ordinary pieces of furniture" (8). Medicine was no exception: "All medical schools in America seem to have at least one computer," he noted, with the size of the computer proportional to the size of the school. In American medical schools, he claimed, analog-digital convertors had become "commonplace," while remote teleprocessing—via Dataphone link—of medical data was "common" too (3). He argued that the main reason for computers' proliferation was the NIH's generous support, and reported with a grain of hyperbole that "in fact all that was necessary at this stage was to let the National Institutes of Health hear that your hospital wished to have a computer, and it was provided— almost to the embarrassment of the research workers." He added: "If a hospital is unable to obtain a computer at the moment for medical work they can usually justify a machine for payroll, billing, inventory control and budgets" (5).[72]

Beyond noting the preponderance of computers in biomedicine, Clark tried to illustrate how they were changing research and healthcare. Echoing the NIH's language, he proclaimed that given what he saw in the United States, the introduction of computers would "create and encourage industry to enter Bio-Medical Engineering." In the United States, he maintained, most biomedical research sites had "bio-engineering activities" of some sort, and the economic and demographic consequences of these activities were profound. "In supporting Medical Computing," Clark wrote, "America has created an industry based on home requirements, which also helps the potential export of computers and medical instruments. This attracts research brains to the country where they are able to see their research ideas realized. Several visiting British scientists would obviously become permanent residents" (9–10).

Clark also took pains to convey that computerization required a costly initial investment, and that the benefits of devoting valuable resources to computing were not immediately apparent. He asked, "Would a computer costing £100,000 go further in the research sense than, say, the provision of 100 sets of apparatus costing £1,000?" (2). The answer in the short term, he conceded, was a resounding no, but he urged his readers to think in a longer frame: "We know, and no-one in America tries to pretend otherwise, that a computer in a hospital is uneconomic in the early stages; but the long-term economic benefits will be enormous." To support his claim that computers yielded long-term economic benefits, Clark pointed to several examples of computers saving hospitals and laboratories money. In hospitals, he found, computer use had reduced EKG costs from $15 to $0.50, food costs by 10 to 20 percent (using menu-planning algorithms), and blood bank waste from 16 percent to less than 3 percent; laboratories, meanwhile, saw the cost of assays drop from $15 to $1.25. Clark also stressed that computers would streamline and economize the bureaucracy of medical care, arguing that computers were seen as the means to mitigate the enormous cost—he estimated 30 percent of the nation's budget—of the Medicare and Medicaid programs (4).

Clark's account of computer use by biomedical researchers and doctors in the United States was not all rosy, however. He lamented that despite broad employment of computers, there was no sign of "a master plan so that all American hospitals can benefit from this investment in technology" (9). Moreover, there was, as far as he could tell, no national plan to manage the increasing complexities of computer-driven healthcare (6). Worst of all, he saw computer work as essentially dull: "There will be little glory in Medical Computing for many years: it is essentially a foot-slogging job." Only in the distant future, he believed, would the area become stimulating and prestigious (12). Nevertheless, after noting IBM's dominance in the field of medical computing, both in hardware and software, Clark asserted that regardless of whether computers would prove to be boon or burden to medicine, "PL/1 [the programming language developed for the IBM 360] would be the medical language of the future" (8).

Massachusetts General Hospital and the Hard Lessons of Medical Computing

In terms of revealing the specific changes and challenges computerization brought to care providers, particularly those working in hospitals, by far the most useful account is G. Octo Barnett's 1966 report to the NIH, "Computer Applications in Medical Communication and Information Retrieval Systems as Related to the Improvement of Patient Care and the Medical Record." The report, which Barnett addressed to his colleagues on the NIH CRSS, detailed Massachusetts General Hospital's attempts to use computer technology to improve patient care and made recommendations based on those experiences. Most of the obstacles to computerization of medicine that Barnett found while heading MGH's computerization effort had not been foreseen by early advocates of computerized medicine. Furthermore, many of these obstacles remain firmly in place in the twenty-first century and continue to hamper computerization efforts.

The main reason Barnett's report stands out among early accounts of computer use in medicine is its blunt clarity. Barnett (b. 1930), a cardiologist by training, ran MGH's Laboratory of Computer Science (LCS) and had a reputation for straight talk. Often prefacing his remarks with "I'm just a country doctor!" in reference to a "backwoods" childhood spent running a "dirt-poor, worn-out farm" in Alabama, Barnett put into plain terms many of the complex problems that plagued hospital computerization projects.[73] Like so many others, Barnett had come to medical computing by accident. While attending Harvard Medical School in the mid-1950s, he lived with a group of MIT electrical engineering graduate students and through that "chance association . . . [he] became acquainted with computer technology and became captivated by it as an idle recreation." He later joked, "I still live in fear that someday it will be discovered that I am getting paid for doing my hobby, and I will have to get a real job."[74] As a resident in medicine at Peter Bent Brigham Hospital (Boston), Barnett's interest in computers caught the attention of Homer Warner, who later recommended him to lead MGH's NIH-funded effort to computerize its medical records system. Bolt Beranek and Newman had initially led the project, but as Robert A. Greenes, a medical researcher who worked in the LCS, explains, "after some of the early enthusiasm died down, it was clear to the leadership at MGH that this project needed physician direction."[75] That physician would be Barnett.

When Barnett arrived at MGH in 1964 to run the LCS—or as he phrased it, to "combine my hobby in computers with the practice of medicine"—he found the hospital was "almost overwhelmed" by the task of data processing. By today's standards, the amount of information managed by hospital staff is aston-ishing given that most of it was handwritten and hand-delivered. On a typical busy day in the mid-1960s, Barnett reported, over five hundred patients were in transit from one part of the hospital to another and "innumerable telephone calls are made between patient care areas, laboratories and various physicians' offices." Each time a patient was admitted, patient information was "sent to 66 different areas in the hospital." Routine treatment of a patient usually re-quired the actions of many hospital staff. For instance, just drawing up a "plan of action" for a common surgical procedure could be a very complex operation, "involv[ing] a large number of individuals from the professional and hospital staff, including such diverse groups as the nursing service, the radiotherapy unit, the operating room and anesthesiology staff, the pharmacy, the blood bank, the diet kitchen, the physiotherapy unit, the social service staff, etc."[76] Carrying out a doctor's order also typically involved generating and sharing much informa-tion. Barnett found that "one simple order (such as the request for a fasting blood test) requires a staggering list of routines." One set of routines for such a doctor's order follows:

> Filling out the laboratory requisition, determining the type and amount of the sample, informing the team which draws the blood, notifying the dietary depart-ment to delay feeding and then to reinstate the feeding schedule after the test sample has been taken, checking to prevent conflict of orders and to ascertain that the patient will be available for the collection of the sample, collecting the sample, transporting the sample with the requisition to the appropriate laboratory by the message service, logging-in the sample in the laboratory, scheduling and perform-ing the test analysis by the laboratory technician, transcribing the test results from the laboratory work sheet to the original test requisition, filing the information to insure that the appropriate charges to the patient will be made, transporting the complete requisition with the test result to the appropriate patient care unit and, finally, sorting all the test results for a given care unit and posting each result in the appropriate patient's medical record. (5)

That was just for one doctor's order. Barnett estimated that "on an average day over 6,000 doctors' orders are written and the Nursing Service administers over 30,000 drugs and treatments." By his reckoning, "at least 50,000 separate items of information are entered into patient records each day, or almost 20,000,000 items each year (4).

At the LCS, Barnett's task was to use computers to help the hospital cope with all of this information. Collaborating with BBN, the LCS set out in 1964 to develop for MGH computerized patient admission/discharge systems and a medication ordering system. Beyond improving patient care, the goal of computerization was to enable "the utilization of the hospital as a laboratory," that is, to use the data collected during treatment to study the effectiveness of drugs, treatment procedures, diet regimens, staff management schemes, and so forth (13). Another advantage of casting the hospital as a laboratory was that computer methods for speeding up experimental work could be applied to hospital settings. The parallel between laboratory experiment and hospital treatment, Barnett explained, was that "any treatment program has some of the characteristics of an experiment and involves the same iterative process of collecting information, analyzing data, formulating an hypothesis, choosing a plan of action and then recycling through the same sequence" (6).

Within months of commencing, the LCS projects met major delays. The most immediate problem was access to the computer: MGH had several terminals for a time-shared DEC PDP-1 computer based at BBN some ten miles away, communicating with it via telephone wires over which data was transmitted at a rate of ten characters per second. More serious was that MGH's priorities clashed with those of BBN. On one side, BBN's computer experts, who operated in a think-tank environment, had ideas about computer use that in Barnett's opinion were "highly creative and had great promise," but they purposefully ignored "questions of priority, time, and cost." On the other side, was MGH, which as Barnett put it, "marched to a different drummer in being more pragmatically oriented." Specifically, the hospital wanted computers to save time and money without being disruptive to hospital operations.[77]

In the working hospital environment, not only did BBN's initial concepts fail, but so did systems that had been carefully tested by the LCS and demonstrated successfully for months in individual departments. During his time at MGH, Barnett "learned to expect that the final program will bear little resemblance to the initial idea and that each program will undergo innumerable modifications." For instance, creating a program that would enable hospital staff to manage the medication cycle (that is, ordering, listing, and charting the effect of medications), took three years of full-time labor by several programmers trained at BBN and MIT. Over that period the program was completely rewritten twice and patched many times. Even after the second rewrite, the LCS had little to show for its work. As Barnett glumly reported, "the cycle [program] at present is little more than a very impressive demonstration and cannot handle many of the procedures or exceptions that actually occur in the normal course of events." The LCS needed "an operational system powerful and reliable enough to cope with the day-to-day functional requirements" to cross the "gap" between demonstration program and everyday tool. "Because of this gap," Barnett found, a third total rewrite would be necessary: "We are starting again from the beginning to examine the medication problem and to re-specify the flow of information and the needs to be anticipated." After this grueling experience, Barnett concluded that "any significant progress in the application of computers to patient care will occur only through an evolutionary process," one that would be "extremely costly in terms of personnel resources and the amount of time expended" (14–15).

By 1966, it was clear to Barnett that hospital computing held a unique set of challenges that had not been anticipated by the NIH, computer manufacturers, or the hospitals themselves. All three parties, according to Barnett, bore a significant portion of the responsibility for the slow rate at which computers were being adopted in hospitals, despite their heavy investment in the new technology. Besides doling out blame, Barnett also suggested ways to more effectively use computer in healthcare settings. Some of these suggestions were followed almost immediately, while others have found currency only in the last decade.

The central problem of hospital computing, as Barnett cast it, was working with the "medical record." "Far more than a dusty volume filed in the tombs of the Records Room," Barnett wrote, "the medical record is a dynamic record of the total physician-patient-hospital encounter . . . it is a collection of all the numerous communications and reports describing the nature and course of the disease process." He noted that the medical record "includes not only the narrative account written by the physician, but also the data on test results from the laboratories, the orders written by the physician, and the record of the patient's response to a prescribed course of therapy" (7). In contrast to the static data computers typically processed in most business, government, or even laboratory settings, the medical record was constantly being revised. Contributed to and negotiated by as many as dozens of different individuals or groups, the medical record for a given patient might change hundreds of times in the course of a hospital stay.

In Barnett's view, any successful effort to introduce computers to hospital operations would need to account for the dynamic nature of the medical record. So far, as of 1965, most of these attempts had met little success and had been built around the assumption that the "application of the computer to medical care involves only the simple transfer of well-defined techniques from the industrial field" (9).[78] While the operations research techniques that had made production and logistics more productive in the 1950s had shown promise in small, controlled clinical environments, such as Homer Warner's cardiology research laboratory in Utah, implementing those techniques across working hospitals proved far more challenging than early advocates like Ledley and Lusted had predicted. Six years after Ledley and Lusted had beseeched physicians to change their behavior in order to reap the benefits of computers had brought to other areas, it was apparent to Barnett that even a small portion of those changes would massively disrupt day-to-day operations at any typical hospital.

Though Barnett and the LCS seemed to have a cozy relationship with BBN, many of the claims BBN developers made—most likely in good faith—to MGH about computers proved unrealistic. BBN was not unique in this regard. After a few years of exposure to marketing by companies like IBM, DEC, and CDC, Barnett concluded that "most industrial organizations have difficulties in appreciating the magnitude and complexity of the problem [of hospital computing] and have a very dangerous tendency to over-simplify and over-sell" (17). Some examples of computer industry's "generalizations which have virtually no basis in demonstrated experience" pointed to by Barnett were: "The advantages of the '. . . . .' will affect virtually all people and functions within the hospital through improved efficiency, cost reduction and better patient care; simplicity of order entry and terminal operation provides greater accuracy and more efficient use of the nurse's time; the nursing staff, as a whole, will show a general tendency to a marked increase in job satisfaction and will be more eager to work in this newly-created atmosphere" (9). Compounding the problem of unrealistic claims by manufacturers was that in most hospitals there was nobody with enough expertise in computing to critically evaluate—let alone do much to realize—these claims. The "common attitude" at hospitals as Barnett saw it, "is one of naive and uncritical acceptance of the computer technology." Once the computer arrived, there were generally no hospital staff able to program or operate the machine, thus "the great majority of hospitals will have to depend upon computer manufacturers to supply most of the programming resources for operational service" (17).

Relying on outsiders to build a hospital's computer system gave rise to another challenge: communication. A newcomer could not simply arrive at a hospital and expect to find organized, written descriptions of hospital operations. Rather, as Barnett pointed out, "many hospitals operate on a day-to-day basis amidst customary but poorly documented procedures." He found that at most hospitals he visited "only staff members with many years of experience have an appreciation of which functions are of concern in the design of a data-processing system and which can be overlooked or investigated at a later time." Without published resources from which to draw, educating computer experts on even simple points of hospital operations required "hours of discussion and explanation," but programmers working against deadlines and physicians with heavy patient loads had little time to spare. In rare instances where computer specialists and hospital staff could spend significant time in discussions, there was the additional problem that they lacked a common language between them. The crux of the matter, according to Barnett, was that "most hospital personnel have had little or no training in the critical analysis of a functioning system; few have had experience in describing all the information-flow requirements of a complex organization such as a hospital" (13).

Without communication between BBN developers and MGH staff, projects failed. In the absence of input from the hospital, BBN developers worked under the mistaken premise that hospital users would resemble computer users elsewhere. As Barnett learned through his experience in the hospital environment, "the hospital user, as opposed to his counterpart in industry, is not a computer scientist or even a trained technician, but is better described as an intelligent individual whose primary concern is the use of the computer as a tool to improve patient care." For the hospital user, the computer's reliability, rather than its potential functionality, was the top concern. The hospital computer, if it was to be a helpful tool, had to be up and running all the time—downtime cost lives once a hospital was committed to using a computer to manage information.

Hospitals had also put demands on computing systems that were not expected by computer makers. Physicians who were too busy treating patients to receive extensive computer training only worked with computers effectively in situations where "the interaction between the user and the system is carried out in a conversational mode using a language similar to English." To accommodate the ever-changing medical record, MGH had to develop "very large files on secondary storage which are rapidly accessible, allowing many users to enter, manipulate and retrieve information on the same data base at the same time." Finally, to use the computers as communication devices that were more effective than telephones or couriers, hospital staff needed a system where "an entry at one terminal causes a variety of messages and reports to be generated at a number of different terminals and where the content of the messages is a function not only of the event prompting the entry at the first terminal, but is also a function of the time and the state of the data base" (10). As of the mid-1960s, even the cutting-edge time-sharing systems developed by BBN did not support real-time communication on this scale.

At the same time the developers were not taking into account the particular needs of hospitals, those same hospitals were also building barriers to computerization. In the case of MGH, Barnett found that a reflexively insular culture undermined his efforts to introduce computers to the hospital. To effectively use new computer technology, hospitals would need to expand their staffs in unconventional ways to access "the talents of several groups of individuals who would normally not be a part of the hospital environment." Indeed, from Barnett's perspective, "Probably the greatest single limiting factor that curtails rapid development in the application of computers to patient care is the unavailability of competent and experienced personnel." In the face of this need, however, Barnett found that established hospital staff took a hostile view of these new workers, who were generally paid "at salary scales much higher than is customary in a hospital." Driving the unwelcoming behavior of hospital personnel was "the existence of an attitude . . . similar to the closed-corporation attitude of the typical trade union, of very circumscribed allegiances and patterns of communication." In this environment it was "almost impossible for an individual from outside the hospital to supervise a co-operative effort involving medical and paramedical staff" (11). In effect, hospital staff would not listen to outsiders, a serious obstacle considering outsiders would be necessary to implement computer systems, and they resisted including computer specialists in their ranks.

Further slowing the adoption of computer technology by hospitals was that hospitals usually took great pains to avoid disrupting their balance sheets. Circa 1966, there was no sign that even the most heavily subsidized computers—essentially gifts from the NIH—would be assets rather than expensive liabilities for hospitals in the long run. "On the basis of presently available evidence," wrote Barnett, "it is very difficult to defend any large-scale hospital information-processing system with the statement that the cost of patient care will be reduced." Beyond the shock of a high sticker price, the apparent long-term expenses of computerization—vis-à-vis not using computers—had discouraged hospital administrators. Mostly this was because up to that point hospitals generally did not document the costs associated with information gathering, processing, and retrieval. "This cost is probably much higher than most hospital administrators appreciate and may be as much as one-fourth of the total operating budget," Barnett reported.

Another—and perhaps the most—discouraging aspect of adopting the new technology from the standpoint of a fiscally conservative administrator was the financial uncertainty associated with computing. Barnett found that in most hospital settings it was "almost impossible to predict the cost of a computer system since the problems are not yet clearly delineated; even where the problems are defined there is little comparable experience in industry that would be useful in predicting costs." Ultimately, computerization would require some tolerance of risk; it would "require a willingness on the part of the hospital to gamble on a development where the economic justification is not defined" (18–19).

Besides computer manufacturers and hospitals, a third party, the NIH, hindered the computerization of hospitals. Ironically, Barnett found, the very same NIH policies that were intended to encourage hospitals to adopt computers ended up preventing that adoption. The main flaw in NIH policy seems to have been that the ACCR and its successors treated hospital computing projects similarly to the way they treated scientific computing projects. What the NIH computerization effort lacked, according to Barnett, were "traditions or procedures to support an internal research and development program in improving the hospital's *raison d'être*—the provision of patient care."

Since early NIH support for hospital computing was oriented toward research, it did not provide the means for most hospitals to use computers on a day-to-day basis to enhance patient care. Without mechanisms to evaluate the effectiveness of computers in improving care, the NIH awarded support based on the viability of a hospital's plans to use computers in research. Even in rare cases where the NIH explicitly funded a computer for the purpose of improving hospital operations, it treated computerization as a research project. In hospitals, this approach proved problematic. Securing NIH support for computers, Barnett found, "require[d] full-time participation of hospital staff who have experience in managing a research effort and who have the ability to understand and deal with the Public Health Service funding mechanisms." Such a high level of involvement was deeply disruptive to the daily running of hospitals—Barnett reported that "in most situations, hospital administration is understaffed and vastly over-committed in the decision processes involved in day-to-day operation and in solving the inevitable crises" (18). Four decades later, Donald A. B.

Lindberg, former CRSS member and present director of the National Library of Medicine, declared that the NIH's lack of engagement with patient care when it came to computerization projects led to "the NIH policy of funding 'research' projects to create practical clinical information systems (frequently under the sham stance that these would support further 'real' clinical research) and then terminating the funding at the end of the initial grant period." Lindberg further asserted that "this policy naturally favored failed efforts that could then 'reset' to a new grant award. It was miserably destructive of research systems that actually straggled over to the side of incipient practical success. How about 2005? Do we not have essentially the same policy?"[79]

In the decades following his 1966 report to the CRSS, Barnett sought to promote the computerization of hospitals by creating software that would accommodate the needs of hospital workers. Under his leadership, the LCS developed the Massachusetts General Hospital Utility Multi-Programming System (MUMPS) programming language in the mid-1960s. "The goal of the MUMPS system," recalled Barnett, "was to combine a simple yet powerful high-level language with an easy-to-use database handling system."[80] To accommodate physicians and other hospital staff who were not familiar with computer languages, MUMPS allowed "a programming session to take the form of a conversational dialogue between the programmer and the terminal device."[81]

Unlike then-popular languages like FORTRAN, MUMPS had powerful string-manipulating commands that facilitated the "management of nonnumerical data which make up the largest part of medical information." MUMPS allowed users to search for records that contained strings of text that resembled—rather than precisely matched—those they had entered. It also enabled complex text searches, that is, for multiple imprecise terms or for the presence or absence of strings of texts in particular data fields. Thus, physicians' notes on patients could be searched and still found if, say, the name of drug had been misspelled. Finally, MUMPS stored data on a centralized computer in such a way that multiple users could access and modify a single record with relative ease. After MUMPS became commercially available in 1969, the language was widely adopted, becoming "the most commonly used programming language in the United States for clinically oriented medical applications during the 1970s and 1980s."[82] Among the many MUMPS-based systems were MGH's COSTAR (Computer Stored Ambulatory Record) and that hospital's DXplain diagnostic decision-support system. MUMPS was also adopted by the Department of Defense and other federal agencies as well as by several large banks.

Starting in the 1990s, MUMPS became more commonly known as M, and its derivatives continue to be widely used in and far beyond medical informatics.

A Foundation for Computing in Biology and Medicine

While biology and medical computing projects drifted apart, Robert Ledley, through the influential nonprofit organization he founded in 1960, the National Biomedical Research Foundation, remained deeply involved in both spheres. Though Ledley tended to view computing in biology and medicine as a single entity, the technologies and resources produced by the NBRF accelerated the division between the two fields. In the decades since the NBRF's founding, it has become increasingly clear that the foundation was also exceptional in that it provided a platform for computing experts to actively shape the work of biologists and physicians rather than simply serving to meet the demands of biomedicine. Today, the NBRF is a marginal and fairly small organization—full-time employees have rarely numbered over thirty, and now there are far fewer—but large swathes of computerized biology and medicine can trace their origins to work conducted at the foundation.

Guided by his father, who was a professional accountant, through the process of setting up a nonprofit organization, Ledley chartered the NBRF in 1960. For the next fifty years, until his retirement in 2010, Ledley would devote his career to directing the NBRF, pursuing research related to the foundation's goals, and editing related journals. From its establishment, the NBRF's priorities reflected those of its founder. Ledley stated that the NBRF's guiding principle would be the understanding that "all natural phenomena could be mathematically derived as consequences of a simple set of fundamental laws of nature." Due to the complexity of biological phenomena, however, the NBRF would not seek "'closed form' solutions" to problems in the life sciences but would rather pursue solutions through "direct numerical computation."[83] This computation-intensive approach would be made possible only with the use of high-speed electronic digital computers, and the NBRF's mission would be to develop such computers and use them in biomedical research.

Rather than merely advocating computer use, Ledley would at the NBRF design and use computers to solve problems in the life sciences. The NBRF started small, using only a portion of the office space the NAS-NRC had loaned to Ledley in 1960, and employed on a part-time basis a half dozen of Ledley's friends and former colleagues. The NBRF treasurer, Louis S. Rotolo, was Ledley's former assistant on the NAS-NRC survey; James B. Wilson, an NBRF research associate, had been one of Ledley's graduate students at GWU; and Margaret O. Dayhoff, a quantum chemist hired by Ledley to lead biomedical computing projects, had grown up with him in Flushing, New York. By the late 1960s, the NBRF had evolved into a large organization with several distinct branches. One was directed by Ledley and specialized in building electronic digital devices for use in biomedical settings, such as the Film Input to Digital Automatic Computer (FIDAC), which was mainly used to conduct rapid chromosome analysis. Another NBRF branch was directed by Dayhoff and specialized in managing sequence databases, most notably the 1965 *Atlas of Protein Sequence and Structure*. In 1970, the NBRF became an affiliate of the Georgetown University Medical Center. In exchange for office and laboratory space, the foundation would apply its research to the care of some Georgetown patients and would bring prestige (and funding) to the university—the NBRF remained physically located at Georgetown until early 2006.

In contrast to his work in the 1950s, Ledley did not attempt to shape the practice of biology or medicine beyond the individual projects in which he was involved. However, it was the enthusiasm for electronic computing that Ledley helped to generate through his early advocacy work that provided the financial resources on which the NBRF depended. In fact, for the first decade of its existence, the NBRF depended almost wholly on funding from the NIH to support its daily operations. As the NIH dedicated more resources to computing, the NBRF's annual budget swelled from less than $50,000 in 1960 to almost $1 million by 1969 (fig 4.1). This income was supplemented by the proceeds of sales of machines the NBRF developed. Often the NIH pointed to work being done at the NBRF as exemplary, which is unsurprising because during this time the agency was in many ways trying to follow Ledley's vision for computerizing biology and medicine. For instance, in 1974 Helen Hofer Gee, head of the NIH's Computer and Biomathematical Study Section (the successor to the ACCR and CRSS), cited the *Atlas* as "a testament to the contributions of computing to one broad area of scientific investigation."[84]

Ledley's first major project at the NBRF, shortly after its 1960 establishment, was to develop machines to automate pattern recognition in laboratory and clinical settings. Initially, the scope of this project was limited to building the Automatic Device for Antibiotic Determination (ADAD), a "laboratory scale" computer that could automatically determine the efficacy of antibiotic drugs.

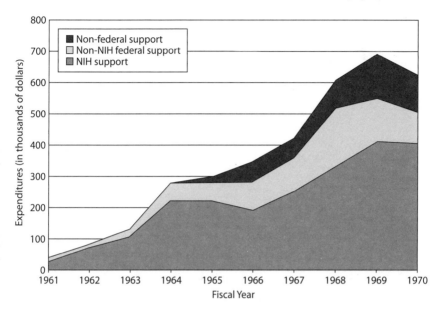

Fig. 4.1. Expenditures of the National Biomedical Research Foundation for the years 1961–70. In all years, most support came from the NIH. By permission of the National Biomedical Research Foundation

The ADAD tested the drugs by measuring how much light passed through bacterial cultures on a petri dish—completely transparent cultures had likely been killed by the antibiotic. This initial project met with limited commercial success, with ADADs sold to the Food and Drug Administration and to large pharmaceutical companies, and was followed by several more attempts to develop devices capable of optical pattern recognition, the best known of which was FIDAC.[85]

Developed, mostly on NIH grants throughout the 1960s, by Ledley, programmer-mathematician James Wilson, and electronic engineer Thomas Golab, FIDAC was designed to "scan" a photomicrograph into its memory and then interface with a larger computer, such as an IBM 7909 or IBM 360, to recognize patterns in that image. To digitize a photograph, FIDAC would divide it into a 700-by-500-point grid—the distance between and size of the points being adjustable—and measure the density of gray-level in each point. Once measured, each point was assigned a number ranging from 0 to 9 based on its density. With the ability to sample one point per microsecond, FIDAC could

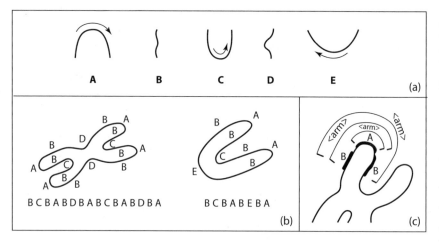

Fig. 4.2. (a) The basic types of curves used for recognizing chromosomes. (b) How curves form shapes representing metacentric (*left*) and telocentric (*right*) chromosomes. (c) How FIDAC assembles curves into an "arm" of a chromosome. By permission of the National Biomedical Research Foundation

generate a complete a 350,000-point scan in under half a second. Users could adjust gray-level thresholds to create a sharp contrast between their objects of study and the background color of the scan.[86]

Beyond creating and providing users with the means to manipulate digital images, FIDAC also automated some aspects of analysis of those images. In the case of scans of chromosomes, FIDACSYS, a program typically run on large IBM computers, could distinguish chromosomes from the background of a photomicrograph scanned by FIDAC, and then count and identify them. This was accomplished by detecting the edge curves associated with particular chromosomes and by measuring the lengths of chromosomes' arms as they extended from the centromere (figs. 4.2 and 4.3).[87]

Using FIDAC and FIDACSYS, a technician could greatly speed up chromosome analysis that hitherto had been performed by eye and hand. Manual analysis of chromosomes required: (1) making a large print of a photograph of each examined cell; (2) cutting the chromosomes out of the photograph, much like one would cut out paper dolls; and (3) aligning the cut-out chromosomes in a prescribed pattern, called a karyotype, to see whether the number and shape/size of the observed chromosomes were normal. This process took a skilled technician about fifteen minutes, whereas someone using FIDAC could perform that same analysis in under forty seconds.[88]

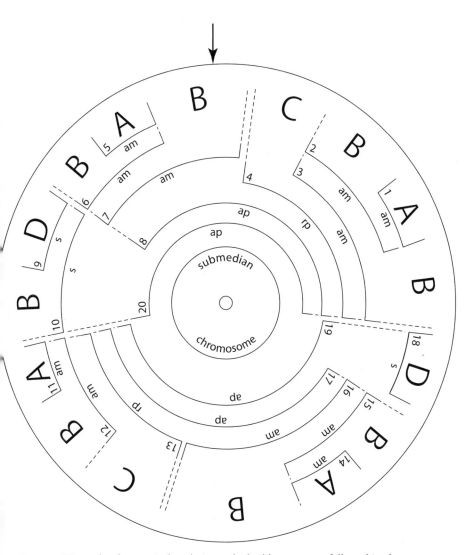

Fig. 4.3. "Example of syntactical analysis, or the build-up process followed in chromo-some recognition." This chart represents the process through which FIDAC assembles curves—see fig. 4.2 (a)—to produce a chromosome the program would recognize as "submedian"—in today's terminology, submetacentric—that is, with arms of unequal length. By permission of the National Biomedical Research Foundation

Ledley initially intended FIDAC to be used mainly to automate chromosome analyses, such as tests for Turner, Klinefelter, or Down syndromes, but it was also used to digitize schlieren photographs (used to visualize the flow of air or fluids) as well as photographs of neurons and Pap smears. Though FIDAC greatly speeded up chromosome analysis, it was impractical for most labs and clinics to use because it required access to a very large, powerful computer in order to run FIDACSYS. On a time-shared IBM 7090 or 360, a FIDAC user might have access for only a few hours a week. Indeed, the NBRF itself did not have such a computer and was forced to seek time on a 7090 at Westinghouse's plant in Baltimore in order to test FIDAC. The organization did not acquire its own large computer until 1968, when it received a large grant from the NIH to buy an IBM 360/44 computer.[89] Because access to a large computer was necessary to use FIDAC, its market was quite restricted. During the 1960s, about a dozen institutions purchased a FIDAC, including: the University of Florida, the Atomic Energy Commission's Lawrence Radiation Laboratory at UC Berkeley, the Health and Welfare Department of Canada, and the Medical Research Council of the United Kingdom. In the early 1970s, in the face of growing demand for an inexpensive machine with the capabilities of FIDAC, the NBRF attempted to develop a much smaller version of FIDAC that could fit into a laboratory. However, when it came to paying for the development of a small-scale chromosome analyzer, the NIH ultimately funded the Jet Propulsion Laboratory (JPL) rather than the NBRF on the grounds that JPL had better chance of quickly developing the machine.[90]

A lasting outgrowth of FIDAC was the journal *Pattern Recognition*, which Ledley founded in 1969. Though FIDAC was developed to digitize and recognize chromosomes, the techniques developed at NBRF could be applied to a variety of domains, and the journal was launched to facilitate the spread of these techniques. In 2008, after years of growth, the journal celebrated its fortieth anniversary, an event attended by fifteen hundred members of the Pattern Recognition Society, whose projects ranged from those close to its biomedical origins, like automating visual analyses of tumors, to broader applications such as text recognition and face recognition, an area that has attracted significant federal funding since the attacks of September 11, 2001.[91] Ledley was succeeded as editor-in-chief of *Pattern Recognition* in 2010 by Ching Y. Suen, who also directs the Montreal-based Centre for Pattern Recognition and Machine Intelligence (or CENPARMI).

In 1973, around the same time the NBRF was passed over for the NIH contract to continue developing a small-scale chromosome analyzer, the foundation also lost the most of its other NIH funding. This "disaster" was a consequence of severe budget cuts that President Richard Nixon made to the NIH. When Nixon froze NIH research funds, grants supporting work at the NBRF were among the first to be cut. In retrospect, Ledley called the loss of NIH support a "stroke of good luck" because in his scramble to generate income he began to develop the device for which he is best known, the full-body CT scanner.[92]

While trying to come up with a way to make enough money to "feed everybody" working at the NBRF, Ledley learned that Georgetown University research physicians wanted to purchase a computerized tomography (CT) X-ray machine from the British firm EMI but had balked at its $500,000 cost. Ledley, seizing on this opportunity, promised Georgetown that NBRF could build a similar machine for about half of what EMI was asking. Drawing on their own expertise in computer imagery, and building on the theoretical work of Tufts University physicist Allan M. Cormack and Veterans Administration neurologist William Oldendorf as well as the early designs of EMI engineer Godfrey Hounsfield, an NBRF team led by Ledley, Golab, Wilson, and draftsman Frank Rabbitt worked around the clock for several months to develop a working prototype. Beyond reducing the price, they sought to fix the major constraint of the CT scanner Hounsfield had developed for EMI, namely that X-rays had to be shone through a water tank enclosing the object to be scanned—thus the EMI machine could only scan patients' heads, which had to enclosed in a rubber bladder that extended into the water tank. This restriction could be fixed, the NBRF team reasoned, by changing the algorithms used to assemble X-rays into a 3-D image. Specifically, the EMI machine had been built around a relaxation (rounding) algorithm, whereas the NBRF sought to employ a convolution algorithm, a moving average of sorts.[93]

Working with Georgetown's machinists and auto body specialists at a local Cadillac dealer, Ledley and his team built their Automatic Computerized Transverse Axial (ACTA) scanner in 1974. ACTA was not only half the cost of EMI's CT scanner, but it required no intermediary between the scanner and the patient and therefore could scan the entire body. The machine was an instant success at Georgetown, after a pediatric neurosurgeon, David C. McCullough, used ACTA—apparently without Ledley's knowledge—one weekend to examine a boy who hit his head falling off a bike. Ledley recalled that McCullough had watched a technician use ACTA, and while trying to detect brain bleeding in his young patient decided to try the machine. As Ledley told it: "[McCullough] says, 'Yeah! And there was a bleed. And I took him down to Surgery and took out the blood, and you [Ledley] saved his life.' It was incredible! He said, 'If I'd waited till Monday, then it would have been over, the kid would have been dead.' "[94]

Following ACTA's initial success, Ledley patented the device, "claiming," as historian Bettyann Kevles writes, "that it was an entirely different instrument from EMI's, that it had roots in the American precedents of Oldendorf and Cormack."[95] Striving to meet to the demand—especially among radiologists—for a full-body CT scanner, Ledley formed Digital Information Science Corporation (DISCO) in 1974 and sold ACTA scanners for about $300,000 each. However, Ledley quickly found that running a hundred-person, multimillion-dollar business "kept me up at night" and sought customers for the rights to ACTA.[96] In 1975, DISCO sold Pfizer the rights to manufacture ACTA for $1.5 million in cash and another (at least) $10 million of guaranteed research funding for NBRF, to be paid out over the course of a decade. Between 1975 and 1977, "the heyday of CT scanning," Pfizer's ACTA 0100 was sold to hospitals worldwide. By the late 1970s, Pfizer had lost much of this market to companies like GE and Technicare, who were selling later-generation scanners, and shortly thereafter exited the medical imaging market.[97] In recognition of ACTA's role in introducing full-body CT scanners, the Smithsonian Institute displayed the ACTA prototype in the National Museum of American History, in Washington, DC, for many years. Ledley also received numerous honors for developing ACTA, including being inducted into the National Inventors Hall of Fame (1990) and being awarded the National Medal of Technology (1997).

In parallel to Ledley's work on medical imaging, another highly influential NBRF project undertaken starting in the 1960s was the *Atlas of Protein Sequence and Structure*.[98] The founder of the *Atlas* was Margaret Oakley Dayhoff (1925–1983), who, having grown up with Ledley in New York, had gone on to graduate school at Columbia University, where she earned a Ph.D. in quantum chemistry under George E. Kimball.[99] Besides being a prominent chemist, Kimball had also been one of the country's foremost operations researchers during the war and was one of the founders of the Operations Research Society of America (ORSA). The George E. Kimball Medal has been awarded annually since 1974 by ORSA and its successor, the Institute for Operations Research and the Management Sciences (INFORMS). While pursuing her degree under Kimball's supervision, Dayhoff used OR methods extensively to collect and analyze research data. She proved so adept at data management that she received a Watson

Computing Laboratory Fellowship, which gave her access to cutting-edge IBM electronic data processing equipment. A biography prepared by Dayhoff's family notes that during the course of her research she "devised a method of applying punched-card business machines to the calculation of molecular resonance energies of several polycyclic organic molecules."[100]

Though Dayhoff would not conduct much quantum chemistry research after completing her degree, her expertise in OR and computing machinery made her a natural fit at the NBRF, which she joined when Ledley founded it in 1960. There, she applied her data management skills—and some of her knowledge of chemistry—to the problem of protein sequencing. Dayhoff's *Atlas*, which appeared annually beginning in 1965, had as its goal to "collect between a single pair of covers as many [protein] sequences and other related data that have been educed by the scientific community."[101] Though Ledley was familiar with protein sequencing from his mid-1950s collaboration with the RNA Tie Club and his late-1950s proposal to automate sequencing, his role was to foster the *Atlas*'s growth—by giving it a home at the NBRF and helping to secure funding for it—rather than participate directly in its development.

Early editions of the *Atlas* had two parts. One contained raw data, cataloging proteins and the sequences of amino acids that formed those proteins. Dayhoff and her team scoured published and unpublished reports from around the world in order to create a comprehensive collection of protein sequences found in all organisms. Dayhoff's group presented the sequences in unified notation, and, where it could, pointed out "alignments," that is, shared sequences, in homologous or related proteins across species. The second part of the *Atlas* contained Dayhoff's research, which used the data to "describe . . . concepts and results in macromolecular evolution utilizing the protein sequences as 'living fossils.'" For instance, by comparing the amino acid sequences of the variant of the protein cytochrome c found in yeast to the variant of cytochrome c found in horses, Dayhoff and Richard V. Eck found that "in 64 of the 104 positions the amino acids in the two chains are identical." When they compared horse cytochrome c to that found in humans, there were only twelve differences in the sequences.[102] "A particularly exciting aspect of this work," proclaimed the NBRF's early 1970s sponsors at the NIH, "is the development of the field of molecular evolution which promises to increase manifold the knowledge of evolution that has heretofore been the almost exclusive domain of the geneticist."[103]

Dayhoff's attempts to trace the evolutionary history of organisms by comparing protein sequences also brought her into collaboration with scientists funded by NASA who were examining how life emerged billions of years ago in the Earth's "primordial soup" and how it could possibly emerge on other worlds. In the latter case, she used Georgetown University's IBM 7090 to simulate the formation of "biologically interesting compounds, such as amino acids" in pre-biological atmospheres and she cowrote a paper in 1967 with chemist Ellis R. Lippincott and astronomer—and soon-to-be-celebrity—Carl Sagan.[104] Though Dayhoff was rising within the community investigating early and extraterrestrial life, funding for this line of inquiry seems to have dried up as public interest in space exploration waned during the 1970s.

The portion of the *Atlas* that served as a comprehensive repository of raw sequence data had a considerably farther-reaching legacy. In its early years, the number of protein sequences listed in the *Atlas* was small enough that the entire *Atlas* was printed in paper books.[105] Copies were distributed by the NBRF to all of the scientists who had produced the sequences, who enthusiastically responded by sending Dayhoff still more sequences to catalog. By the mid-1970s the *Atlas* had become the major repository of sequence data. As more and larger proteins were sequenced, the *Atlas* grew too big to print and was distributed on magnetic reels, and eventually floppy diskettes and CD-ROMs. During the 1980s, historian Bruno Strasser points out, the *Atlas* served as a model for the nucleic acid sequence databases such as GenBank as well as the Protein Data Bank.[106]

The *Atlas* was a template for what became indispensible tools in large portions of DNA or protein-related biomedical research, but Dayhoff was marginalized by the community of sequencers her *Atlas* helped to bring about. When the NIH awarded the contract to manage GenBank in the early 1980s, the agency passed over the NBRF in favor of Walter Goad at the Los Alamos National Laboratory. Strasser contends that experimental scientists disdained Dayhoff's role as a compiler and disseminator of data, and despite relying on her *Atlas* for their research did not include her in their ranks.[107] One source of this attitude may have been sexism, another the clash of Dayhoff's values with those of the sequencers. By setting up the *Atlas* as an almanac, Dayhoff assigned little importance to authorship and priority, and in so doing she had run afoul of the prevailing values of experimental sciences. Strasser explains that by the early 1980s, sequences came to be considered highly proprietary knowledge and publishing them would bring considerable esteem to an individual author or laboratory. Submitting sequence information to a commonly accessed database, by contrast, did not establish priority or authorship, both of which brought recognition and scientific credit.[108] Taking a broader historical perspective, Strasser places Dayhoff's approaches to property and priority, so incongruous with experimental science, in the older collection- and cooperation-oriented tradition of natural history.[109]

In 1983, shortly after losing the GenBank contract to Los Alamos, Dayhoff died of a heart attack at the age of fifty-seven. Less than a week before she died, however, she had proposed to the NIH an online version of the *Atlas*, called the Protein Identification Resource (PIR), which would enable researchers who had computers to access NBRF protein sequence databases via a modem connection or TYMNET.[110] Initially led by Ledley and Winona C. Barker, who both stepped in after Dayhoff's death, and supported by the NIH's Division of Research Resources, the PIR (now known as the Protein Information Resource) has been a public repository of sequence data for more than a quarter century. The PIR is today run by staff based at the University of Delaware and Georgetown University, and is part of the NIH-sponsored UniProt consortium.

Beyond providing instruments and resources, the NBRF also promoted computing in biology and medicine via the peer-reviewed journals it managed. In academic and medical institutions where hiring and funding were based on the production of scholarly articles rather than building instruments or creating algorithms, these journals provided not only discursive space but also the means for many biomedical computing specialists to gain employment and compete for grants. Some of these journals grew out of specific instruments, while others were more general. The journals *Pattern Recognition* (1969) and *Computerized Medical Imaging and Graphics* (1976) grew out of FIDAC and ACTA respectively. *Computers in Biology and Medicine* (1969) began as a more general forum for sharing ideas, in the form of traditional articles, algorithms, and descriptions of instruments, related to biomedical computing. *Computer Languages, Systems and Structures* (1972) was from its establishment oriented toward computer science rather than biomedical applications. Ledley remained editor of all these journals until early 2010.

5

Martians, Experts, and *Universitas*

Biomedical Computing at Stanford University, 1960–1966

Perhaps the best way to understand how computers changed the study of life and vice versa is to take a close look at the formation of a major center of biomedical computing. One such center, at Stanford University, had by the late 1960s emerged as a leading nexus for the exchange of ideas between life scientists and computer scientists. Out of this exchange grew widely used resources like the Stanford University Medical Experimental Computer–Artificial Intelligence in Medicine (SUMEX-AIM) network, novel approaches to computing such as expert systems, and a template for a new relationship between universities, the federal government, and private enterprise. These phenomena, in turn, all had deep roots in Ledley and Lusted's vision for computer use and also in Clark's revolt from centralized computing.

Stanford's rise to early and continued prominence in biomedical computing was by no means a tale of cascading triumphs. Rather, it is a story of convergences—some fruitful, others painfully disappointing. Interacting were the ambitions of young scientists who wanted to transform their fields, deans and provosts attempting to restructure an ailing university, federal administrators eager to use information technology to advance biology and medicine, and computer manufacturers seeking a lucrative new market. Each of these parties had its own strong motivations for devoting enormous energy and resources to establishing Stanford as a center for biomedical computing. When their interests did not align, multimillion-dollar projects were canceled and promising career paths abandoned. When, however, common causes were recognized and acted upon, a new world of possibilities was opened.

Stanford was at once exceptional and exemplary. By today's norms, many of the major projects pursued there might seem quixotic or downright bizarre. Using computers to study amino acids on Mars or to automate the formation of scientific hypotheses would indeed seem unconventional in the twenty-first century. However, the ways in which early Stanford life sciences computing projects were run have been emulated many times around the world in the decades since. These 1960s projects had four characteristics that are found in most modern American efforts to bring information technology to bear on biological and medical problems: interdisciplinary collaboration, federal sponsorship, heavy involvement of computer manufacturers, and the extreme devotion of those involved to the project itself and to the whole enterprise of biomedical computing.

Building *Universitas*

As the site of the largest, most comprehensive efforts to computerize biology and medicine, Stanford University was where much of the early rhetoric about computers transforming intellectual and institutional aspects of life sciences research was put to the test. In the 1960s rush to computerize biology and medicine, Stanford, was a latecomer. By 1961, Stanford's rival in Los Angeles, UCLA, was running two multimillion-dollar NIH-funded biomedical computing facilities while Stanford had not even submitted a grant application for the purpose. Yet as the 1960s drew to a close, Stanford had become the dominant center of biomedical computing on the West Coast and arguably in the whole world.

Stanford's late arrival to biomedical computing and then its intensive activity in that domain were both consequences of the transformation the university had been undergoing since the end of World War II. In the decades following the war, Stanford president John Ewart Wallace Sterling (1906–1985), and academic dean, then provost Frederick Terman (1900–1982) undertook an aggressive and sustained effort to reorient the university toward interdisciplinary and federally supported research. In so doing Sterling and Terman created an environment at the university that made plans for massively computerizing life sciences research seem feasible. Indeed, without their unprecedented institutional support for large-scale, interdisciplinary, and federally funded projects, there would have been little to distinguish Stanford's attempts to computerize biology from the enthusiastic but nevertheless limited efforts of other universities to devote computing resources to life sciences research.[1]

Were one to have visited Stanford before the Sterling-Terman era, the university would have seemed an unlikely venue for pursing major biomedical research projects at all, let alone computerizing them. The late 1940s and early 1950s had been lean years for Stanford. The excitement, breakneck productivity, and generous funding that marked World War II and its immediate aftermath had dissipated, leaving the school in the intellectual doldrums as well as in dire financial straits. In the life sciences, departments and disciplines tended toward isolation, from each other as well as the broader university and national research communities.[2] Moreover, these researchers, having settled in their niches, showed little interest in sacrificing any of their autonomy for the purpose of drawing resources from burgeoning civilian federal funding agencies like the NIH or NSF. Yet by the late 1960s this state of affairs had been completely reversed, to the point where Stanford prided itself as the archetype of integrated, federally funded research. Computers were instrumental in this reversal.

In the last few years, much scholarship has been devoted to Stanford's postwar transformation.[3] These scholars devote most of their attention to Terman, now widely remembered as the "Father of Silicon Valley," pointing out that he pushed the life sciences toward interdisciplinary collaboration and federally supported research just as aggressively as he famously integrated Stanford applied physics and engineering research with federal monies, basic sciences, and local private enterprise in order to help create Silicon Valley. Thus far, however, there has been little discussion of one of the major forces that enabled—and in turn was enabled by—Terman's vision for biological and medical research at Stanford: *computerization*. Indeed, the persistence of the new orientation of Stanford life science depended primarily on access to powerful computing facilities, the availability of which, in turn, was contingent upon massive support from both the university administration and the federal government.

When Terman left his wartime post as head of Harvard's Radio Research Laboratory to become Stanford's Academic Dean in 1946, he immediately tried to reorient Stanford toward federally directed and funded research, but he met extensive resistance. A political progressive and an engineer by training, Terman saw federal support, national coordination, and the use of new technologies as essential to the university's survival as a center of important research. However, for the bulk of Stanford's faculty, such an approach was anathema to what they regarded as a very successful mode of research.[4] During the war, Stanford researchers had made significant contributions to many areas, ranging from engineering projects to atomic energy to a major penicillin production program, and there was a general sense of satisfaction on campus that the university had served the nation well.[5] Once the war ended, many Stanford researchers, like their peers at many other American universities, believed it would be quite reasonable to retreat to their individual labs and again pursue their particular interests.[6] As Eric Vettel shows, they generally wanted to revert to the prewar status quo of conducting isolated, self-directed research.[7] For many, the independent nature of Stanford research had been the university's defining quality. Among them, biologist George Beadle came to Stanford for the express purpose of conducting laboratory work unfettered by officious federal fund managers or unscientific entrepreneurs; he had left Caltech for Stanford because he believed that "applied research" on behalf of San Joaquin Valley farmers "tainted the purity of his own work."[8] For Beadle's collaborator, Edward Tatum, the separation of Stanford's Palo Alto campus from the School of Medicine in San Francisco was appealing specifically because he believed it would protect his research from time-consuming and distracting "clinical needs."[9]

School of Medicine faculty, meanwhile, took pride in their school's strong tradition of rigorous pedagogy, and they feared that introducing too many research activities would deprive the region of its largest source of quality physicians. Isolated from the main campus, the School of Medicine faculty seldom interacted with the university's scientists and resisted introducing coverage of basic life sciences to their curricula. Instead they focused on training physicians as healers, not scientists. Through the mid-1950s, the School of Medicine was geared toward producing such doctors. As university administrators described it, "The program of education for medicine at Stanford University is organized around the student's need to learn and the patient's need for care in order that the physician—whether he be practitioner, teacher, administrator or investigator—will be prepared to meet the responsibilities of medicine as a social as well as natural science."[10]

After surveying the situation in the life sciences departments and the School of Medicine, Terman concluded that if the faculty had its way Stanford would be "destined for mediocrity."[11] While researchers at other major universities tended toward coordination and conglomeration, Stanford's faculty had turned inward and its departments had balkanized. To his alarm, Terman saw very little interest in—and indeed much active resistance to—drawing from burgeoning sources of civilian federal patronage such as the NIH. During this time the vast majority—some years exceeding 90 percent—of government-sponsored research at Stanford was funded by the Department of Defense.[12]

Beyond Stanford researchers' reluctance to adapt to the presence of large bureaucracies in science was the greater and much more imminent threat posed by the university's financial woes. In short, Stanford's School of Medicine was going broke. Housed in a crumbling facility in San Francisco, it was hemorrhaging $400,000 of university funds each year.[13] By eschewing research in favor of raising funds via providing clinical services, Stanford was missing out on the significant federal and philanthropic support for research activities that other major American medical schools were receiving.

By 1950 it was clear the School of Medicine was never going to be able to generate enough funds to break even, let alone pay for the desperately needed multimillion-dollar renovation of its physical plant. That year, with the university facing the possibility that the School of Medicine would have to close, the Committee on Future Plans of the Medical School was formed to determine what needed to be done in order to keep the School of Medicine alive. Led by Henry Kaplan, then director of radiology, the committee conducted a survey in 1951 and 1952, looking especially to other leading medical schools for new approaches to funding and administration.[14] From their survey, the committee recommended that the school undertake a major renovation of its facilities, increase annual financial support, and create a $15 million endowment and a $15 million short-term fund to support reconstruction.[15] What the committee did not offer, however, was any new means to enable the School of Medicine to obtain support from federal funding agencies.

With $30 million at stake, Sterling's administration decided that it could not afford to throw good money after bad and concluded that if such money were to be spent on the School of Medicine, it might as well be built anew, this time on Stanford's main campus. The aim of the move, in their words, "is the creation of a university atmosphere in which the whole scholarly body of the institution, teachers and students of all levels of maturity, learn together and together advance knowledge. This is but a return to the early concept of *Universitas*, a community of masters and scholars."[16] Terman, AnnaLee Saxenian maintains, saw Europe's earliest universities as a template for Stanford's *Universitas* and envisioned a "community of technical scholars" based in northern California that would serve as a modern counterpart to the centers of medieval scholarship in Oxford, Heidelberg, and Paris.[17] Sterling also spoke several times along this vein; for instance, at the 1959 dedication of the new medical facility, he proclaimed: "This key relationship of medical education and science to other scientific fields can best be strengthened and advanced by bringing the medical school into the closest possible physical and intellectual relationship to the whole university."[18]

To realize the vision of *Universitas*, the Medical Council's Committee on Curriculum, working under Sterling's guidance, called for a "new [School of Medicine] curriculum [that] will emphasize the essential unity of biology and the basic medical science, and the interdependence of medicine and other university disciplines."[19] This unity, upon which Sterling expounded during his 1959 dedication address, was vital to the advancement of both science and medicine: "Central to this new Stanford program is the concept that future progress of the medical sciences is inextricably linked with progress in the physical and biological sciences and increasingly with progress in the social sciences."[20] By integrating the School of Medicine with the main campus, Sterling also intended to run it the same way he ran the rest of the university: it would be oriented toward federally funded research and interdisciplinary collaboration. Success would be measured primarily by the "ability of faculty to receive federal funding to support their work."[21] Instead of serving local needs, the School of Medicine would be reoriented to serve Sterling and Terman's goal of building Stanford into one of the country's major universities.[22] Consequently, Sterling called for School of Medicine faculty to be treated like the university's other researchers: "The Medical Faculty will become true university professors, devoting full time to their university functions of teacher and researcher."[23]

In June 1957, ground was broken for the new Palo Alto home of the School of Medicine, the Stanford Medical Center (SMC). With the backing of the university's trustees, Sterling began implementing the institutional changes he believed would be necessary to transform the School of Medicine into a research center that would "open eyes."[24] Two months prior to the SMC groundbreaking, Sterling appointed Robert H. Alway to replace Windsor Cutting as Dean of the School of Medicine. In contrast to Cutting, Alway's top priority was research, not direct care. Under Alway's leadership, School of Medicine faculty would be full-time researchers, and one of his earliest moves was to set a policy to force them to support their work with university or federal funds rather than clinical fees.[25] Twenty professors who obstructed the move from teaching to research were fired. With the exception of Kaplan, the administration forced every School of Medicine department head to resign by the end of August 1958.[26] Faculty who had split their time between the School of Medicine and private practice were asked to devote themselves wholly to one or the other, a move that further depleted the school's ranks.

In their place, Sterling and Terman encouraged Alway to hire top scientists whose work they believed would advance both medical and scientific research, as well as open new areas to private enterprise.[27] In 1959, Alway recruited Arthur Kornberg to head the new Department of Biochemistry, offering to move his whole Washington University department en masse to Stanford.[28] He also recruited Nobel laureate Joshua Lederberg to establish and lead the Department of Genetics. Lederberg's work, in contrast to what had been undertaken at the School of Medicine in decades past, was highly mathematical, strongly associated with the physical sciences (because it relied on mass spectrometry techniques), had absolutely no clinical component, and was sponsored by federal bodies like NASA and the NIH.

During the move, the School of Medicine's curriculum was overhauled as well. Taking advantage of the new faculty and the SMC's proximity to Stanford's various science departments, the new curriculum introduced mandatory courses in basic physical and life sciences. To absorb this new material, Stanford increased the medical student's normal length of study from four to five years. Time spent studying science came at the expense of clinical training, and Terman was harshly and publicly criticized in the early 1960s for putting research ahead of providing healthcare training. Administrators siding with Terman retorted that by treating medical students as research-oriented graduate students he was providing them the best possible education and the means to fundamentally improve medicine.[29]

In the late 1950s and early 1960s, as part of restructuring the university, Terman and Sterling also encouraged departments to hire experts in new technologies like cyclotrons, transistors, and electronic digital computers. At the Department of Mathematics, one such hire was numerical analyst George Elmer Forsythe (1917–1955), who during the early to mid-1950s had worked extensively with the NBS's Standards Western Automatic Computer (SWAC), the West Coast counterpart to the SEAC. When Forsythe arrived at Stanford in

1957, he found little interest among his colleagues in computers, and he subsequently launched an effort to raise that interest on campus. With support from university administrators, Forsythe was able to offer interdepartmental courses in computer programming. The university also stepped in when Forsythe called for a means to provide students with "general-purpose mental tools" after he had observed that traditional training in mathematics and engineering would not suffice to produce students capable of conducting meaningful work on computers. In 1961, using funding and space provided by the university, Forsythe founded the Division of Computer Science within the Department of Mathematics in order to better train Stanford students and faculty to use computers and also to provide institutional support for talented computer experts.[30]

In the early 1960s, Forsythe also promoted computers as a means to realize the ideals espoused by Terman and Sterling, particularly when it came to the life sciences. Computers, he asserted, would not only give researchers greater capacity to manage and analyze data, but using—or even planning to use—these machines would also attract positive federal attention, qualitatively improve the intellectual process of biomedical research, and render disparate fields of inquiry accessible to each other and indeed anyone who understood computers. In short, Forsythe had found a technical means of achieving the administrators' vision of *Universitas*, and consequently he was given the leading role in the task of computerizing Stanford's community of biologists and physicians.

Forsythe's Other Battle: Stanford's First Attempt at Biomedical Computing

When George Forsythe died suddenly in 1972 at the age of fifty-five, he was remembered not only as the founder of Stanford University's Computer Science Department but also as a prolific author of algorithms, professional letters, and essays promoting computer science as a discipline among mathematicians, scientists, and government planners. That summer, Donald Knuth, author of the definitive *Art of Computer Programming* series of computer science texts and the creator of the TeX typesetting system, eulogized Forsythe: "It is generally agreed that he, more than any other man, is responsible for the rapid development of computer science in the world's colleges and universities."[31] Knuth went on to hail Forsythe as "almost . . . the Martin Luther of the Computer Reformation," recalling that "George argued the case for computer science long and loud, and he won; at Stanford he was in fact the producer and director, author, scene designer, and casting manager of this hit show."[32] Forsythe's outreach met with resounding success, especially in terms of establishing computer science as a top priority for major universities. But Forsythe's greatest effort of the early 1960s, promoting computer use in biology, which went unmentioned by his eulogists, was met with indifference and bewilderment on the part of biologists and their sponsors, ending in a rare and bitter defeat.

Forsythe's passionate efforts to bring computer technology to biology should be seen as part of his better-known attempts to establish computer science as a discipline distinct from mathematics and also worthy of serious attention and funding. In 1991, Gio Wiederhold, who was hired by Forsythe in 1965 and whose primary work was in biomedical computing, would reflect that "Forsythe's global contribution was recognizing and helping to define computer science as a broadly inclusive new field."[33] As early as 1961, the year Forsythe founded the Division of Computer Science within Stanford's Mathematics Department, he sought to include biomedical applications when he delimited the realm of computer science. That year, Forsythe wrote, "Enough is known already of the diverse applications of computing for us to recognize the birth of a coherent body of technique, which I call computer science. Whether computers are used for engineering design, medical data processing, composing music or other purposes, the structure of computing is much the same."[34] Forsythe's inclusion of biomedical computing in his vision for computer science became manifest in his hard-fought but ultimately unsuccessful 1962–63 attempt to convince the NIH to grant Stanford about $1 million toward supporting an IBM 7090 that would be used primarily by biologists.[35]

In his quest to introduce computers to Stanford life sciences, Forsythe teamed up with Keith F. Killam Jr. (1927–1998), Associate Professor of Pharmacology at the School of Medicine. As R. Wade Cole, associate director of operations at the Stanford Computation Center and Forsythe and Killam's lieutenant in this effort, later related, the specific priorities of the venture—as well as the intensity of Forsythe's passion—evolved during the course of applying for NIH funds: "Our own sense of mission in bringing computing to Life Science at Stanford grew on us during the time we were preparing our request and during the time our request was being processed by the NIH."[36]

Their initial aims were both immediate and far-reaching. "The immediate goal," they proposed, "is to provide researchers in the biomedical sciences access to currently available high speed digital processing equipment." They regarded this near-term goal as but the "the first phase toward fulfillment of a long range plan which is to provide researchers with on-line, real-time use of high speed digital computing equipment during the course of experiments."[37] To implement their plan, Forsythe and Killam requested a $1 million, five-year grant from the NIH for funds to rent an IBM 7090, a tape-driven x-y plotter, specialized analog-to-digital conversion equipment, and the full-time services of a professional programmer.

Killam was to be the direct beneficiary of the project, but the effort to acquire computer equipment for Stanford's biomedical researchers was largely Forsythe's initiative. Evoking what he termed "the Computer Revolution," Forsythe had called on universities and their sponsors to "respond with far-reaching changes in educational structure."[38] To bring the "Computer Revolution" to Stanford biomedicine, Forsythe planned to introduce the machines to neurophysiology, a domain that had seen extensive computer use as of 1962, and then expand the user base to include the rest of the biomedical sciences. As Forsythe and Killam argued in their grant application statement, the necessary first step toward computerizing biomedical research would be to acquire the capacity to overcome the difficulties posed by the problem of translating analog biological signals into a digital output that could be interpreted by a computer. Without a general-purpose computer of their own, they noted, researchers in biomedical sciences could digitize—or "reduce" as they called it—data they gathered during experiments only through using special-purpose equipment or by undertaking laborious transcription by hand of analog data from strip charts onto punched cards for subsequent processing at a centralized computing facility—or "digital facility" (2).

The second stage in Forsythe and Killam's plan to computerize biomedical research would be to augment researchers' ability to manage and manipulate their data. Specifically, the designers sought to "include among the possible modes of data presentation automatically prepared graphs." They hoped that "with reasonably short turnaround times, a researcher can gather data during an experiment, edit the data, convert it to digital form, carry out appropriate computations to reduce the data and display his results in easy-to-interpret graphical form." They further noted that such techniques had been successfully implemented in the missile and spacecraft industries and would "certainly provide immeasurably expanded facilities for biological medical research" (6).

Initially, access to the computer would be limited to the general computation center staff and research scientists working in neurophysiology and cardiovascular research; emphasis would be placed on processing electrophysiological phenomena. Besides Killam, immediate beneficiaries of the presence of such a system were to include Kao Liang Chow and Frank Morrell, both neurology researchers; Karl Pribram, professor in the Departments of Psychiatry and Psychology; and Lincoln Moses, statistician and Professor in Preventative Medicine. All of these researchers were facing the prospect of abandoning promising projects because of "inadequate processing capabilities for data gathered in analog form" (5).

The trio of Chow, Killam, and Morrell had by this point also applied for a LINC in order to conduct pilot experiments that they argued would help them "improve the efficiency of design of experiments for use of large scale computer facilities for analysis of research data." However, the LINC was by Forsythe's reckoning "a limited capacity computer" and would not suffice as a data processor once researchers accumulated the amounts of data their studies called for. Only direct access to a machine with much greater processing power would enable them to analyze their data in a timely manner—on the order of hours, not months. Pribram, meanwhile, intended to utilize a large computer as part of a plan for "developing an interdepartmental curriculum of graduate study in brain research [that would] focus heavily in information theory and processing as applied to brain research." As Forsythe and Killam described it, the program's computer-oriented direction would embody "the feeling of the group that tomorrow's research worker in brain research must be trained in computer technology as well as in the classical training offered heretofore" (9).

Forsythe and Killam envisioned that after a few months of use by the neurology researchers the computer center would be ready to broaden its base of users so as to serve as "the foundation for a future general medical data processing center embracing all aspects of medical problems." They expressed confidence that such a center would "establish an intellectual bridge between the computation facility and the medical center, bringing into focus the problems of quantification peculiar to biological systems and also serve to build a reservoir of talent who would be familiar with modern computational facilities on the one hand and the kinds of problems facing medicine on the other" (5).[39]

The grant request authored by Forsythe and Killam was submitted to the NIH in early June 1962. Reports of NIH's reception to the proposal trickled back to California starting in November, and the news was not good. On November 12, 1962, Wade Cole wrote to Forsythe that he had heard that Stanford's NIH proposal was in trouble (his words) because the ACCR was "unwilling to game so much money in equipment and personnel on an 'unproved'" approach to the general problem of processing medical data."[40] Indeed no such system had ever been implemented in a biomedical environment; the only precedent for large-volume analog-to-digital conversion was set by the McDonnell Aircraft Corporation's Automation Center, in St. Louis), where McDonnell had invested millions in developing devices for this purpose, and which had only met with limited success in this endeavor. Moreover, Cole had heard of NIH grumblings concerning what they saw as slow progress at the computational centers they had sponsored at UCLA, with A-D conversion appearing to be the major bottleneck for those using large computers.[41]

Forsythe and Killam reacted quickly, and within a week were preparing a modified proposal calling for a contract arrangement in which several research centers (Stanford University, Washington University, Massachusetts General Hospital) would use federal funds to pay the McDonnell Automation Center to process their biomedical data. Most of the data pertained to neuro-pharmaceutical problems, and Forsythe expressed hope that computers would better enable researchers to "employ neurophysiological and psychological methodology in an investigation of the mechanisms of action of drugs affecting the central nervous system."[42] Consequently, Stanford's Computation Center would only be "incidentally involved," and plans calling for the center to bring computational power to the rest of the university's biomedical research community were dropped. Yet, with the possibility of access to more powerful equipment, Forsythe and Killam only broadened their ambitions. Indeed, the McDonnell "McAuto" equipment—about $10 million worth of top-of-the-line IBM and CDC digital computers and custom-built A-D conversion equipment—was so much more powerful than anything biomedical researchers could then access or even formulate problems for, that Forsythe and Killam concluded, "The limits to the new horizons are unbounded and are sharply defined and useful according to the individual investigator's ingenuity."[43]

With access to the McDonnell equipment, Forsythe and Killam saw the possibility of establishing a new intellectual framework for approaching biomedical research. The new goals of the project were expanded "to investigate the problems of putting all biomedical data into a processing form, and to demonstrate the practical usefulness by analyzing the data in a number of ways." Specifically they hoped to formalize, and ultimately mechanize, the process through which biologists went about—as they put it—"sanitizing" the data they had accumulated in the course of their research. As they explained, biologists had needed a new way to display and manage their data: "In the past, since biology has been predominantly descriptive, the display of accumulated data has been visual, necessitating the intervention of a trained specialist to interpret and correlate the results."[44] Such expertise would be unnecessary if the data could be organized in a way that computers could filter out the noise. Nonetheless, with there being no formal system for sanitizing the data, and given that computer experts had no experience in this area either, Forsyth and Killam cautioned that in the near term, "One cannot turn over to or expect the machine to perform the non-verbal trained selection of real from artifactual data performed by the investigator."[45]

At the heart of the problem, they argued, was communication: "Even the better trained representatives from biology and systems engineering have difficulty communicating at an intellectual level." Nevertheless, by giving life sciences researchers access to the McDonnell machines, they proposed to "extend interaction [between biologist and engineer] at the bench level." By working alongside engineers on the McDonnell computers, Forsythe and Killam hoped biologists would develop "an appreciation of what would be called in a broad sense operations research." Furthermore, they saw this interaction as a potential boon for biology in general. If biologists used OR methods, Forsythe and Killam argued, "Data would be provided as to the efficient handling of biomedical data, what costs in terms of hardware are needed to implement varying degrees of efficient systems, and what the manpower investment would be to maximize the interchange between a biological laboratory and a computational center."[46]

Just days after the counterproposal was submitted, Forsythe and Killam received word that NIH had formally rejected both their initial and modified proposals. The NIH's official reason for turning down Stanford was that the NIH felt the project was too tightly focused on Killam's research, with there being no apparent mechanism to expand the project's scope beyond neurophysiology.[47] Furthermore, the NIH argued that Killam had already received a small grant for computing equipment, which they believed was sufficient to enable his work. Forsythe in particular was dispirited by NIH's "complete refusal of an extremely well thought-of plan," and he wondered in one memo, "Do they really understand computing at NIH?" From his perspective, Stanford's computer experts, who had enjoyed generous funding from federal sources, had put forward their best plan. "I don't believe," he said, "any proposal or report we have ever made was so much thought about, or involved coordination with so many people." And then it was rejected for mysterious reasons. Wrote Forsythe, "I feel quite disappointed about this" before adding "it's unclear what the NIH wants."[48] At this point he confided to Wade Cole that he was entertaining the possibility of simply abandoning the effort to bring computers to the life sciences: "I think we must ask . . . [Dean Al Bowker] whether it's worthwhile to think any more about biomedical computing."[49]

Forsythe remarked in late November 1962 that he was "pretty bitter about this matter," but he and Cole did not give up, and instead launched a "two-man crusade" to introduce computers to Stanford biologists and physicians.[50] Their new aim was to achieve, using existing resources, "a satisfactory marriage at the working level between the Computation Center and the Medical School."[51] Now armed with the knowledge that the ACCR was concerned that researchers would avoid a computer if they did not have ready access to it or the means to convert their data into digital form, Forsythe proposed to the Stanford administration a plan to ask the NIH for $1.5 million to support for three years an annex of the Stanford Computation Center (SCC) located physically inside the Stanford Medical Center and packed with A-D conversion equipment. The hope was that putting a computing center in the SMC would eliminate many questions about access and availability, and that the Computation Center's involvement would ensure that the computer was well run.[52]

In early December, however, when Forsythe and his assistants began canvassing Stanford for more biomedical researchers to lend their support to his plans to acquire a major computer with NIH funds, they found that they were much more dedicated to the endeavor of computerizing biology than many of the biologists were. For instance, when Cole met with biostatistician Lincoln Moses to muster support for another pass at the NIH, Moses said little to encourage further efforts to advance biomedical computing at Stanford. For Moses, who would have been one of the rejected system's primary users, the possibility of biologists being overwhelmed by data they needed to digitalize was not a particularly pressing issue—he found that Stanford's Radio Science Laboratory handled his A-D conversion needs sufficiently. As far as Moses was concerned, any further efforts to court the NIH may as well be dropped unless Stanford (and researchers in general) could prove broad need for biomedical computational resources.[53]

Such talk frustrated Forsythe, who along with Cole, had by that point become "firmly convinced that computing in life science research will ultimately be an absolutely essential ingredient for the rapid growth of fruitful investigations."[54] Moreover, Forsythe did not want to model Stanford's biocomputing efforts after those undertaken by other universities. Rather, he insisted that Stanford, with its singular collection of computing experts should be the bellwether, not a follower. He specifically pointed to faculty like John McCarthy, whom he had just recruited to Stanford from MIT, whose expertise in designing time-sharing computer systems he believed could be harnessed to develop a system that would let scientists put consoles in their labs and use them in real time with their experiments. "At Stanford," explained Cole to the NIH, "we are firmly committed to the principle that more computation can be bought per dollar through a centralized computing agency."[55]

Belatedly appealing to the administration's emphasis on aggressive innovation, Forsythe attacked Moses's plan to wait for demand to emerge before trying to acquire more computer equipment as a potential lost opportunity: "If we wait until everyone at Stanford is begging for the installation of equipment which at that time will exist at many other institutions, there will be no pioneering effort involved." In Cole's blunt words to Forsythe: "Since Moses probably won't support another NIH attempt, we should get someone here who will, if it's decided that Stanford wants to pursue life science computing."[56] Pushing further, the solution Forsythe settled on was to encourage Stanford to import, à la Kornberg, Dean Clyde's entire University of Miami Biometrics Laboratory, but this never came to pass.

As Forsythe ran out of options at Stanford, he found that like minds were meeting similar resistance at the NIH. In early December 1962, he received word via Killam that the ACCR was far from unanimous in their decision to deny his project funding and that there were several on the committee who strongly sympathized with his vision. There were two forces at work within NIH hampering Stanford's efforts to secure funding. On one side there was staunch opposition to investing in computing among the leaders of most of NIH's research institutes. On the other side were members of the ACCR who believed that the Stanford proposal did not go far enough in terms of spreading computer technology in the life sciences.

Within the NIH, Forsythe's most vocal supporter was Thomas J. Kennedy Jr., then an associate director at the Division of Research Facilities and Resources (DRFR). Though a powerful figure within the NIH, Kennedy did not exert much influence on the ACCR, which ultimately made the decision whether or not to fund Stanford. He could make useful observations, however, most of which were crafted to encourage Forsythe and Killam to conform to the ACCR's agenda. Overall, Kennedy painted a gloomy picture of the prospects of the NIH funding biomedical computing projects and made clear to Forsythe that at the NIH the ACCR was the only party active in promoting the extramural funding of computing.[57] In December 1962, Kennedy wrote to Cole, "There appears to be a rather striking resemblance between the obstacles encountered in both our institutions in furthering computation in the life sciences." Pointing to hostility toward computers on the NIH campus, Kennedy conceded, "I am not too sanguine over the prospects that our biomedical research community will be excited over our proposals, and I have no real assurance that the Director [James Shannon] will take vigorous action in the face of the antipathy of our community." From Kennedy's perspective, resistance to computerization was not so much intellectual or even institutional, but rather the blame lay in the "'cultural' problems associated with introducing computer technology into the mainstream of life science research."[58] What Forsythe and Killam needed to do but had not done was to directly address life scientists' opposition to computing.

In the case of the Stanford grant, which Kennedy had strongly supported, time had been the main factor in rejecting the application. Whereas proponents like Kennedy empathized with Forsythe and Killam's suggestion that the initially supported system would be the "modest start of a larger project," the project's opponents on the ACCR saw it as too narrow and too difficult to expand.[59] When the debate continued right up to the deadline, the committee was forced to err on the side of caution and reject the Stanford proposal. Afterward, the ACCR's executive secretary, Bruce Waxman, related to Killam that "there were apparently second thoughts among some members of the committee who suddenly realized that they had not turned down Podunk College but Stanford University. The feeling is that if [Stanford's] request were made again, it would be granted."[60]

Working against Forsythe's effort to court the NIH were the far-reaching ambitions for computing held by the ACCR's leadership, especially Lee Lusted and Waxman (see chapter 2). Forsythe learned of these priorities only after Killam travelled to Bethesda, Maryland, to exchange ideas with Waxman. It was during this exchange that the NIH first articulated to Stanford what would be the core goals of its computing policy. As Killam reported to Forsythe, "It seems that the NIH seeks to sponsor active computation centers rather than passive ones. By active they mean vigorous proselytizing of biomedical researchers in the use of computing." By the NIH's measure, Forsythe and Killam had been "passive" rather than "active." Specifically, NIH-ACCR site visitors expressed dissatisfaction with their hosts' response to the question of "how a potential user gains access to the Computation Center." In answering that question, Forsythe and Killam had envisioned a process wherein scientists would, by their own volition, approach the Computation Center or the Department of Mathematics with a proposal to use the computer. However, the NIH wanted them to take a more aggressive approach and be "out constantly knocking on doors and selling computation." The committee also seemed hostile to plans to associate a biomedical computing center with any other campus activities or to have that center run as an adjunct to a larger campus facility. When ACCR site visitors arrived, fresh from having heard Wesley Clark's attack on time-sharing, they proved unreceptive to Forsythe's promotion of the notion that life scientists could effectively use time-shared mainframes. The visitors bombarded their hosts with stories of underutilization of centralized facilities at Tulane University and UCLA, leaving Forsythe to wonder if the NIH "has a basic dislike of the notion of a strongly centralized data processing center." To a confused Forsythe, it appeared that same the NIH committee that had promoted the establishment of large biomedical computer centers was now favoring computing along the lines of the relatively small LINC, where the biologists always had direct control over all aspects of computing, thus giving them the capacity to deal with changing parameters, even if such control came at the cost of efficiency and access to processing power.[61]

By January 1963, it was evident to Forsythe and Killam that the NIH grant application was a lost cause. Facing insurmountable resistance from both Stanford biologists and NIH administrators, not to mention ever-changing expectations for computing among both of these parties, Forsythe abandoned his formal effort to promote computer use in biomedical research. Forsythe's enthusiasm for broadening the scope of computer science was, however, unabated; and the next thirty-six months were arguably the most intensive and fruitful of his career. In 1964, he began his two-year term as president of the Association for Computing Machinery (ACM), and in 1965 he established the Computer Science Division as a formal Stanford department.[62] Meanwhile, Killam joined the ACCR. Waxman, who had regretted the decision not to fund the Stanford project, used his powers as executive secretary to appoint Killam to the committee in early 1963. While there were no formal guidelines for selecting committee members, it is likely that Waxman selected Killam because of his hard-won expertise in the arena where those who promoted computing in the life sciences had battled, and because Waxman wanted to maintain a good relationship with Stanford. Killam served on the ACCR until it became the CRSS in 1964.

The NIH also granted to Killam—off the records—what they called a phantom LINC so that he and his colleagues could begin to computerize their work.[63]

As of 1963, Stanford had no computing facility for biomedical researchers, and the principals of the effort to acquire that facility had all moved on to other projects. However, just three years later, Stanford would host the world's largest and most expensive center for biomedical computing. Though Forsythe and Killam had not succeeded, Stanford administrators and NIH grant evaluators still desired to transform Stanford into a major center for biomedical computing. What had been missing from the first effort was a desire among the biologists and physicians themselves to computerize their work. But among the new medical center hires brought in as part of Sterling and Terman's efforts to restructure the university was a young geneticist who fervently believed that computers were necessary to advance his own research as well as science and medicine in general.

Earth Computers and Martian Life: Lederberg's Computing Agenda

Joshua Lederberg wanted to know how life worked on Mars.[64] In the late 1950s, the existence of Martian life seemed much more likely than it does today, and he sought to apply his expertise in molecular genetics and bacteriology to the task of exploring "the possibility of finding another branch of evolution."[65] Then in his mid-thirties, Lederberg already had two major breakthroughs to his name. First, in 1946, he had discovered bacterial conjugation—that is, the conclusion that some bacteria share genetic information through sex, for which he shared a Nobel Prize in 1958. Second, in 1952, he discovered transduction, the phenomenon where some bacteriophages—viruses that infect bacteria—could carry not only their own genes but also bacterial genes from one bacterium to another. Lederberg, who had grown frustrated by his University of Wisconsin, Madison, colleagues' disdain for the molecular approach to biology and their close ties to the agricultural industry, came to Stanford in hopes of leading a group that would apply the newest bacteriological and molecular genetics research to medicine.[66]

Lederberg's agenda at Stanford was to aid medicine by creating a framework to expand what Berkeley biochemist Cornelius Bernardus van Niel called "comparative biochemistry," or the comparison between terrestrial and extraterrestrial life.[67] Specifically, he sought to find and study organic macromolecules on Mars. Lederberg understood that "the odds . . . were very long," but he believed that the potential yield of extraterrestrial biology—or "exobiology," as he called this branch of the study of life—was so great that he devoted most of his time and energy in 1958 and 1959 to rallying other elite scientists and the newly formed National Aeronautics and Space Agency (NASA) to his cause.[68]

It worked. By early 1959, Lederberg's West Coast Committee on Extraterrestrial Life (WESTEX) had attracted the founding figures of California's nascent molecular biology and biochemistry communities as well as high-profile scientists working within more traditional biology and chemistry disciplines. Early members included prominent biophysicists, biochemists and early molecular biologists such as Gunther Stent, Melvin Calvin, Harold C. Urey, Matthew Meselson, Norman Horowitz, and Roger Stanier. As historian Audra Wolfe notes, the committee's agenda reflected the excitement surrounding the molecularization of biology. "According to WESTEX," she wrote, "an exobiology that stressed analysis at the level of the molecule could inform scientific debates on evolution, comparative microbiology, and theoretical biology. The transnational search for the so-called unity of life, as it was unfolding through contemporary experiments in molecular genetics and biochemistry, lent a certain prestige to the field."[69]

WESTEX hoped that by discovering "the composition of the indigenous amino acids" they would acquire the means to resolve their debates concerning the origin of life's building blocks.[70] On the one hand, in 1953 Stanley Miller and (early WESTEXer) H. C. Urey had "demonstrated the production of amino acids by action of electric discharges on gas mixtures containing the hydrides NH_3, OH_2 and CH_4."[71] On the other, a more widely accepted contemporary theory held that complex organic macromolecules were ubiquitous byproducts of the same condensation of the universe's lighter elements (including H, C, O, and N) that produced the nebulae from which stars formed. These and other 1950s theories of the formation of life, however, failed to provide an experimentally verifiable mechanism for "the actual formation of a *replicating* polymer in such a morass."[72]

WESTEX's great hope was that something on Mars would furnish just such a mechanism. Consequently, they believed that they and America's burgeoning space program had much to offer each other. "All the projected space flights and high costs of such developments would be fully justified," claimed Miller and Urey, "if they were able to establish the existence of life on either Mars or

Venus. In that case, the thesis that life develops spontaneously when conditions are favorable would be far more firmly established, and our whole view of the problem of the origin of life would be confirmed."[73]

Having agreed on the importance of extraterrestrial organisms, Lederberg and his colleagues began to fear for the safety of their hypothetical Martians. Henceforth, WESTEX's primary concern was not to lobby governments to send probes to look for life but rather to "rigorously exclude terrestrial contaminants from our spacecraft."[74] Besides worrying about the more destructive facets of the Cold War space race, namely US and Soviet plans to detonate thermonuclear devices on the Moon, WESTEX railed against the general principle of manned space programs on the grounds that they: (1) were politically—rather than scientifically—oriented; (2) had as their goal the transport of bacteria-ridden human beings to hitherto pristine environments; and (3) represented a threat to humanity because organisms brought to Earth—intentionally or not— could be dangerous. NASA's mission, WESTEX insisted, should be to win the race to discover life beyond Earth, and to win in such a manner that both terrestrial and extraterrestrial life would be safe from contamination by the other.[75]

Beyond establishing a policy of sterilizing exploratory vessels before they launched and quarantining them upon their return, WESTEX did not succeed in convincing NASA to change its priorities. Moreover, Lederberg's alarmist articles and speeches on the dangers posed by extraterrestrial contamination had agitated the general public to a point where plans to return samples of lunar and Martian soil to Earth had become politically unfeasible.[76] If WESTEX wanted to study Martian amino acids, they would have to do so remotely, which meant figuring out to how land a well-equipped biochemistry laboratory on Mars at a time when NASA struggled to fire rockets past the Earth's atmosphere, let alone send them to other planets.[77]

Although the prospects of being able to examine an extraterrestrial organism had grown more remote by late 1959, Lederberg and the other early exobiologists could take solace in the steady stream of credible, optimistic studies regarding the possibility that such organisms indeed existed. One of the most prominent such studies, encouragingly titled "Further Evidence of Vegetation on Mars," appeared in the November 6, 1959 issue of *Science* and posited that mass spectrometry analysis had possibly solved the mystery of the migrating dark patches on Mars that Palomar Observatory astronomers had been tracking for decades: the patches were composed of vegetation, waxing and waning with the seasons.[78] What captured Lederberg's imagination, however, was not just the piece heralding the likelihood of Martian plant life but also the preceding article, "Digital Electronic Computers in Biomedical Science," Robert S. Ledley's pitch to biologists to mathematize their experimental agendas and consolidate their small laboratories in order to harness computer technology.[79]

Immediately after reading Ledley's article, Lederberg enrolled in his first computer-programming course, thus joining the tiny but growing community of biologists trying to adopt computer technology.[80] Lederberg's newfound interest in computers would first complement his Mars-related activities, then eclipse them. At roughly the same time he founded WESTEX, Lederberg was also establishing Stanford's Department of Genetics, an endeavor that drew him into Stanford's academic community, which, owing to Terman's priorities, was oriented much more toward the development of electronics than space exploration.[81] Further cementing Lederberg's commitment to computing was that he had, upon settling in Stanford, sworn off travel; as the 1960s progressed, he became increasingly involved in Stanford's intellectual life and academic politics at the expense of extramural activities.[82] Consequently, Lederberg's interactions with Stanford's growing community of computer scientists drew him first toward regarding computers as a means to overcome the challenges of studying Martian life and then toward the realization that they were tools to advance biology and medicine in general.

Ledley's article may have prompted Lederberg to begin using computers, but it was not a bolt from the blue in terms of his intellectual development. Programmable, digital computers were a natural fit to his broader ambitions as well as to the general thrust of his career. Since early childhood, Lederberg noted, he "had fantasies that echo Leibniz' dream of a 'universal calculus' for the 'alphabet of human thought,' that all of knowledge might be so systematized that every fact could be tagged with a code."[83] As an undergraduate at Columbia University, he had broken from the traditional biology curriculum and enrolled in several philosophy courses in logic and the scientific method because he was "eager to have some understanding of the epistemological roots of science." The philosophers at Columbia encouraged him to read the work of George Boole, Bertrand Russell and A. N. Whitehead, as well as J. H. Woodger's *Axiomatic Method in Biology*, an attempt to unify via mathematics all that was known of genetics and development. Lederberg did not employ electronic computers in the course of his Nobel-winning work on bacterial conjugation with Beadle and Tatum or his 1951 transduction experiments, but he had by the mid-1950s become interested in "information theoretic formulations of genetics" and was sufficiently versed in theories pertaining to automata that artificial intelligence pioneer Marvin Minsky visited Wisconsin to consult him in 1955.[84]

The exobiology work itself also provided a spur for Lederberg to computerize his research. At the NASA-funded Instrumentation Research Lab (IRL), which Lederberg established in 1960 to pursue exobiology, his primary mission was to design the Automated Biology Laboratory, a twenty-five-ton, fully automated laboratory that was to be flown to Mars in future decades for the purpose of studying life there.[85] However, when he and his fellow exobiologists attempted to build instruments to manage the "immense amount of information . . . still locked up in spectra" of their extraterrestrial subjects, they ran into a major obstacle. He explained, "As any experienced hand would have predicted, many of the 'bright ideas' we have developed, either as requirements for instruments, or as their designs, have bogged down when the construction and debugging of the devices took months instead of weeks."[86] As a result, Lederberg's group was so exhausted from building the instruments that they had lost sight of the purpose of their devices' design. Ironically, these instruments, instead of making a project feasible to pursue, had brought about "hypercaution when deciding to go ahead [with] a given project."[87]

Lederberg's solution to the challenges posed by building instruments was to try to acquire one of the dozen LINCs the NIH initially offered to researchers in 1963. As Lederberg saw it, the little LINC, with its unrivaled A-D conversion capabilities and its low operating costs, could be inexpensively programmed to emulate many of the instruments the IRL was struggling to build. In "An Instrumentation Crisis in Biology," Lederberg's successful petition to acquire a LINC for the IRL, he cast the LINC as the remedy to "the inadequacy of current art in biomedical instrumentation [that] was brought home to us in our efforts to meet the mission requirements of exobiological studies."[88] This crisis within the exobiology community, Lederberg insisted to the NIH, was replicated in more traditional areas of biology as well, and its resolution was, he claimed, "equally pertinent to present efforts in the terrestrial biochemical and microbiological laboratory."[89] The crisis was exacerbated by what he felt were counterproductive practices among biomedical researchers and their sponsors. First, he decried a "lack of flexibility" concerning considerations pertaining to the use of instruments. Namely, he found that he was unable to convince his colleagues and patrons to set aside significant time and resources to improve or develop new instruments. Worse, he found a "practical attitude of disdain for preoccupation with instrumentation displayed by most members of the biochemical scientific fraternity."[90] For instance, he observed that biochemists looked down on those who concerned themselves deeply with "mere instruments, tools."[91]

To overcome this crisis, Lederberg believed that all biologists needed access to a new sort of instrument, one that would allow them to pursue their research without becoming overly distracted by the vicissitudes of building and using equipment. The solution, he argued, came in the form of digital computers, which he believed would give life scientists "increased leverage in the solution of complex problems."[92] Like Wesley Clark, LINC's architect (see chapter 3), Lederberg regarded difficulties related to data acquisition and analog-to-digital conversion as the main barriers to biologists making good use of digital computers. Consequently, the LINC very much fit Lederberg's call for a computer that would enable "the investigator to deal directly with the large data file in real time, while his attention is still concentrated on the problem at hand and in the formulation of new hypotheses for prompt testing."[93] With Sterling and Terman's support, Lederberg would take more substantial further steps; first, by using computers in the course of analyzing the molecules of possible extraterrestrial organisms, and then by attempting to computerize all of Stanford biomedical research.

In the early 1960s, as his involvement in computing deepened, Lederberg was also mulling his precocious success as an experimentalist. "My own laboratory research," he wrote, "was a very mixed bag of theoretical formation and empirical encounter. I had been extraordinarily lucky on several occasions—but I didn't want to be a hostage to chance." Why, Lederberg wondered, had not genetic recombination in bacteria been examined forty years earlier? Lederberg had no answer, but his inquiry did raise "serious questions about the rational direction of science."[94] One such question he asked himself was: "Should there not be a more systematic strategy of problem formation? And if one could do that, problem-solving might be a throwaway."[95] Before he could pursue experimental biology's shortcomings, though, the Space Race heated up, and he became preoccupied with his exobiology projects. Nevertheless, Lederberg retained the desire for a more rational, ordered approach to biology throughout his early Stanford years.

A New Kind of Artificial Intelligence for Biomedical Research

Lederberg began working with computers in earnest in 1961, when he and library information science pioneer Eugene Garfield developed a computerized citation index for articles pertaining to genetics.[96] The next summer, Lederberg learned BALGOL (Burroughs Algol) by enrolling in one of the first programming courses offered on Stanford's campus. Thenceforth, Lederberg explains, "I quickly succumbed to the hacker syndrome . . . this was reinforced by the relentless rectitude of the machine in rejecting my errors—always so obvious in retrospect." By "hacking" Lederberg meant writing programs and configuring hardware for the purpose of exploring the capabilities of a computer system rather than any scientific end. During one of his hacking sessions on Stanford's Burroughs 220 (one of the last vacuum-tube computers), Lederberg met John McCarthy, then freshly recruited by Forsythe from MIT, who introduced him to the "possibility of engaging in Artificial Intelligence research" and to the new real-time interactive mode of computing embodied by the DEC PDP-1, which dispatched with punch card stacks and tiny blinking lights in favor of keyboards and CRT displays. Mainly, they played the game Spacewar and pontificated about the possibilities of interactive computing, but Lederberg had seen enough to become convinced that "computers were going to change the whole style of scientific investigation."[97]

Having seen the potential of the PDP-1, and soon afterward the LINC he acquired from the NIH, Lederberg sought ways to incorporate interactive computers into his exobiology research, with the specific hope they could help him overcome a data-management crisis that had arisen during his attempts to adapt mass spectrometry to the study of alien organic compounds. When he was not wrestling with the Burroughs 220, Lederberg collaborated with Stanford chemist Carl Djerassi (b. 1923) to develop a way to efficiently translate mass numbers to molecular formulas. If anyone could help Lederberg do this, it was Djerassi. Nicknamed "El Supremo" by colleagues and graduate students who admired his mastery of methods of determining organic molecular structure from raw mass spectrometry data, Djerassi had written the bible of mass spectrometry, and he was best known for synthesizing the first oral contraceptive for women in 1951.[98]

The specific issue confronting Lederberg and Djerassi was that mass spectrometers produce data that is ambiguous. A brief overview of mass spectrometry should suffice to illustrate the challenge Lederberg and Djerassi faced. A mass spectrometer is an instrument that breaks down molecules of a sample material into ions that are accelerated and measured one by one. Setting aside the possibility of further fragmentation and the fact that atoms' mass numbers do not precisely match their atomic masses, the ions can be added up to provide researchers with the total atomic/molecular mass (m) of the sample. The exact composition of that sample, however, must be determined using the mass numbers of atoms (for, say, hydrogen, m = 1; carbon, m = 12; nitrogen, m = 14; oxygen, m = 16) and valence rules (hydrogen can only bond once, oxygen twice, nitrogen three times, carbon four, and so on). For instance, a substance with m = 18 is almost certainly water, because H + O + H is the only stable configuration that satisfies all of the above mass and valence rules. For molecules where m < 500, a chemist could consult published tables (~570 pages of print) that sorted by mass and valence considerations all possible combinations of atoms.[99] But for the complex organic substances (m > 3000) that interested Lederberg, no such tables existed, which meant that a great deal of trial-and-error computation was required to determine their composition. With the help of an expert chemist such as Djerassi, Lederberg could apply a large set of rules of thumb generated by contextual information (that, say, there are constraints on the number of single-valence H atoms given the mass of the molecule; or that molecules demonstrated to be hydrophobic or hydrophilic have characteristic structures) in order to "prune the tree of possibilities."[100]

Even when Lederberg had determined the exact molecular makeup of a substance, he still needed to take into account the fact that mass spectrometry yields no information about the topological connectivity of the constituent atoms, or isomerism. The medically important example of isomerism Lederberg liked to give to computer scientists was that of C_2H_6O (m = 46), which has two very common configurations: CH_3CH_2OH (ethanol) and CH_3OCH_3 (dimethyl ether).

Here again, the knowledge of an expert like Djerassi came to the rescue. Typically, chemists try to distinguish one isomer from another by searching for the presence of radicals (for example, ethanol's -OH), which can be detected by mixing the sample material with a substance that reacts to the presence of radicals. In the case of dimethyl-ether and ethanol, the substances also have different smells. Unfortunately for Lederberg, shipping chemists' noses or tubes of reagents to Mars was out of the question; therefore, he could rely only on obtaining mass spectrometry data. Distinguishing isomers using only this data was, in the early 1960s, not a practice governed by written rules or even understood rules. "It is remarkable," Lederberg noted, "that while hundreds of thousands of students of elementary organic chemistry are challenged in this way every year, no algorithm for generating and verifying complete lists of isomers has hitherto been presented. Each student is left to work out his own intuitive approach to this problem, which may account for the bafflement with which very many students approach this subject upon their first exposure to it."[101] Nevertheless, Djerassi had found that the molecular ions produced by mass spectrometers sometimes left characteristic "fingerprints" from which he could infer the configuration of atoms that comprised the molecule. Furthermore, as in the case of determining the molecule's composition, Djerassi drew from a vast body of rules of thumb to narrow down the possible choices he would make. It was this procedure that Lederberg wanted to model and automate.

The first concrete step Lederberg took toward creating an automatic machine that could replicate Carl Djerassi's work was to figure out how to represent organic molecular structures in a form that could be efficiently processed by a computer. To that end, he sought the guidance of George Pólya, then nine years into his thirty-two-year career as an emeritus professor at Stanford. It was through this consultation that Lederberg came to understand both the immensity of his task and that a heuristic approach could be effectively employed to formulate workarounds for more difficult problems.[102] Beyond the challenge of determining a molecule's structure using only mass spectrometry information, there was the issue of organic chemistry not having a mathematically consistent system for representing molecules. For a century (since Berzelius), chemical structure had been represented by an undirected graph whose nodes are atoms and whose edges are chemical bonds.

In the 1930s, Pólya undertook a systematic inquiry of these representations and toyed with the idea of applying his enumeration theory and his knowledge of combinatorics to problems of chemical topology. As Lederberg tells it, chemistry problems were regarded by mathematicians as superficial and set aside, while chemists lacked the mathematical training to see what combinatorics offered their field. "Partly in consequence," Lederberg argued, "the taxonomy, i.e., nomenclature, notation, homology, of the field lags behind its substance, which impedes communication, whether this be information retrieval or professional education. Hence the mystification often provoked by the proper name of a new drug."[103]

Lederberg devoted much of 1963 and 1964 to trying to map organic structures onto standardized geometric forms in order to simplify and rationalize their description. For instance, he found that he could represent pyrene ($C_{16}H_{10}$) as a prism, which could easily be described to a computer (fig. 5.1).

Chemists do not appear to have rushed to adopt Lederberg's proposed system, but his mappings of chemical graphs onto geometric forms laid the foundation of his efforts to design algorithms that could efficiently express the

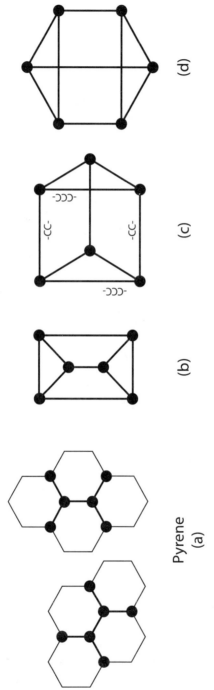

Pyrene
(a)

(b)

(c)

(d)

Fig. 5.1. Pyrene becomes a prism. Lederberg explains the transformation: "For topological analysis of a ring the linear paths and vertices connecting them are first identified. The vertices are simply the branch of points, that is, the atoms with three or more links to the rest of the ensemble. For these purposes, a double or triple bond is a single link. The paths are then the intervals between the vertices. A path may be a simple link or linear string of tandemly linked atoms. For example, marking the paths of pyrene (a) gives the diagram (b), which is readily recognized as isomorphic to the prism (c) and its formal graph (d)." Joshua Lederberg, "Topological Mapping of Organic Molecules," *Proceedings of the National Academy of Sciences* 53 (1965), 136–37

structure of organic molecules.[104] Lederberg first attempted to write a computer program capable of simulating Djerassi's induction of molecular structure from mass spectrometry data in early 1964, but he quickly found that despite having mastered BALGOL programming, his skills were not up to the task.[105] He needed somebody who knew computers, programming languages, and heuristics well enough to coax a machine into actually inducing the way Djerassi could. That someone was Edward Feigenbaum.

Edward A. Feigenbaum (b. 1936) "had never heard of mass spectrometry in [his] life" when he met Joshua Lederberg. Nevertheless, when the conversation turned to the simulation of inductive processes, the two men "vibrated sympathetically" and realized with delight how much they had to offer each other. Feigenbaum usually protests when chroniclers describe his initial encounter with Lederberg as serendipitous, and he portrays their meeting as the inevitable convergence of two complementary bodies of knowledge. Indeed, an examination of Feigenbaum's path to Stanford, reveals that despite the vast gulf between their fields (computer science and biology), the two researchers drew heavily from the same ways of thinking about how scientific problems should be constructed and solved. Yet chance also did indeed factor heavily into Feigenbaum's decision to dedicate much of his career to developing a new computer technology called an expert system.

Like Lederberg, Feigenbaum showed an early interest in both science and epistemology. A precocious student, Feigenbaum, dreamed of conducting important scientific research at an Ivy League university, but a misinformed high school guidance counselor and parents who wanted him to pursue a "practical" career as an engineer conspired to send him to the Carnegie Technical Institute (now part of Carnegie Mellon University). Despite his parents' wishes, Feigenbaum gravitated toward courses that emphasized "theory and thinking" instead of those that would teach him the skills necessary to land a secure job. His first major influence at Carnegie was James March, a professor at the institute's School of Industrial Relations (specifically the Industrial Administration program). In a course called "Ideas and Social Change" March introduced Feigenbaum to von Neumann's work, and the young Feigenbaum was sufficiently taken by game theory that he started to pursue a career in studying human behavior from a mathematical perspective.[106]

Feigenbaum's interest in mathematical applications to psychology also led him to take the 1955 graduate seminar on mathematical models in social sciences offered by Carnegie professors Allen Newell and Herbert Simon. At the time Feigenbaum met them, Simon and Newell were developing a theory of human problem solving that would help them more accurately model the process of decision making; they had just reached the conclusion that computers could enable them to simulate human cognition when they offered the seminar. When the class convened in January 1955, Simon announced to the students: "Over Christmas vacation Allen Newell and I invented the thinking machine!" and handed each of them a manual for the IBM 701 (aka, the Defense Calculator), an early-1950s computer designed primarily to perform repetitive arithmetic operations for engineers developing jet engines for the military.[107] Although the class had no access to an actual computer, Feigenbaum was so stimulated by the manual that he stayed up all night to finish it and decided at the break of dawn that he wanted to master this new technology.

Immediately following his graduation from Carnegie, Feigenbaum interned at Columbia University's Watson lab, where he learned to operate the IBM 650 (the business-oriented version of the 701) and later the IBM 704, a mainframe designed for scientific use, especially for physicists performing calculations that required voluminous simple arithmetic operations. When he returned to Carnegie to pursue a graduate degree—in cognitive psychology—an IBM 650 was waiting for him when he arrived, and he became involved in most projects that utilized the machine because he was one of only a handful of people at the university who could program it. For a young, skilled computer programmer interested in simulating human thought, 1956 was a tremendously exciting year: that summer the Dartmouth Conference was held; and Noam Chomsky had just published his description of a computational approach to linguistics. When it came time to settle on a dissertation project, Feigenbaum chose to work with Simon on the problem of simulating verbal learning behavior.

The vast implications for psychology and artificial intelligence (that is, the study and design of intelligent agents) of Simon and Feigenbaum's project, the Elementary Perceiver and Memorizer (EPAM), lie beyond the scope of this book, but the approach to problem-solving that Feigenbaum developed under Simon's tutelage merits discussion here because it would shape how the young man would come to see both scientific research and AI. Early in the project, Simon imbued Feigenbaum with two notions: AI is an experimental—as opposed to theoretical—science; and science, despite vigorous assertions to the contrary by its practitioners, is by and large an exercise in inductive reasoning.[108] Simon also encouraged Feigenbaum not to dismiss incomplete but useful solutions to complex problems, and turned him on to Pólya for further grounding in heuristics. Feigenbaum later explained to Pamela McCorduck how his unconventional training shaped his research priorities: "I began to get interested in a set of problems that it seemed to me hadn't been well explored by earlier AI work, namely tasks of empirical induction—given a set of data elements, construct the hypothesis that purports to explain that set of data. And I viewed empirical induction as being prototypic of scientific behavior."[109]

Upon receiving his doctorate in 1960, Feigenbaum applied for a position at Stanford's Psychology Department, and despite Simon's efforts on his behalf, he was promptly rejected. Consequently, he backed away from pure psychological research and wound up at the UC Berkeley School of Business, where he intended to develop computer models of decision making that would be useful to economists and businessmen. He also moonlighted as a consultant for the Research and Development (RAND) Corporation. Besides the rejection from Stanford, Feigenbaum had another reason for avoiding psychology: he believed that Simon and Newell had exhausted all of the interesting ideas in the field, and he wanted to make his name elsewhere. Moreover, by time he settled in Berkeley, Feigenbaum had begun to drift away from EPAM, mainly because his ideas were coolly received by psychologists.

What Feigenbaum really wanted to do was to "work on empirical induction in science, within the methodology that [he] had learned from Newell and Simon, i.e. work on a concrete task domain, not in the abstract."[110] What he lacked, however, was a concrete task domain. During his early years in California, Feigenbaum considered modeling baseball as a possible domain; in a nutshell, he wanted to create a system that could induce a model of the rules of baseball from the flow of events in the game. Feigenbaum never got around to modeling baseball, namely because he was preoccupied by his work for RAND, which involved extensive traveling, but also because he was generally unenthusiastic about baseball as a problem domain. He wanted to create a model that would help scientists just as much as computer scientists.

Feigenbaum's professional break with psychology and EPAM came when John McCarthy recruited him to Stanford for a joint position as a professor in the university's Computer Science Program (within the Mathematics Department, but soon an entity unto itself) and the administrator of the university's new Computing Center.[111] In early 1964, he was also tapped to serve on the NIH's CRSS, whose energy and vision he described as "comparable to Wiener's cybernetics group at MIT." For Feigenbaum, participating in the CRSS was "like getting another Ph.D." At the NIH the task at hand was how best to harness computers for the advancement of medicine, and Feigenbaum was in a position that allowed him to survey how biomedical researchers intended to do this. The experience, while edifying, left him with the impression that biologists did not understand the potential of the machines they wanted to bring into their laboratories. Primarily, from his perspective, they wanted to use computers to crunch numbers, not assist them in the more creative aspects of research, such as theory formation and the selection of which problems to examine.[112]

Back at Stanford, Feigenbaum had by April 1965 become a regular at neurologist-psychologist Karl Pribram's Saturday morning seminars on "Mind and Machines." Joshua Lederberg was also a devoted attendee, and his familiarity with both biological problems and computers caught Feigenbaum's attention. Once they got talking, it transpired that Lederberg's attempt to automate the induction of molecular topology from mass spectrometric data was just the kind of domain Feigenbaum had been trying to find for years. On their meeting, Feigenbaum remarked, "I needed a domain, a sandbox; and Lederberg provided it."[113] He recalled, "We were not in conversation more than ten minutes before we were in complete agreement about the interest in the problem and the reasonableness of the approach."[114] Further attracting Feigenbaum to Lederberg's project was its potential as an AI venture that was unhindered by the fixation among many AI workers on replicating either all aspects of a human thought process or none at all: "[Lederberg] had no intention whatsoever of building a psychologically valid model of a chemist, because we would have had to include all the wrong things they do. We wanted to do better."[115]

Once Lederberg and Feigenbaum had been introduced, the luxury afforded by their circumstances allowed the two men to begin collaborating immediately. Procuring equipment, for instance, was never much of a challenge because Feigenbaum ran Stanford's Computing Center; and because neither man had any major research projects competing for their time, they did little besides develop their new computer system.[116] Moreover, they could take advantage of the early time-sharing systems McCarthy had developed for Stanford starting in 1962; these shared resources enabled them to program from their offices and debug the program almost whenever they desired, which was quite often.[117]

After spending a week or so being brought up to speed on mass spectrometry by Lederberg, Feigenbaum began the process of coding. His first move was to translate the primitive algorithm Lederberg had written in BALGOL into Lisp, a much more difficult but also more versatile programming language that McCarthy had just designed. He also had the advantage of not having to "unlearn" much chemistry in order to think in terms of Lederberg's geometric approach to describing molecular topology. Finally, the combination of Feigenbaum's connections to RAND, ARPA, and the NIH, and Lederberg's to NASA ensured that generous funding was plentiful.[118] By the end of April 1965, DENDRAL was becoming a reality.

Lederberg and Feigenbaum planned to begin with relatively simple amino acids and work their way up toward complex organic molecules. In modern computer science parlance, they developed what is a called a *legal move generator* in that they had a set of about two dozen valence rules for determining the structure of amino acids using only mass spectrometry data, and an algorithm that was capable of generating a large number (hundreds or thousands) of topologically legal structure candidates using these rules. Once a set of candidate structures had been proposed, the program drew from a set of rules of thumb, called a *knowledge base*, to eliminate all candidates that were not "chemically plausible," usually leaving under ten possible structures, which a researcher could print out and study further.[119] As one of Lederberg and Feigenbaum's later collaborators crisply put it, "In the knowledge base lies the power!"[120]

Likening the process of generating candidate structures to the growth of branches of a tree, and the process of eliminating those structures to pruning most of those branches, they called their system the Dendritic Algorithm, or DENDRAL.[121] Though DENDRAL was capable of matching some amino acids to their spectra, it was "incompetent" when it came to the spectra of ketones or alcohols because it "knew almost nothing about the mass spectrometry of these families."[122] To teach DENDRAL how to induce the structure of ketones and alcohols from spectra, Lederberg and Feigenbaum reenlisted Carl Djerassi, and hoped that he would endure the long process of trying to figure out how to translate his knowledge into lines of Lisp code.

Djerassi was initially hesitant, but once he saw that his input enabled DENDRAL to evolve from a program that could not distinguish a ketone from an inert gas to one that could induce the structure of ketones from mass spectrometry data about as well as he could, he became hooked. Gratified by the experience of seeing DENDRAL improve in its ability to apply his techniques to mass spectrometric problems, Djerassi immersed himself in the project and organized a "carefully orchestrated sequence of organic chemical families" for DENDRAL to attack: ethers, thioethers, then amines. Within months, Djerassi had taught DENDRAL most of the tricks in his bible of mass spectrometry.[123] With these rules in its knowledge base, DENDRAL could automatically eliminate most "chemically implausible" structures, usually producing a hand-ful of possible structures that could then be tested for validity by non-experts. If DENDRAL was consistently incorrect about the plausibility of a structure candidate, this could be remedied by entering into the knowledge base a new criterion for removing a candidate.

In late July 1965, just as the DENDRAL project was beginning to make tangible progress toward meeting Lederberg's original goals, the team received devastating news: NASA's Mariner 4 spacecraft had flown by Mars and found that the planet was barren and appeared to have been that way for eons. If Mars could sustain life, there was no sign of it on the surface. Though Lederberg had not been expecting to find Mars teeming with advanced organisms, he neverthe-less disappointed by the finding that Mars seemed to resemble the sterile Moon more than the Earth. In the face of this setback, however, he gave up neither his ambitions for performing comparative biochemistry nor the DENDRAL project, whose implications were spreading far beyond exobiology.[124]

Despite having no apparent Martian organic compounds to study and no ride to Mars, the DENDRAL project persisted, albeit with much more emphasis on advancing AI research and the experimental practice of biochemists than on solving potential problems of exobiology. With the focus shifted to AI, though, a problem that had been plaguing the DENDRAL project all along quickly became acute. Even from the project's outset, it was clear to Lederberg that the equipment on which DENDRAL was running, first an IBM 7090 modi-fied for time-sharing then a PDP 6, would not—even if somehow pooled into a single shared system—suffice to test and retest DENDRAL as it attempted to determine the structure of the compounds it was examining. In a 1964 plea to NASA for more funding, Lederberg and McCarthy had already noted that the $450,000 the IRL and the Artificial Intelligence Group of the Computer Sci-ence Division could jointly hope to expect from NASA was far too little to get them the system the IRL needed. To pursue the mission and other functions of the Mars-bound automated laboratory, they predicted they would need a "large system," including two processors, 256K of memory, and a time-sharing system with multiple displays. The price tag for the system they needed was about $3.5 million.[125] NASA support for this large computer did not materialize, leaving the NIH as the only federal agency able and willing to spend that kind of money on a computer for biologists.

ACME: The Computer atop the Peak of Excellence

Earlier in 1965—even before Mariner 4 flew past Mars—Terman and School of Medicine Dean Robert Alway had noticed Lederberg's interest in computers and his success in competing for one of the NIH's LINCs. Consequently, they selected him to lead the School of Medicine's newly formed Computer Policy Committee (CPC). Now that Mars seemed barren and his exobiology was so much less feasible for the time being, Lederberg threw himself into CPC work. Motivated to find a permanent home for the DENDRAL project and to build a community of computer-using life scientists at Stanford, Lederberg undertook an effort to acquire a state-of-the-art computer for the Stanford Medical Center.

Using Forsythe's project as an example, Lederberg set to work crafting a grant proposal that would appeal to both the NIH and Stanford's administration.[126] In several ways, Lederberg's goals for Stanford biomedical computing echoed those of Forsythe. Both men saw computers as the means to unify and fundamentally improve the study of life, and both promoted the interdisciplinary cooperation and engagement of federal patronage bodies that were the core of the Sterling-Terman vision. Unlike Forsythe, however, Lederberg explicitly cast biomedical computing as a catalyst of Sterling and Terman's most ambitious plans for the newly restructured medical school. Keeping with the Sterling-Terman vision, the committee's ostensible mission was to use computer technology to further Stanford's "conscientious self-dedication to far-reaching communion of medical research and education with university life, based on the principle of mutual interdependence of medicine with the physical sciences and with human affairs." Moreover, as the CPC put it, "in future outlook, computers will be central to communication within the University, and this motive alone reinforces a policy of the feasible convergence with the central facility for the University, serviced by the Stanford Computing Center."[127]

The CPC's first mission was to determine what hardware would be needed to enable the computational fusion of the various branches within the medical center, and then of the medical center with the broader university research community. They decided very quickly that they would need access to processing power several orders of magnitude greater than what Forsythe and Killam had requested from the NIH. What they wanted was for the medical center to purchase its very own IBM 360—then still in development—akin to the one that the university planned to install as the Computing Center's primary mainframe. Although numerous life scientists used mainframes in the course of their work,

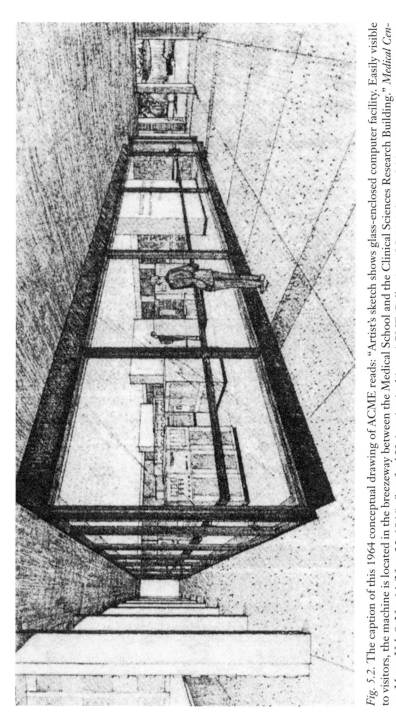

Fig. 5.2. The caption of this 1964 conceptual drawing of ACME reads: "Artist's sketch shows glass-enclosed computer facility. Easily visible to visitors, the machine is located in the breezeway between the Medical School and the Clinical Sciences Research Building." *Medical Center Memo,* Vol. 8, No. 14 (Nov. 25, 1966). Stanford University Archives, ACME Collection (SC 236), box 1, folder 16

nothing remotely as large or expensive had ever been requested for the *exclusive* use by biomedical researchers.

There was in 1965 much excitement that the IBM 360 was qualitatively different from other large computer systems. Even by 1960s standards, the development of the System/360 was a gigantic project. *Fortune* magazine famously called the 360 "IBM's $5 billion gamble"—the only larger contemporary endeavor in technology development was the Apollo Program. The aim of the 360 was to unify IBM's diverse and diverging product line. Henceforth, all IBM computers would be built on the same architecture and would use the same command set. It was left to the users to decide how powerful (and therefore expensive) their computers would be. IBM's plan was for the 360 to become the standard computer of the corporate and scientific worlds, the difference between business and research use coming down to a matter of configuration. IBM also sought to build on its dominance in the realm of biomedical research, and was looking for a way to establish the 360 there.[128]

Over the next year, Lederberg's committee would convince Terman's administration that such a machine would bring to fruition their vision of a research-oriented medical school integrated with the rest of the university. The project's name, ACME (Advanced Computer for Medical Research), played on Terman's appeals to "build what [he] used to call 'spikes of excellence, peaks of excellence.'"[129] Beyond serving as a computing resource, ACME would, according to Lederberg, be the centerpiece of the entire Stanford Medical Center. His plans called for it to be highly visible, centrally located, and otherwise an integral part of daily biomedical activities, be they research-related, care-oriented, or administrative. One conceptual drawing put ACME in the breezeway between the SMC's teaching building and its research building, so that even visitors would instantly recognize the 360's importance to the institution (fig. 5.2).

With the School of Medicine requesting an IBM 360, the question emerged as to why its faculty did not simply do what many other biomedical researchers around the country did, and make use of existing facilities, such as the 360 planned for the Stanford Computation Center (SCC). The committee acknowledged that the SMC's having its own 360 would lead to redundancies but stressed that the SCC computer would not meet their needs: "Medical research does have special requirements and challenges, and there is bound to be a significant gap, at least in time, between the level of service that the SCC can offer the University as a whole and the technical possibilities of the art."[130] They further argued that because the SCC would be preoccupied with addressing campus-wide concerns, it would be unwilling or unable to meet biomedical researchers' rather time-consuming needs. Particularly galling was SCC's refusal to offer real-time analog-to-digital conversion service, despite high demand on the part of biomedical researchers. Only unfettered access to a machine as powerful as the 360 would overcome "the unwillingness or inability of SCC to offer complete problem-solving services" and meet the researchers' demand, which Lederberg argued would only increase if the School of Medicine were to fulfill Sterling and Terman's vision of it conducting pioneering research.[131]

The committee also desired a 360 on the grounds that if all medical school research were conducted on one giant machine, they would not again face the issues of hardware and software incompatibility that were then hampering their work. At the time they proposed the 360 to the administration, SMC workers were using four LINCs and a PDP-8 in their laboratories as well as the SCC's IBM 7090/1401 combination and a Burroughs 5500. On the 7090, they programmed in SUBALGOL, LISP, and FORTRAN, while the Burroughs machine generally used BALGOL; none of these languages was easily translated to or from routines written for the LINCs or PDPs. Sending data from one machine to another also proved difficult. When, for instance, Lederberg decided he wanted to use the IBM 7090's superior processor to analyze mass spectrometry data in real time that he could only collect using the LINC's A-D conversion apparatus (and interface), it took more than two frustrating years to successfully establish a wire connection between the two machines.[132] As Lederberg put it: "From a user's standpoint the utter incompatibility of languages on the two computers appears like a calculated source of frustration."[133]

Yet another advantage of the 360 would be its potential to eliminate the need for the special-purpose analog equipment computers that could be found all around the SMC.[134] Such machines were relatively inexpensive compared to general-purpose digital computers, but they were generally not programmable and little of the knowledge acquired in mastering one analog computer could be applied anywhere else. Consequently, advances in analog hardware came very slowly, which irked those who reasoned that the vast majority of the tasks performed by such machines could also be carried out by digital programmable computers. Access to a 360, according to Lederberg, thus presented, "in some measure the possibility of leapfrogging over a good deal of analogue hardware that should have been developed, but has not been."[135]

Institutionally, Lederberg asserted that the 360 would catalyze both Terman's vision of a medical school integrated with Stanford's research community and the NIH's call for the broadest possible promotion of computer technology in the life sciences. His plan was for Stanford to treat the Computer Policy Committee as an "ad hoc department of medical research computation" in line with the university's "well-established tradition of flexible, ad hoc Ph.D. programs in interdisciplinary studies."[136] The committee, which was comprised of representatives of life sciences departments around campus, would render itself accessible to any biologist or physician who wanted to pursue research-related computing. Furthermore, it would help the university offer interdisciplinary courses that depended on access to computers, such as statistics for epidemiology or inductive logic and linguistics in health science. Finally, all initial NIH funds for ACME would be spent exclusively on introducing new users to computing: "experienced users will be expected to arrange to finance these charges from their project grants."[137]

A model of the way a project would be organized once the School of Medicine had its 360 could, according to Lederberg, be found in the exobiology work being conducted at his own lab, the IRL. Endeavors like DENDRAL, he wrote, "demand the capability to program and reprogram an experiment in biochemistry or microbiology," which required the expertise of computer scientists, life scientists, and engineers. Already, the lab had forged "especially close relationships with [Computer Science] Professors McCarthy and Feigenbaum." Shifting the emphasis away from inquiries into Martian life, Lederberg cast the IRL work as having applications in automation of many kinds of life sciences laboratories, especially in terms of integrating laboratory instruments (such as spectrometers) with computers. He pointed out that since the IRL's work was a boon to medical researchers, the lab was able to supplement its NASA funding with grants and equipment (for example, the LINC) from the NIH.[138] The implication here was that having a 360 would enable projects that would attract funding from multiple agencies even if the projects themselves were highly esoteric.

In short order, the NIH approved Lederberg's proposal. After several site visits by CRSS members in 1965, the DRFR's Special Resources Branch, then led by Bruce Waxman, agreed to provide enough funding to purchase, maintain, and operate for several years an IBM 360.[139] Though the NIH had been stung by failure of biocomputing centers to live up to expectations (such as at UCLA) or to take root at all (such as at MIT), Lederberg's project was different in that it had the staunch support of Stanford's administration. Moreover, Lederberg's status as a very young Nobel Prize laureate bestowed a degree of prestige to the project that similar large-scale computing endeavors at other institutions lacked. Finally, IBM was more enthusiastic about ACME than about previous attempts to use its large digital computers in biology and medicine, mainly because it saw in ACME's success the means to create a lucrative market for its new 360 line. Indeed, well before ACME was ever turned on, IBM made big promises about how the system could help its users. In a special issue of its *Scientific Marketing Newsletter* dedicated to biomedical computing, IBM stressed that the 360's true benefit was not found in what could be accomplished using it but what could be accomplished in the time saved by using it. "Even more important than what a computer can do directly is what it can do for the scientist indirectly," IBM claimed. "It can give him more time to plan, think, reason, conclude, present, devise, propose, and hypothesize, while at the same time accelerating his research by from 50% to 600%. The computer can measurably aid science and the scientist in achieving the primary goal: new knowledge, hopefully for the good of mankind."[140]

As the groundwork was being laid for ACME, DENDRAL's mission also changed, taking Lederberg into the world of AI research. In the first months following the Mariner 4 flyby, the DENDRAL team began to recruit postdoctoral fellows for the tasks of refining Feigenbaum's original Lisp code and helping Djerassi build up the system's knowledge base. Among the new postdocs was Bruce G. Buchanan, who came to the project with ambitious plans of his own, and who was largely responsible for implementing DENDRAL's forays into realms that had long been the exclusive domain of philosophers of science.

Like Lederberg and Feigenbaum, Buchanan was from an early age both highly mathematical and inquisitive about issues of epistemology. Unlike his senior collaborators, however, Buchanan supplemented his computer skills with formal, graduate-level training as a philosopher. His 1966 Michigan State University doctoral dissertation, *Logics of Scientific Discovery*, was among the first to formally consider the implications of the impact of computer technology on experimental practice. Buchanan's special interest was hypothesis formation, because he believed that act to be the heart of discovery. Moreover, he believed that even this most creative aspect of science could be automated, if only its exact mechanisms were better understood.[141]

Buchanan was brought into DENDRAL by happenstance: Feigenbaum had heard about his dissertation through a colleague at RAND, where Buchanan held occasional programming jobs, and then pitched the project to him. When Feigenbaum explained to Buchanan the aims of DENDRAL, Buchanan "dropped everything, including defending his dissertation and looking for a real job, so he could join the project."[142] Looking back on his snap decision to move to Stanford, Buchanan recalls that DENDRAL's potential to address questions raised by philosophy of science was immediately apparent: "DENDRAL in many areas went well beyond what philosophy of science had to say because it [DENDRAL] had to get specific about discovery processes, whereas most of philosophy of science deals with verifications processes."[143] Donald Michie, the Bletchley Park cryptographer and AI pioneer, saw this potential too in DENDRAL, and upon reading about the project for the first time, exclaimed: "It's Bacon come alive! It's an instance of a living piece of the scientific method that you can study in detail."[144]

Buchanan's ambitions may have found fertile ground in DENDRAL, but a system that generated and pruned candidate trees of possible structures based on mass spectrometry data was a far cry from the automatic hypothesis former Buchanan wanted to create and study. Buchanan was not so much interested in a system that could hypothesize the structure of a molecule by choosing from a library—that is, the system's knowledge base—of known structures as he was in a system that could hypothesize a *novel* structure by applying its knowledge base to the mass spectrometry data.[145] As suggested, he wanted the system to make discoveries on its own, not just help humans make them.

When Buchanan presented this plan to Feigenbaum and Lederberg, they were both enthusiastic but also somewhat skeptical as to whether he could pull it off because he "had no deep knowledge of chemistry." Enthusiasm carried the day, because for Buchanan, Feigenbaum, and Lederberg alike, the raison d'être of the DENDRAL project was not to solve a chemistry problem but rather to demystify the human process of discovery. After building DENDRAL, they had concluded, "We could consider discovery to be merely successful guessing" and saw as the next step "program[ming] a machine to perform random genera-tion of hypotheses—perhaps restrained within the correct subject area." Their proposed machine "could test each random hypothesis against the criteria of success and stop when a hypothesis met the criteria of reasonableness."[146] This follow-on project they called "Meta-DENDRAL," and they saw its potential success as an automatic hypothesis maker as tantamount to the disproof of "the widely held view that there is no method underlying the creation of new terms in the language of science." The particular position they hoped to attack by build-ing Meta-DENDRAL was articulated by philosophers like Jacob Bronowski, who argued, "We do not know; and there is no logical way in which we can know. . . . The step by which a new axiom is added cannot itself be mechanized. It is a free play of the mind, an invention outside the logical process."[147]

Finally, having dispensed with the unquantifiable human element, or at least having replicated it through Meta-DENDRAL's guesswork, the DENDRAL team called for the recognition that the heuristic method formed the basis of the scientific method. As they put it, "The problem of giving rules for producing true scientific statements has been replaced by the problem of finding efficient heuristic rules for culling the reasonable candidates for an explanation from an appropriate set of possible candidates."[148] Should the above statement hold true, there seemed to be absolutely no reason computers could not participate directly in the process of discovery.

Thus, work began on Meta-DENDRAL, which was designed to induce new rules of thumb, which could, in turn, be added to DENDRAL's repertoire. Meta-DENDRAL worked as follows: DENDRAL would attempt to induce the structure of an unknown molecule, then Meta-DENDRAL would "accept known mass spectrum / structure pairs as input and attempt to infer the specific knowledge of mass spectrometry that can be used by DENDRAL to explain new spectra."[149] In other words, Meta-DENDRAL would come up with new rules of thumb and DENDRAL would test their applicability.

Buchanan had a beautiful plan but found it impossible to implement, mainly because he did not know enough chemistry. First, he tried creating the program without learning chemistry, focusing exclusively on simulating how mass spectrometers produce output. He remembered, "I spent a lot of spare time in those days, without ever telling Ed [Feigenbaum] or Josh [Lederberg], trying to axiomatize mass spectroscopy. I thought that surely I could find some small set of axioms from which to build a good mass spec simulation, but it was frankly a waste of time." Having reached a dead end, Buchanan "resigned" himself to learning Djerassi and Lederberg's chemical techniques. Buchanan "immersed himself in chemistry" during these years (1965–67), often "working at Djerassi's knee" in order to give himself the grounding he needed to bring his program to fruition.[150] A much simplified account of Buchanan's 1966 breakthrough follows.

With much input from Lederberg, Feigenbaum, and Djerassi, Buchanan wrote a Lisp algorithm that would look for patterns in the raw mass spectrometry data and suggest to DENDRAL a rule of thumb. For instance, it may find a positive correlation between the molecular mass of an organic compound and the relative amount of carbon in the molecule; and even though this was not a rule known to or accepted by chemists, DENDRAL would then be instructed to discard all non-carbon-rich structures when it set about eliminating candidate structures. Usually the rules of thumb Meta-DENDRAL proposed were already known to scientists, but occasionally it would produce new rules that seemed valid, or at least ones that appeared useful. The DENDRAL team published their findings in a long series of articles in the *Journal of the American Chemical Society* called "Applications of Artificial Intelligence for Chemical Inference," which ran from the late 1960s to the late 1970s, in hopes that a chemist would understand the mechanism behind Meta-DENDRAL's proposed rule. Usually that mechanism was found, but by the mid-1970s, Meta-DENDRAL had generated several useful rules of thumb that could not be accounted for by any laws of chemistry known even to Carl Djerassi.

Meta-DENDRAL was but one of many projects making use of ACME. While Buchanan was developing algorithms for generating rules of thumb, dozens of other researchers and some physicians were using the same computer for their own purposes. Setting up ACME had not been easy, though. Securing support from Terman and funding from the NIH turned out to be by far the least challenging part of the ACME project. The IBM 360/50's installation was plagued with delays caused both by Stanford and IBM. The university fell months behind schedule in building the new computing facility at the medical center, which meant housing the machine in a huge, climate-controlled tent for its first year. IBM, meanwhile, had sold to Stanford several 360 components that turned out to be faulty, and it encountered difficulties in interfacing the 360 with laboratory equipment. Additionally, IBM raised the price by 25 percent (amounting to several hundred thousand dollars) halfway through the installation of what turned out to be defective equipment.[151] Lederberg scrambled for more funds, calling the project "the most vexatious" of his career.[152] Indeed, by the late 1960s he and other biologists had learned to leverage IBM by appealing to the NIH, which, as the main sponsor for biomedical computing projects, was effectively IBM's largest customer in this area.

By the beginning of 1966 ACME was operational. The first group to use the IBM 360 were the medical center's administrators. This transpired because most existing software on the IBM 360 had been developed for business administration and therefore it took the least effort to begin to use the machine for the medical center's administrative tasks. For the purposes of the biomedical researchers, however, the existing 360 software did not suffice, nor did its essentially batch-processing architecture. Thus, before Lederberg's vision of the 360 serving as the medical center's centerpiece could be realized, some major changes to the machine had to be made.

The task of transforming the IBM 360 into a machine capable of allowing dozens of researchers—such as Buchanan—to use it in real time fell to Gio Wiederhold (b. 1936). Born in Italy and educated in the Netherlands before coming to the United States, Wiederhold had been recruited from the aeronautics industry (and IBM) in 1965 by Forsythe to his new Computer Science Department. By this point, Wiederhold was established as an expert in writing compilers, which are programs that transform code written in a higher level programming language (in his case FORTRAN), into machine code instructions executed by a computer's central processing unit.[153] At Stanford, Wiederhold's initial interest had been working with McCarthy to implement a time-sharing system. When he heard about ACME, he saw that time-sharing was essential to meeting the researchers' needs, and proposed to develop a means of "real-time data-acquisition control and data analysis using coupled computers for clinical research."[154]

While designing the ACME time-sharing system, Weiderhold met an obstacle that he and other developers of time-sharing had not encountered before: extreme and unpredictable variations in demands on the system by the users. Traditional time-sharing schemes, Wiederhold found, could not "accommodate all of the laboratories in the Medical School with their widely varying data rates."[155] For instance, in the course of one hour one lab might be running a real-time simulation while another lab was using ACME to tabulate data; the next hour, both labs might be running simulations. Simply assigning labs predetermined time slots was out of the question, because one of ACME's major missions was to meet biologists' need to quickly adapt their programs to changing experimental parameters by giving them on-demand real-time computer use. In this regard, Lederberg saw no reason why the 360 could not be treated just like the LINC, even going so far as to suggest to Torbjörn Caspersson, a visiting microbiologist from the Institute of Cell Research at the Karolinska Institute, that his lab should consider renting access to ACME at a rate of $20,000 per month rather than investing $75,000 in a LINC and its peripheral devices.[156]

Operating under these conditions, Wiederhold's design for ACME ended up as a compromise between a computer that provided the total real-time control sought by Wesley Clark and a time-sharing system along the lines of what Licklider and McCarthy had envisioned. He did this by transforming how the

360 assigns slices of time. On a normal IBM 360, the amount of processing time allotted to each user was fixed per a given period. For example, one user might be given twenty milliseconds of processing time every second; for users who were not undertaking resource-intensive tasks, the experience of using this system was indistinguishable from that of using the whole computer in real time. This scheme, however, would not suffice for users who were running programs that interacted graphically in real time, such as those that generated x-y plots of a phenomenon while it was being measured. If those users were deprived of total control of the system, they would notice a lag when the computer did not respond to their input in a reasonable amount of time. Wiederhold's solution was to determine "the amount of time required by [a user] to acquire and process one data point."[157] The data point was an arbitrary unit of measure. For a user entering text into ACME, it was a single character displayed on the CRT; for a researcher digitizing analog signals (such as EEG), it could be the average measured strength of a signal over one-tenth of a second; for a biologists running a graphical simulation it might be one frame of the simulation—the resources required would depend on the complexity of the simulation. Thus, users undertaking more complex, memory-intensive tasks were given appropriately larger slices of time.

Usually this system worked, but in many cases real-time tasks were so complex that ACME gave particular users control over the entire machine for seconds or even minutes at a time. In order to know when ACME was being appropriated by a single heavy user, and was therefore not available, users had in their offices or labs a small console, which Wiederhold called a "light box," to inform them of ACME's status. Thus, Wiederhold let Lederberg have his cake and eat it too; everyone had access to a time-shared computer over which they could have complete operational control if they needed it.[158] Wiederhold had, in short, given Lederberg and the other biologists the means to satisfy their experimental agendas as well as their institutional priorities. Developing ACME's programming language, PL/ACME, went relatively smoothly, using input from potential users as well as Stanford computer scientists who were interested in improving the interface of time-shared systems.[159]

Operationally, the system was designed for use by both experts and novices. One could use ACME to write programs or simply to run programs written by others. Nevertheless, getting new users—especially medical students who may not have been as motivated to use the machines as scientists—to actually sit down at the terminals and work for prolonged periods of time proved difficult.

The main problem was fatigue: most medical students, few of whom had much experience typing, were quickly worn out and frustrated by searching for keys; this on top of having to learn new commands. As David Clark, who visited Stanford in 1966, reported, "One medical unit, using such a system [remote access terminals] for the training of medical students in computer science, discovered that when a student is first introduced to such a system he can only manage about one hour on the terminal a day; the machine tends to exhaust him." Clark noted, however, that "after a few months he is able to spend up to 5 hours a day on the terminal doing medical work."[160] To Clark's surprise, he observed that a large number of students had adjusted well to using computers. "What was a shock," he wrote, "was to discover the number of medical students using the computer . . . the younger generation—the future doctors—are certainly getting acquainted with it." Such acquaintance was not merely casual, he found, noting that curricula at Stanford and other US medical schools were in the mid-1960s beginning to teach "not just how a computer works and a few calculations, but how to use it as an information storage device and how to develop models of medical problems on the machine." For Clark, students' heavy involvement with computers was a sign of what would come; he predicted, "Although this was only the start, it was anticipated that by 1980 half of the medical graduates would have a knowledge of computing science, mathematics and electronics."[161]

The diversity both of biomedical researchers using ACME and of ways in which the computer was used was striking. By 1970, four years after the system became operational, ACME was used intensively by cardiologists "to monitor prospective open-heart surgery patients," geneticists "to inquire into the structure of the molecules that define our genetic makeup," and kidney transplant teams "to compile information for potential kidney donors." Lederberg reported that other uses of ACME included "analysis of EEGs, the study of mechanisms of normal breathing, studies of effects of environments such as air pollution on humans, studies related to brain function and mental development, and the collecting of medical information in such a manner that documentation will be available to support decision making in health care."[162] Besides the NIH, IBM took notice of the extensive—and simultaneous—use of the 360 by such a wide variety of researchers and physicians, and held up the system as exemplary. To capitalize on this success, IBM showcased ACME in two short films, produced in the late 1960s and distributed widely to universities and medical schools.[163]

In terms of reorienting Stanford biomedical research toward federal funding sources, the effect of using ACME was much more pronounced. In order to use ACME, each project had to raise funds to pay for access to the computer. In all but a few cases, laboratories, projects within laboratories, and individual researchers would apply for an NIH grant to pay for time on ACME.[164] The grant applications did not go directly to the NIH but were instead channeled through the ACME Policy Board, which had been set up in 1966 for the purpose of regulating ACME's use. One could under almost no circumstance use ACME without support from the NIH and the necessary approval of the ACME Policy Board. The only use of ACME paid for directly by the university was that related to the instruction of students.[165]

A Networked World of Experts: The Legacies of DENDRAL and ACME

DENDRAL and ACME each became victims of their own successes. By the early 1970s, DENDRAL had become a template for expert systems, programs that simulate the behavior of human experts when they make rough guesses based on partial information. It also spawned what Feigenbaum called "knowledge engineering," which aimed to demystify the process of the process of expert reasoning through the construction of a computer program that would emulate that reasoning. "Ultimately," Feigenbaum hoped, "the construction of such programs becomes itself a well-understood technical craft."[166] ACME, meanwhile, by providing to a large community relatively easy access to a powerful computer, created among its users—including DENDRAL's developers—a thirst for even more computing power. As early as 1969, before ACME had even been operational for a thousand days, Lederberg, citing demand for faster processing and more memory, had declared the system obsolete and had begun to lobby the NIH for support to upgrade components of the 360 to a Xerox Data System Sigma 5.[167]

To expand both DENDRAL and ACME, Lederberg launched a project intended to meet the anticipated needs of each. Called the Stanford University Medical Experimental Computer–Artificial Intelligence in Medicine (SUMEX-AIM), the project aimed to provide a large population of researchers the resources they needed to computerize their daily work and build expert systems modeled after DENDRAL. The drawback of a system of such awesome capability, however, was cost. Initially, Lederberg proposed that Stanford acquire two DEC PDP-10 supercomputers and various peripheral equipment, costing in the low tens of millions to purchase and roughly $1.3 million per year to staff and maintain. When Lederberg floated his plans for this system in the early 1970s, the NIH balked.[168] At the time, the agency was under great pressure from the Nixon administration to cut its budget, and the DRFR Special Resources Branch, which had directly funded ACME, was now led by the budget-conscious William Raub instead of the more risk-inclined (and extremely sympathetic to Lederberg) Bruce Waxman. Thus, if Lederberg wanted to expand ACME and DENDRAL on the NIH's dollar, major changes had to be made.

By 1973, after intense negotiation between Lederberg, Stanford administrators, the NIH, and DEC, a compromise was reached that more or less satisfied all involved parties. The compromise was to turn SUMEX-AIM into a "national resource." Rather than just being accessible by Stanford researchers, some 40 percent of SUMEX-AIM's resources could be accessed, typically via a telephone-line connection but also via ARPANET, the military-developed predecessor to the modern Internet, by researchers all around the country. Beyond developing AI projects, a new goal for SUMEX-AIM became "exploration of the use of computer communications as a means for interactions and sharing between geographically remote research groups engaged in biomedical computer science research."[169]

For all involved, casting SUMEX-AIM as a national resource was a regarded as a boon. For the now frugal NIH, the project's new character enabled the agency to justify the massive expense of SUMEX-AIM on the grounds that it served a large community and that funds were not being monopolized by Stanford. Rather than being perceived as a zero-sum situation, the decision to invest in SUMEX-AIM could now been viewed as a boon to non-Stanford researchers as well. SUMEX-AIM also got the NIH's foot in the door in the military's ARPANET project. For Lederberg, sharing SUMEX-AIM was not necessarily a sacrifice; though Stanford AI researchers lost some access to processing power, they gained access to a large population of experts now able to contribute to the process of building expert systems. To be a model expert, one no longer had to be physically located near the computer programmer at Stanford. Among Stanford administrators, the project was well received, despite Stanford's loss of complete control over a computer located on its grounds, because it provided a steady source of federal funding and it established Stanford as a central node of an emerging network of research computing facilities.

In April 1974, the hardware for SUMEX-AIM was delivered, and the system became operational for users that summer. NIH funding was guaranteed for five years. Once it was up and running, SUMEX-AIM did indeed become the focus of efforts to build expert systems related to life sciences research. On the new system, DENDRAL evolved into the Heuristic Programming Project, which encompassed expert systems related to both biology and medicine. On the biology side, there were the original DENDRAL project; Meta-DENDRAL; Crysalis, which interpreted 3-D electron density maps used in protein crystallography; and MOLGEN, the task of which was to "provide intelligent advice to a molecular geneticist on the planning of experiments involving the manipulation of DNA" and in which the expert system could help design the experiment from scratch or based on constraints. Also under the rubric of HPP was several medical projects: Ventilator Management (VM), which gave real-time advice to physicians on when to remove a patient from a ventilator; RX, which was designed to help physicians track chronic diseases through populations using the records from the American Rheumatism Association Medical Information System (ARAMIS); PUFF, which analyzed spirometer outputs to determine whether or not a patient had a particular lung ailment; and MYCIN, which helped physicians diagnose meningitis and blood infections.[170]

As if to cement Frederick Terman's vision of Stanford biomedical research that was both federally oriented and deeply involved in local private enterprise, in the 1980s Feigenbaum founded IntelliGenetics Inc., which sold expert systems and computer hardware to run those systems to molecular biologists. Primarily, the IntelliGenetics system would automate the process by which a molecular biologist would match a particular string of nucleotide bases to sets of genes, proteins, or regulatory mechanisms. For instance, a biologist user who found a sequence could use the system to see if there were matching sequences in the NBRF Protein Atlas, NIH's GenBank, or the European Molecular Biology Laboratory database. Then the system would initiate a dialogue with the user, asking questions such as "Is this sequence found in an AC- or GC-rich region?" and "Do you think this sequence is near a binding site?" To further help molecular biologists identify sequences, IntelliGenetics offered software tools to "search [the sequence] for hairpins, repeats, and symmetries within a sequence [homologies], symmetries and regions of hybridization within sequences." Software that allowed researchers to build customized databases from the NBRF, GenBank and EMBL data were also provided.[171]

The way IntelliGenetics planned to make money is telling in terms of how far biology had come in two decades. The profit was not to be found in selling the initial hardware and software package, but rather it was in subscriptions to an updating service. As new discoveries were made and dogmas challenged, the rules of molecular biology changed; and as the speed of computers improved, so did researchers' capacity to process data. The expert's expertise, after all, had to be maintained. Researchers who did not keep abreast of both would fall behind, and by 1983 over five hundred laboratories had secured the services of Intelli-Genetics. The company's self-proclaimed objective was simple: "to insure that your molecular biology research tool is not made obsolete."[172]

As expert systems and other tools initiated on SUMEX-AIM transformed into widely used research tools and occasionally commercial successes, Lederberg drifted away from computing and back toward more traditional biology research. In 1978, he accepted Rockefeller University's offer to become its fifth president and served in that capacity until 1990. Without Lederberg to tether the AI research to life sciences, many SUMEX-AIM developers rapidly applied their knowledge engineering skills to a wide variety of nonbiology, nonscientific domains. For his contribution to the development of expert systems, Feigenbaum received the 1994 ACM Turing Award, along with Dabbala Rajagopal "Raj" Reddy, "for pioneering the design and construction of large-scale artificial intelligence systems, demonstrating the practical importance and potential commercial impact of artificial intelligence technology."[173]

Since the early 1980s, thousands of expert systems have been developed, and they are used on a daily basis by millions. Well-known examples include the Mavent Expert System, used by Fannie Mae to automatically screen loan applications for compliance with various mortgage laws and its own policies; Intuit's popular TurboTax program, which helps non-expert users emulate the response of a trained accountant to a particular set of financial circumstances; and many of the "AI" routines that govern the behavior of computer-controlled opponents in computer games. In short, the community of biologists, physicians, and computer scientists at Stanford had, in its efforts to digitize the study of life, created many of the tools later used to digitize everyday life in America and beyond.

Conclusion

There was a young Doc from Atlantic
Whose data was all automatic
To go on a house call
Computer and all
He needed a bag most gigantic

LEE B. LUSTED

Not only do physicians today tote machines that are explicitly computers, but many of their instruments also have tiny computers embedded within them. When Lee Lusted scratched out the above bit of "doggerel" on his way to a conference in 1962, the notion of fitting a computer into a physician's bag was absurd. Indeed, one tends to forgot that, just a half a century ago, the prospect of using computers meant accommodating machines that took up entire rooms and that required extensive knowledge of mathematics and engineering to operate. Apparent then, as now, however, was the potential of computer technology to give the life scientist and medical worker control over vast volumes of information produced by the enormously complex and chaotic natural world. For the likes of Lee Lusted and Robert Ledley, the life sciences did not seem ready for computers, thus these thinkers regarded transforming the research practices and institutional priorities of biology and medicine as a necessary investment to reap the benefits of computing. The NIH too saw computerization and the mathematization of the life sciences as means to each other, and made effecting this transformation one of its top priorities in the 1960s. Today, though, computers are ubiquitous in the life sciences and the

NIH remains a strong supporter of biomedical computing, but there is little sign that the study of life has espoused the changes the early computer advocates sought.

What surprised those who wanted to restructure the life sciences to meet the needs of computer technology circa 1960 were the rapid changes within the technology they were trying to harness. As early as 1963, the LINC was providing biomedical researchers the means to use computers without necessarily retraining as mathematicians. With its interactive, graphical interface that reported results in real time, the LINC enabled researchers to evaluate data as experiments progressed and make changes according to what they observed; essentially, it allowed them to continue working without establishing universal, mathematical axioms to describe biological phenomena. Granted, several LINC users testified that the process of programming the computer forced them to arrive at a "clear and careful formulation of a problem," but many of the broader changes, particularly the emergence of a mathematized, standardized biomedicine, sought by the initial visionaries and sponsors of the computerization of the biologist's laboratory, did not materialize.[1]

Instead, computerization brought profound change of a different sort. At Stanford University and many other major locales of biomedicine during the mid-1960s, using computers (like the LINC and the ACME IBM 360) locked researchers into agendas that required constant access to the machines and therefore steady support from entities that were paying their laboratories' computer bills. For the manufacturers of the computers, meanwhile, the life sciences emerged as a lucrative market, a circumstance they did their best to perpetuate. Using computers, in short, brought many biomedical researchers inextricably into contact with the federal funding infrastructure and made them major clients of the burgeoning computer industry. Further reinforcing the triangle of researcher, government funder, and manufacturer in biomedicine were new technologies like ARPANET. Using ARPANET, Stanford's SUMEX-AIM and its successors have made it possible for life scientists to collaborate globally without significantly disrupting their local research environments, yet continually accessing to such networks usually requires that researchers obtain grants to buy new computers and improve communications infrastructure.

In the more care-oriented areas of medicine, the path to computerization was quite rocky. Indeed from the perspective of the early visionaries, the progress in this area has not been impressive. For instance, in 1962, Lusted looked forward to a distant future, 2012 to be exact, where computers and electronics had radically altered medicine. He predicted that within fifty years from the beginning of the computerization of medicine, the following feats (among others) would have been accomplished: (1) "nearly all of the body organs can now be replaced by compact artificial organs with built-in control systems"; (2) "the ability to find the correct nerve circuits and to trace the circuit like a telephone repairman"—this, he claimed, would be "developed in the 1990s"; (3) "high speed computers . . . and recently developed new mathematical techniques now help identify the exact composition of the nucleic acids and a host of enzyme systems"; (4) "parents can now choose to have a boy or a girl (with about 90 per cent probability of success)"; and (5) "people have become accustomed to the regular health checkup most of which they can have in their own homes"—he listed 2000 as the date when this last circumstance would come about. Lusted, however, conceded that, "the cause of some types of cancer have been discovered by 2012 a.d., but some are still an enigma."[2] To date, only some of Lusted's predictions have been realized. Researchers today do indeed have at their disposal computers and techniques that allow them to quickly determine most of an organism's DNA sequence. However, computer-controlled artificial organs and engineerable "nerve circuits' still remain distant prospects. In the clinic, Ledley and Lusted's vision of automated diagnosis by computers has not come to pass, and the notion that computers would automatically perform regular home-based checkups for healthy people verges on the fanciful.

As Octo Barnett made so clear in 1966, just four years after Lusted's bright piece of futurism, computerizing medical practice, especially in hospitals, was considerably more difficult than computerizing laboratory science. Hospitals were bigger operations than labs, physicians and administrators more hostile to computers, and patients somewhat wary of computers as medical devices. In the intervening decades, hospitals have adopted computers both for administration and diagnosis. In the former category, no major hospital in the United States today functions without a computerized medical information system. In the latter, computerized devices like the full-body CT scanner, in large part pioneered and disseminated by Ledley and the NBRF, or Edward Feigenbaum's PUFF, an expert system embedded in a spirometer, are integral parts of routine clinical care. Referring to CT, Lee Rogers wrote, "What was once amazing is now mundane."[3] Nevertheless, physicians still resist computers in many ways too. As Nathan Ensmenger points out in "Resistance is Futile? Reluctant and Selective Users of the Internet," physicians are highly Internet savvy—some 97 percent have access—but the vast majority do not use e-mail to communicate with patients or perform remote diagnosis using popular communications tools. Ensmenger found that an array of economic, legal, ethical, and cultural factors constrained doctors' use of the Internet, and that many such factors will not disappear simply if computer technologies become more accessible.[4] Thus, as long as efforts to computerize medicine remain focused almost exclusively on the computers themselves, progress toward the lofty goals of the early 1960s will likely remain slow.

Although many care providers have been slow to adopt computers, practitioners of evidence-based medicine (EBM) have been quite enthusiastic computer users. EBM, which is grounded in data produced by controlled and randomized clinical trials, grew out of Archie Cochrane's advocacy in the UK during the 1970s to make use of data from such trials as well as the work of epidemiologists John Wennberg (USA) and David Sackett (USA/Canada/UK). For these parties, "evidence" can be, in the words of Milbank Memorial Fund President Daniel M. Fox, essentialized as "the antonym of authority derived from experience and opinion."[5] In more mechanistic terms, EBM has been described by its advocates as "the process of systematically finding, appraising, and using contemporaneous research findings as the basis for clinical decisions . . . and harnessing that information for everyday clinical practice."[6] Unlike the way medicine is traditionally practiced in most settings, where it is up to the individual physician to make decisions about diagnosis and the course of treatment, EBM calls for care providers to adhere to standards and protocols derived from the analysis of large amounts of data. To analyze that data, EBM makes heavy use of computers.

In the USA, Utah's Intermountain Healthcare system has been a leader in applying EBM on a clinical level. Since the 1990s, Intermountain's data-driven (and computer-dependent) effort to improve patient care has met considerable success, and has become a focus of national attention during debates surrounding the Obama administration's attempts to shape the future form of healthcare in the United States. In his special address on healthcare to a joint session of Congress in September 2009, President Obama pointed specifically to Intermountain as an example of a system that would provide inexpensive yet high-quality care, and it is plausible that adopting the practices found at Intermountain nationwide may be crucial to Obama's proposal that "reducing the waste and inefficiency in Medicare and Medicaid will pay for most of" his trillion-dollar plan to reform healthcare.[7]

The roots of Utah's application of EBM can be found in two areas. One is the work of quality control expert W. Edwards Deming, which Brent C. James, Intermountain's Chief Quality Officer and the leader of its efforts to implement EBM, describes as the source of his idea to use the tools of quality control to improve medicine.[8] The other area is Ledley and Lusted's 1950s and 1960s efforts to automate diagnosis and introduce computers to medicine.

At Intermountain, James was working in an environment that had been shaped by Ledley and Lusted's ideals. There, he could develop EBM with relative ease, because the organization already had a long-running computerized system for managing patient data and because he could work from within, rather than impose, a clinical culture sympathetic to his vision of optimizing physicians' behavior, having them follow guidelines generated through the quantitative analysis of medical data. The roots of these conditions can be seen in the 1960s work of Homer Warner, the physician and cardiology researcher working at the Latter-Day Saints Hospital in Salt Lake City, which was absorbed into the Intermountain system in 1975. Warner was a prominent early adopter of Ledley and Lusted's methods, and he was also Lusted's handpicked successor as the head of the NIH's national computerization effort. As early as 1959, inspired by Ledley and Lusted's writings, Warner employed OR-derived methods to improve the efficiency of some of his hospital's operations. Warner gradually built an environment in Utah in which intense use of computers was encouraged. When James arrived in 1986, Warner's Hospital's Health Evaluation Through Logical Processing (HELP) computer system had long been in place and was generating the data that serves as "evidence" in EBM.[9]

While many of the early advocates' visions remain unrealized or are only now beginning to come to fruition, there also have been some quite unexpected developments in biomedical computing. In the case of the DENDRAL project, computers began to be employed in domains of mental labor that traditionally had been the realm of human experts, transforming not only practices in Joshua Lederberg's exobiology work but in areas far beyond. An additional consequence of the development of expert systems at Stanford was the emergence of an industry that sold biologists the means to automate much of this mental labor. IntelliGenetics, for instance, provided a way to organize information in local experiments and to examine that information in the context of the ever-expanding contents of sequence and bibliographic databases. Broadly, to integrate themes from chapters 1 and 5 of this book, systems like DENDRAL amounted to a break from OR-inspired procedural programming methods. Whereas OR was built around very simplified but nevertheless exact models of the real world, the kind of AI found in expert systems like DENDRAL is built around complex and highly nuanced approximate models. As Herbert Simon explains, "AI methods generally find only satisfactory solutions, not optima . . . we must trade off satisficing [a portmanteau coined by Simon in 1956 combining the words *satisfy* and *suffice*] in a nearly-realistic model (AI) against optimizing in a greatly simplified model (OR)." Simon concluded that "sometimes one will be preferred, sometimes the other."[10] Indeed, each seems to have found niches in both biology and medicine, and exploring how these niches formed would tell historians a great deal about the assumptions that go into model building in many areas of the study of life.

Another area of broadly unanticipated development—though Lusted did vaguely predict it—was that DNA sequencing became thoroughly computerized. A central challenge of recent decades has therefore been to provide computers capable of interfacing with ballooning volumes of sequence data. The techniques for managing data developed by Dayhoff and her NBRF colleagues in the 1960s and 1970s subsequently became indispensible tools in fields like genomics and proteomics in the subsequent decades. Today, the emergence of massive computerized databases as a crucial tool for life scientists is only beginning to be examined by historians, though early efforts are promising. In his investigation of Margaret Dayhoff's *Atlas*, Bruno Strasser holds that reports of the demise of the natural historical tradition of collecting and distributing information for its own sake may have been premature. The enormous sequence databases did not grow on their own but had to be supplied with information and actively managed. Consequently, information managers like Dayhoff became crucial components of a great many molecular biology projects; experiments could not proceed without them. But as Strasser illustrates, the values of molecular biology experimentalists were not compatible with their reliance on information managers such as Dayhoff, resulting in several moves to diminish the worth of Dayhoff's work as a collector, organizer, and distributor of information.[11]

When one surveys the changes between the mid-1960s, where this book's main coverage ends, and today, many worthy questions emerge. One is the absence of European-based researchers (with the notable exception of Kendrew) from almost all accounts of the early history of the computerization of biology and medicine. Many observers attributed the lack of biomedical computer projects in Europe simply to intellectual and institutional backwardness; for instance, in 1967 the UK Ministry of Health's David Clark, fresh from touring over seventy US laboratories and hospitals that were employing computers, complained that "as far as medical computing is concerned, England is in the dark ages."[12] Nevertheless, as German biomedical computing pioneer Jochen Moehr remarked, even though there were relatively few European projects, they were unsurpassed in terms of computerizing the entire process of the production and analysis of data: "less of the leading edge of technology advancement was achieved in Europe, but greater success with more comprehensive approaches was realized."[13] As Moehr saw it, there emerged in the 1960s a distinctly European model for biomedical computing, one motivated by patient care and supported by organizations, namely the Max Planck Institute and the Kaiser Wilhelm Institute, whose aim was to steer research in the long term. Although Moehr trained several cohorts of undergraduate students, and although his program served as a model for similar endeavors in North America, his efforts to gain European support and recognition for medical informatics (qua discipline) foundered. By 1980, though, he had emigrated, eventually settling in Canada. How such inhospitable conditions came about remain to be investigated.

Another question raised by this account is: what happened next? Given that most of the actors here were still professionally active and influential through the 1980s, there is much work to be done on the matter of how the early developments discussed in this book shaped the convergence of the life sciences and computing in the 1970s and 1980s. Wesley Clark's post-1965 work illustrates what a historian exploring biomedical computing in the 1970s would encounter. After the LINC users departed from the final meeting of the LINC Evaluation Program, Clark, Charles Molnar, and the others at Washington University's Computer Systems Laboratory continued their mission of designing "personalizable" computer systems throughout the 1960s. Besides support from the NIH, the CSL received several multimillion-dollar grants from ARPA starting in 1967 for the development of the "macromodules" that had been the pretext for the NIH grant that supported them during the years 1965–67. Compared to even LINC, the macromodules project was enormously ambitious. Clark's goal was to enable biologists not just to design their software but design and build their own machines, from the logic up, without needing to know very much about computer architecture. The idea, as he later put it, was: "You [the biologist user] build your own real-time interactive environment, to your specifications—we provide the tools so you can do it easily."[14] Investigating the macromodules project also provides access to the origins of asynchronous computing (or "clockless" computing), a technology that has only recently come to prominence.

Finally, there is the matter of the great hope invested in computer technology. For all the speculation and hype found in the 1950s and 1960s, today's consensus is similarly sanguine. It holds that the use of computers in biology and medicine is only just beginning in earnest and that enormous potential lies ahead for those who combine computing with the study of life. Probably Freeman Dyson best captured this excitement when he wrote in 2009, while surveying the past and future of science, that "if the new Romantic Age is real, it will be centered on biology and computers, as the old one was centered on chemistry and poetry."[15]

NOTES

Introduction

Epigraph. Theodor D. Sterling and Seymour V. Pollack, *Computers and the Life Sciences* (New York: Columbia University Press, 1965), 1. Sterling and Pollack conceded that from the perspective of 1965, robotized science was only in its nascence: "We are still at a very early state of creation. If computers are to be compared in status with other artifacts, they might be called the Model T's or the Flying Jennies of robots."

1. CNN Transcript, President Bill Clinton, British Prime Minister Tony Blair Deliver Remarks on Human Genome Milestone, June 26, 2000, http://transcripts.cnn.com/TRANSCRIPTS/0006/26/bn.01.html, accessed Jan. 12, 2011.

2. US Department of Energy, "Human Genome Project Budget," www.ornl.gov/sci/techresources/Human_Genome/project/budget.shtml, accessed Jan. 12, 2011.

3. The 1980s and 1990s also saw advances in sequencing technology, such as Leroy Hood's automatic DNA Sequencer, which greatly facilitated the HGP.

4. Genome News Network (J. Craig Venter Institute), "Genetics and Genomics Timeline," www.genomenewsnetwork.org/resources/timeline/2000_human.php, accessed Jan. 12, 2011.

5. Kaushik Sunder Rajan makes explicit the causes and immediate effects of some of the forces that brought about the NASDAQ bubble in *Biocapital* (Durham, NC: Duke University Press, 2006). James Shreeve, meanwhile, brings to light the personal motivations driving the exuberance related to biotechnology in the 1990s in his journalistic account of Celera's history, *The Genome War: How Craig Venter Tried to Capture the Code of Life and Save the World* (New York: Ballantine Books, 2005).

6. Richard Dawkins, "Genetics: Why Prince Charles Is So Wrong," *The Times* (London), Jan. 28, 2003. The article's subheading reads: "Genes work just like computer software, says this writer—which is why the luddites don't get it, but their children probably will."

7. Christopher Vaughan, Incyte Genomics "Featured Scientist" interview: "Leroy Hood: Inside Genomics," http://wayback.archive.org/web/*/http://www.incyte.com/insidegenomics/int/int/int_int_0011/int_int_0011_18.shtml, accessed July 13, 2011.

8. Joris Evers, "Two Words from Bill Gates: Computer Science," *PC World*, October 2004, www.pcworld.com/article/118029/two_words_from_bill_gates_computer_science.html, accessed Jan. 12, 2011.

9. Ashlee Vance, "Merely Human? That's So Yesterday," *New York Times*, June 12, 2010.

10. NIH Acting Director Raynard S. Kington, quoted in "NIH Announces American Recovery and Reinvestment Act Funding Opportunities" Mar. 11, 2009, News Release, www.nih.gov/news/health/mar2009/ncrr-11.htm, accessed Jan. 12, 2011.

11. NIH Research Portfolio Online Reporting Tools (RePORT) database, http://report.nih.gov/, accessed Dec. 21, 2010.

12. Francis S. Collins, "Statement for hearing entitled, "NIH in the 21st Century: The Director's Perspective," Testimony before the Subcommittee on Health Committee on Energy and Commerce, United States House of Representatives, June 15, 2010.

13. Andrew Pollack, "Awaiting the Genome Payoff," *New York Times*, June 14, 2010.

14. Merck has been particularly aggressive in drawing attention to its investment in IT. Kevin Davies, "Merck's Informatics Mission," *Bio-IT World*, May 8, 2008, www.bio-itworld.com/issues/2008/may/cover-story-merck-informatics.html, accessed Jan. 12, 2011.

15. Barack Obama, Remarks by the President to a Joint Session of Congress on Health Care, Sept. 9, 2009, US Capitol, Washington, DC.

16. David Leonhardt, "Making Health Care Better," *New York Times Magazine*, Nov. 3, 2009.

17. Stefan Timmermans and Marc Berg, *The Gold Standard: The Challenge of Evidence-Based Medicine and Standardization in Health Care* (Philadelphia: Temple University Press, 2003), 19.

18. Jerome Groopman, "Diagnosis: What Doctors Are Missing," *New York Review of Books* 56, no. 17 (Nov. 5, 2009).

19. A widely read recent example is Megan McArdle, "Paging Dr. Luddite: Information Technology Is on the Brink of Revolutionizing Health Care—If Physicians Will Only Let It," *Atlantic Monthly*, December 2010.

20. Vannevar Bush, "As We May Think," *Atlantic Monthly* 176, no. 1 (July 1945): 101.

21. Joshua Lederberg, "Computers and the Life Sciences," *Science* 150 (1965): 1577.

22. Michael S. Mahoney, "The Histories of Computing(s)," *Interdisciplinary Science Reviews* 30, no. 2 (2005): 119.

23. Explicitly cybernetic research received little funding, with the great exception being the work led by Heinz von Foerster at UIUC. His singular career and work is discussed in detail in Albert Müller and Karl H. Müller, ed., *An Unfinished Revolution? Heinz von Foerster and the Biological Computer Laboratory (BCL) 1958–1976* (Vienna: Edition Echoraum, 2007).

24. Subjects of this book Wesley Clark, Charles Molnar, J. C. R. Licklider, and Edward Feigenbaum all recalled being stimulated by Wiener's writings and talks when they thought about the possibilities of human-computer interaction, but none considered himself a cybernetician or explicitly drew from cybernetics concepts in their published work.

25. The best known piece of such futurism was Norbert Wiener's popular 1950 book, *The Human Use of Human Beings: Cybernetics and Society* (Boston: Riverside Press, 1950).

26. High expectations for the future influence of technology on biomedicine are crisply articulated in 1950s published material and internal memoranda generated by the NIH, ARDC (US Air Force), and the NAS-NRC. These hopes are discussed at length in chap. 2.

27. Martin H. Weik, *A Survey of Domestic Electronic Digital Computing Systems*, Ballis-

tic Research Laboratories Report No. 971, (Aberdeen, MD: BRL, 1955), ed-thelen.org/comp-hist/BRL-e-h.html, accessed Jan. 12, 2011.

28. Martin Campbell-Kelly and William Aspray, *Computer: The History of the Information Machine*, 2nd ed. (Boulder: Westview Press, 2004), 89.

29. I. Bernard Cohen notes, "Howard Aiken is often quoted as having declared that only a very small number of computers would be needed to serve the needs of the whole world—perhaps a dozen, with eight or ten for the United States. Sometimes the number is given as six or even two or three. Documentary evidence confirms that Aiken did indeed once say that one or two "computers" would suffice, but he does not seem to have been thinking of all the possible uses of computer power. The context shows that his remark did not have the general meaning that might be supposed and that it was not, therefore, as outrageous as it might appear." I. Bernard Cohen, *Howard Aiken: Portrait of a Computer Pioneer* (Cambridge, MA: MIT Press, 1999), 283.

30. One of the most accessible yet still technically sound discussions of ENIAC-like computers is Martin Mann, "Want to Buy a Brain?," *Popular Science* 154, no. 5 (May 1949): 148–52.

31. Kevin Maney, "In '52, huge computer called Univac changed election night," *USA Today*, Oct. 26, 2004. Max Woodbury, the mathematician consulted by Eckert and Mauchly to help them write the algorithms used to predict the 1952 election results, would become active in the NIH effort to introduce computers to biology and medicine in the early 1960s.

32. Campbell-Kelly and Aspray, *Computer*, 127.

33. Paul E. Ceruzzi, *A History of Modern Computing* (Cambridge, MA: MIT Press, 2003), 27. Characterizing early computer use in the mid-1950s, Ceruzzi wrote that "the Information Age had dawned."

34. David Halberstam, *The Fifties* (New York: Villard Books, 1993), x.

35. William L. O'Neill, *American High: The Years of Confidence, 1945–1960* (New York: Free Press, 1986), 291.

36. Ibid., 138.

37. National Institutes of Health, Office of Budget, "Appropriations History," officeofbudget.od.nih.gov/approp_hist.html, accessed Jan. 12, 2011.

38. Morris Frank Collen, *A History of Medical Informatics in the United States* (Bethesda: American Medical Informatics Association, 1995), 40; see 38–43 for a useful discussion of the etymology of "medical informatics."

1. Putting Molecular Biology and Medical Diagnosis into Metal Brains

1. Arnold W. Pratt, "Computers in Biomedical Research," in *NIH: An Account of Research in Its Laboratories and Clinics*, ed. DeWitt Stetten (New York: Academic Press, 1984), 460.

2. Robert Ledley, "Preface" to *NBR Research Accomplishments 1960–1970* (Washington, DC: NBRF, 1973), xv.

3. Harold Dorn, "Purchase Cost of IBM 650 Equipment," memorandum, March 29, 1957, NIH Electronic Data Processing Collection (RG 443 G2A 64, box 90, file 52), National Archives.

4. Frederick S. Brackett qtd. in Committee on Uses of Electronic Computers in Biological and Medical Sciences Collection, National Research Council, "Round Table

Conference on a Symposium on the Use of Computers in Biology and Medicine" (Washington, DC: National Academy of Sciences–National Research Council, 18 January, 1957), National Academy of Sciences Archive.

5. Robert Watson-Watt, quoted in Erik P. Rau, "Technological Systems, Expertise, and Policy Making: The British Origins of Operational Research," in *Technologies of Power: Essays in Honor of Thomas Parke Hughes and Agatha Chipley Hughes*, ed. Michael Thad Allen and Gabrielle Hecht (Cambridge, MA: MIT Press, 2001), 219.

6. Ibid., 223.

7. Ibid., 243.

8. E. C Williams, "The Origin of the Term 'Operational Research' and the Early Development of the Military Work," *Operations Research* 19, no. 2 (June 1968): 112.

9. Joseph F. McCloskey, "British Operational Research in World War II," *Operations Research* 35, no. 3 (May–June 1987): 453.

10. E. C Williams, "The Origin of the Term 'Operational Research' and the Early Development of the Military Work," 113.

11. McCloskey, "British Operational Research in World War II," 453.

12. Herbert A. Simon, *The Sciences of the Artificial* (Cambridge, MA: MIT Press, 1969), 27.

13. Ibid.

14. This model held that vital processes in cellular reproduction and growth could be explained by the presence of protein-based self-duplicating autocatalytic enzymes. Wendell Stanley's 1935 work with tobacco mosaic virus (TMV) crystallization served as "proof" for this enzyme theory of life. See Angela Creager's *The Life of a Virus: Tobacco Mosaic Virus as an Experimental Model, 1930–1965* (Chicago: University of Chicago Press, 2002).

15. Max Delbrück, qtd. in Gunther S. Stent, "That Was the Molecular Biology That Was," *Science* 160 (1968): 392. As Werner Lowenstein saw it, "Delbrück dug out Aristotle's ["who had been consigned to the trash-heap"] biological information and restored it in his essay "Aristotle-totle-totle." Lowenstein, *Touchstone of Life: Molecular Information, Cell Communication, and the Foundations of Life* (Oxford: Oxford University Press, 1999), 337.

16. Delbrück qtd. in Gunther S. Stent, "That Was the Molecular Biology That Was," 393.

17. Stent, "That Was the Molecular Biology That Was," 392.

18. Ibid., 395.

19. Ibid. 391.

20. Ibid., 390.

21. Nikolai W. Timoféeff-Ressovsky, Karl G. Zimmer, and Max Delbrück, "Über die Natur der Genmutation und der Genstruktur," *Nachrichten von der Gesellschaft der Wissenschaften zu Göttingen: Mathematisch-Physische Klasse* 6, no. 13 (1935): 190–245.

22. Daniel J. McKaughan, "The Influence of Niels Bohr on Max Delbrück: Revisiting the Hopes Inspired by 'Light and Hope,'" *Isis* 96 (2005): 510. McKaughan notes that Delbrück "shared Bohr's hope that scientific investigation would vindicate the view that at least some aspects of life are not reducible to physico-chemical terms."

23. Stent, "That Was the Molecular Biology That Was," 392.

24. For their work on the bacteriophage, Delbrück, Luria, and Hershey were awarded the Nobel Prize in Physiology or Medicine in 1969.

25. Erwin Schrödinger, *What Is Life?* (1944; repr. Cambridge, UK: Cambridge University Press, 1992), 69.

26. Ibid., 5.

27. Ibid., 30.

28. Stent, "That Was the Molecular Biology That Was," 392.

29. Schrödinger, *What Is Life?*, 21.

30. Joyce M. Wheeler, "Applications of the EDSAC Programming Systems," *IEEE Annals of the History of Computing* 14 (1992), 31. Wheeler explains why this process was so arithmetically laborious: "The spatial arrangement of atoms in a molecule can be found by studying the X-ray diffraction pattern of its crystals, each spot in the pattern corresponding to a train of waves running through the crystal. The distribution of matter in the crystal can be inferred by measuring the amplitude of the reflections."

31. Soraya de Chadarevian, *Designs for Life: Molecular Biology after World War II* (Cambridge, UK: Cambridge University Press, 2002), 113.

32. Robert O. Gould, "Cover Story: Arnold Beevers at 90," *Crystallography News* 65 (June 1998): 38–39, http://bca.cryst.bbk.ac.uk/bca/CNews/1998/Jun98/Beev90.html, accessed Dec. 3, 2010.

33. Henry Lipson, "Reminiscences and Discoveries: The Introduction of Fourier Methods into Crystal-Structure Determination," *Notes and Records of the Royal Society of London* 44 (1990): 257–58.

34. R. O. Gould, "The Mechanism of Beevers-Lipson Strips," *Crystallography News* 65 (Dec. 1998).

35. Ibid.

36. Gould, "Cover Story: Arnold Beevers at 90," 38. Gould maintains that depictions of Rosalind Franklin employing such machinery were apocryphal because Franklin's arithmetical acuity allowed her to dispense with the machines. He opined: "In fact a BBC documentary of a few years ago showing Rosalind Franklin with a box of strips laboriously cranking them into a mechanical calculator was almost certainly apocryphal. She would not have wasted time on that!"

37. Ibid., 39. Gould reports, "Over 500 sets [of Beevers-Lipson strips] were sold between 1948 and 1970."

38. Wheeler, "Applications of the EDSAC Programming Systems," 31.

39. de Chadarevian, *Designs for Life*, 107–8.

40. Martin Campbell-Kelly, "The Airy Tape: An Early Chapter in the History of Debugging." *IEEE Annals of the History of Computing* 14, no. 4 (1992): 16. Campbell-Kelly explains that Wilkes took a "conservative approach to design. For example he opted for a pulse-rate of 0.5 MHz when 'any electronic engineer worth his salt' would have accepted the challenge of working at 1 MHz. The reason for this attitude was that Wilkes was motivated not only by the engineering challenge, but also by 'the desire to get a machine on which we could try out programmes, instead of just dreaming them up for an imaginary machine.'"

41. Ibid., 18.

42. Ibid.

43. John M. Bennett and John C. Kendrew, "The Computation of Fourier Synthesis with a Digital Electronic Calculating Machine." *Acta Crystallographica* 5 (1952): 109–10.

44. Ibid. Bennett and Kendrew explain that "Some of the first methods [of one- and

two-dimensional Fourier synthesis] were developed by one of us (J.M.B) [Bennett] in collaboration with Mr. H. E. Huxley of the Cavendish Laboratory."

45. Ibid.

46. Ibid., 109. This article was published several years before the myoglobin problem was actually solved.

47. Fred Hoyle, *The Black Cloud* (New York: Harper, 1957), 32. Unlike his rival, George Gamow, Hoyle had little to do with life scientists (or even physicists venturing into the life sciences).

48. de Chadarevian, *Designs for Life*, 115.

49. Wheeler, "Applications of the EDSAC Programming Systems," 37.

50. Ibid., 31.

51. Bennett and Kendrew, "Computation of Fourier Synthesis," 115. Each contour took between half an hour and an hour to plot.

52. de Chadarevian, *Designs for Life*, 127.

53. Ibid., 133.

54. Bennett and Kendrew, "Computation of Fourier Synthesis," 109.

55. de Chadarevian, *Designs for Life*, 132.

56. Ibid., 119.

57. Ibid., 121.

58. EDSAC was notorious for suffering mechanical failures during the course of calculations, and determining where the failure took place required one to have intimate knowledge of the system.

59. W. Peyton Cunningham, Denys Freeman, and Joseph F. McCloskey, "Of Radar and Operations Research: An Appreciation of A. P. Rowe (1898–1976)," *Operations Research*, 32, no. 4 (Jul.–Aug., 1984): 963.

60. de Chadarevian, *Designs for Life*, 119–20.

61. Ibid., 120–21.

62. Ibid., 132.

63. Ibid., 118–19.

64. Ibid., 123–24.

65. David Edgerton, *Warfare State: Britain, 1920–1970* (Cambridge, UK: Cambridge University Press, 2005), 205.

66. John Krige, *American Hegemony and the Postwar Reconstruction of Science in Europe* (Cambridge, MA: MIT Press, 2006), 248.

67. The fate of OR in Britain after the war has been explored by John Agar and Brian Balmer in "British Scientists and the Cold War," *Historical Studies in the Physical and Biological Sciences* 28, no. 2 (March 1998): 209–52.

68. David E. Clark, "Computing Requirements of the Hospital and Medical School," Jan. 23, 1967, Medical Computing Unit, University of Manchester, United Kingdom, 9. Box 1, folder, 9, Stanford University Archive, ACME Collection (SC 236).

69. de Chadarevian, *Designs for Life*, 305–6.

70. Rau, "Technological Systems, Expertise, and Policy Making," 243.

71. Krige, *American Hegemony and the Postwar Reconstruction of Science in Europe*, 230–31.

72. Philip M. Morse, "The Growth of Operations Research in the Free World," lecture given at the Operations Evaluation Group 20th Anniversary Conference on Opera-

tions Research," May 14–16, 1962. Qtd. in Krige, *American Hegemony and the Postwar Reconstruction of Science in Europe*, 232.

73. Frederic Lawrence Holmes, *Meselson, Stahl, and the Replication of DNA: A History of "The Most Beautiful Experiment in Biology"* (New Haven: Yale University Press, 2001), 40. Holmes relates that Kendrew was well aware of Watson's difficulties at Caltech, asking him in a November 1953 letter, "Have you reconciled Max [Delbrück] to the DNA structure?"

74. Crick did not formally articulate the "dogma" until 1958, but its underlying notions had been explored by Crick and members of the Phage Group starting in 1953.

75. Lily E. Kay, *Who Wrote the Book of Life?: A History of the Genetic Code* (Stanford: Stanford University Press, 2000), 174. Giovanni Boniolo asserts that one should take Crick's 1958 statement "By information I mean the specification of the amino acid sequence of the protein" at face value. Essentially, Crick is employing "information" in a semantic sense, not a syntactic sense or Shannonian sense. "Biology Without Information," *History and Philosophy of the Life Sciences* 25 (2003): 258.

76. Kay, *Who Wrote the Book of Life?*, 174–75. As Kay put it, "In single masterly stroke Crick encapsulated the ideology and experimental mandate of molecular genetics: genetic information, qua DNA, was both the origin and universal agent of all life (proteins)—the Aristotelian prime mover—as Delbrück suggested."

77. Holmes, *Meselson, Stahl, and the Replication of DNA*, 33.

78. Gamow spelled it "RNATIE Club" (see fig. 1.10).

79. Gamow to Watson, Dec. 6, 1954, reproduced in James D. Watson, *Girls, Genes, and Gamow: After the Double Helix* (New York: Knopf, 2002), appendix.

80. Judson, *Eighth Day of Creation*, 256.

81. Robert S. Ledley, "Medical Informatics: A Personal View of Sowing the Seeds," in *A History of Medical Informatics: Proceedings of Association for Computing Machinery Conference on History of Medical Informatics*, ed. B. Blum and K. Duncan (New York: ACM Press, 1990), 92.

82. Ibid., 89.

83. Ledley's father had attempted to obtain an advanced degree in physics but was discouraged by the lack of lucrative employment opportunities in related areas.

84. Although Ledley was unaware of it at the time, Rabi and many of his other instructors (including E. Fermi, H. Bethe, W. Lamb, H. Yukawa, J.A Wheeler) were initially at Columbia under the auspices of the Manhattan Project.

85. Ledley, "Medical Informatics: A Personal View of Sowing the Seeds," 89.

86. Robert S. Ledley, interview with the author and Bruno Strasser Jan. 27, 2006.

87. Morse and Kimball coauthored what is perhaps the most widely read American book on OR, *Methods of Operations Research* (MIT Press, 1951). Dover Publications still prints the book.

88. Ledley in Robert S. Ledley and Joseph A. November, "A Lifetime of Biomedical Computing: A Conversation with Robert S. Ledley," NIH public science lecture, Feb. 21, 2008.

89. Ledley's wife, Terry, was also excluded by the corpsmen's wives when the assignments were posted. Terry Ledley, interview with the author Feb. 7, 2008.

90. Robert S. Ledley interview with author Jan. 27, 2006.

91. "Mathematics Now Protects False Teeth," *Los Angeles Times*, May 4, 1952.

92. Robert S. Ledley interview with author Feb. 14, 2006.

93. Robert S. Ledley interview with author Jan. 27, 2006.

94. Atsushi Akera, *Calculating a Natural World: Scientists, Engineers, and Computers During the Rise of U.S. Cold War Research* (Cambridge, MA: MIT Press, 2007), 153–55.

95. Terry Ledley interview with author Feb. 7, 2008. Terry Ledley left her job in 1954 in order to raise her and Robert's sons, Fred and Gary.

96. Robert S. Ledley interview with author Feb. 14, 2006.

97. Ledley, "Medical Informatics: A Personal View of Sowing the Seeds," 90.

98. Ibid.

99. Robert S. Ledley, "Mathematical Foundations and Computational Methods for a Digital Logic Machine," *Journal of the Operations Research Society of America* 2, no.3 (Aug. 1954), 249. Ledley assigned each n-lettered sentence a "designation number" in binary notation, which would be entered into a Boolean lattice with n elementary elements (that is, a lattice with n generators).

100. Ibid., 273. Ledley's description of his proposed machine read: "The operations such a logic machine might contain are: simplification in either the simplest sum of products or product of sums form; transformation to the absolute simplest form; checking statements for consistency, contradictions, redundancies, implications, or tautologies; generating all implications from a given hypothesis; making changes of variables; and solving logical equations."

101. Raymond J. Nelson, review of Robert S. Ledley, "Mathematical Foundations and Computational Methods for a Digital Logic Machine," *Journal of Symbolic Logic* 20, no. 2 (1955): 195–96. The "mathematical computer theory" to which Nelson referred was articulated in Alan M. Turing, "On Computable Numbers, with an Application to the Entscheidungsproblem," *Journal of Symbolic Logic* 2, no. 42 (Mar. 1937): 42–43, and Arthur W. Burks and Jesse B. Wright, "Theory of Logical Nets," *Journal of Symbolic Logic* 19, no. 141 (June 1954): 141–42.

102. C. Stewart Gillmor, in his *Fred Terman at Stanford: Building a Discipline, a University, and Silicon Valley* (Stanford: Stanford University Press, 2004), relates that these changes at the NBS also wrecked the Institute for Numerical Analysis (INA) at UCLA, which was supported by an NBS contract. George E. Forsythe was among those who left INA; he went to Stanford.

103. Ledley, "Medical Informatics: A Personal View of Sowing the Seeds," 90. The Johns Hopkins University Operations Research Office was located in Chevy Chase, Maryland. Ledley, who was raised in New York City, also explained that he was hesitant to relocate to IBM offices in relatively rural Poughkeepsie, NY.

104. Robert Steven Ledley, CV, 1960, NBRF Archive.

105. Robert S. Ledley "Digital Computational Methods in Symbolic Logic, with Examples in Biochemistry," *Proceedings of the National Academy of Sciences* 41 (July 1955): 511. The article was communicated by Gamow. There is a small error in the article—20! = 2,432,902,008,176,640,000 (or 2.4329×10^{18})—which means that Ledley made an arithmetic error while preparing his paper. He likely got this figure from Gamow because of the elegant comparison to the age of the universe. Despite the error, Ledley was correct to contend that the brute-force solution would be grossly impractical. To put into perspective the growth of processing power since 1955, the top supercomputers in 2010 can perform a quadrillion floating point operations per second (FLOPS)—and could theoretically complete the task Ledley described in a few hours.

106. Ibid., 508.

107. Ibid., 505.

108. Ibid., 506.

109. In September 1956, Sydney Brenner sent to the RNA Tie Club "On the Impossibility of All Overlapping Triplet Codes," his proof that triplets could not overlap entirely. Kay remarks, "[Brenner's] proof was dazzling in its directness and generality, a validation of the superiority of the mind over a computing machine, as Crick might have put it" (Kay, *Who Wrote the Book of Life?*, 161).

110. Gamow to Watson, Nov. 28, 1954 (reprinted in James Watson, *Girls, Genes, and Gamow*, appendix).

111. Kay, *Who Wrote the Book of Life?*, 158–59.

112. Robert S. Ledley, "Biomedical Computer and Biomathematics Research Center," Application for Research Grant, National Institutes of Health, B-RG-2075 (formerly RG 7323), Nov. 1, 1959, Robert S. Ledley Papers, National Biomedical Research Foundation, 58. This was probably the first formal proposal to use computers to sequence proteins. Indeed, Ledley claimed at the time, "As far it is known to us, there has never before been an attempt to develop a digital computer aid to the analysis of the amino acid sequences of protein" (59).

113. Ibid., 57.

114. Ibid.

115. Ibid., 59.

116. Robert S. Ledley, "A Format and Computational Aid for Operation Simulation," *Operations Research* 4, no.3 (June 1956): 400.

117. Ibid.

118. Ledley also gave a third paper that was strictly related to war gaming.

119. Robert S. Ledley, "Operational Simulation in Medicine," *Operations Research* 4, no.3 (June 1956): 392.

120. Ibid.

121. Robert S. Ledley, "Logical Aid to Systematic Medical Diagnosis," *Operations Research* 4, no. 3 (June 1956), 391. McBee cards were widely used in university libraries to track circulation starting in the early 1960s.

122. Ledley, "Medical Informatics: A Personal View of Sowing the Seeds," 93. Ledley also noted, "Of course, the cards did not truly carry out the logic that was required, and of course no probabilities were involved."

123. Ledley, "Logical Aid to Systematic Medical Diagnosis, 391.

124. William J. Horvath, "An Operations Research View of Medicine and Public Health," *Operations Research* 4, no.3 (June 1956): 390.

125. Lusted grew up in Iowa, where his father was a Methodist minister and his mother a voice instructor. His two brothers also became physicians.

126. Lee B. Lusted, "Some Roots of Clinical Decision Making," in *A History of Medical Informatics: Proceedings of Association for Computing Machinery Conference on History of Medical Informatics*, ed. Bruce I. Blum and Karen Duncan (New York: ACM Press, 1990), 395.

127. Lusted, "Some Roots of Clinical Decision Making," 395–96.

128. Ibid., 396.

129. AIL was founded in 1945 by Columbia University, Harvard University, and MIT scientists and engineers to commercially manufacture electronic instruments they had developed for the war effort. Primarily they sold defense-related equipment such as

avionics, radio antennas, and radar, but they also built electronic equipment and non-electronic measurement devices (for example, slide rules) that could be used in medicine.

130. Lusted, "Some Roots of Clinical Decision Making," 397.

131. Lee B. Lusted, "The Proper Province of Automatic Data Processing in Medicine," *Annals of Internal Medicine* 57, no. 5 (Nov. 1962): 856.

132. Lusted, "Some Roots of Clinical Decision Making," 397.

133. Ibid., 398.

134. Ledley, "Medical Informatics: A Personal View of Sowing the Seeds," 92.

135. Lee B. Lusted, "The Clearing Haze: A View from My Window," *Medical Decision Making* 11, no. 2 (Apr.–June 1991): 77.

136. Lusted, "The Clearing Haze," 77.

137. Ledley and Lusted noted that a small number of physiologists and physicians utilized punch cards in their research and diagnostic work. For instance: C. F. Paycha, "Mémoire diagnostique," *Montpellier méd* 47 (1955): 588 ("Punched Card Symptom Registration for Differential Diagnosis of Ophthalmological Diseases"); "Diagnosis by Slide Rule," *What's New (Abbot Labs)* 189 (1955); "Differential Diagnosis: An Apparatus to Assist the Logical Facilities," *Lancet* 1 (1954), 874; E. Baylund and G. Baylund, "Use of Record Cards in Practice, Prescription, and Diagnostic Records," *Ugeskrift Laeger* 116, no. 3 (1954); M. Lipkin and J. D. Hardy, "Mechanical Correlation of Data in Differential Diagnosis of Hematomological Diseases," *Journal of the American Medical Association* 166, no. 2 (1958).

138. Among the article's readers was Alan N. Schechter, MD, then about to begin medical school and now chief of the Molecular Biology and Genetics Section, NIDDK. Schechter cites the article as the beginning of his decades-long interest in using computers to solve biomedical problems (Schechter e-mail to author May 5, 2008).

139. Ledley and Lusted, "Reasoning Foundations of Medical Diagnosis," *Science* 130 (July 3, 1959): 21.

140. Robert G. Hoffman, "Computers in Medicine," *Science* 131 (1960): 472, 474, 564.

141. Lusted, who had just been introduced to Bayes' theorem, later claimed to have been unaware of the criticism. Ledley was aware of the criticism but ignored it on the grounds that there were many medical cases to which the theorem could be productively applied despite its flaws.

142. Lusted, "The Clearing Haze," 78.

143. Ledley and Lusted, "Reasoning Foundations of Medical Diagnosis," 21.

144. Edward A. Feigenbaum interview with author June 20, 2004.

145. H. R. Warner et al., "A Mathematical Approach to Medical Diagnosis. Application to Congenital Heart Disease," *Journal of the American Medical Association* 177 (1961): 177–83.

146. Homer R. Warner, "History of Medical Informatics at Utah," in *A History of Medical Informatics: Proceedings of Association for Computing Machinery Conference on History of Medical Informatics*, ed. Bruce I. Blum and Karen Duncan (New York: ACM Press, 1990), 359.

147. Ibid., 363. Warner recalled in 1987 that "this program has served us well over the years. We've done 35,000 sequential Bayesian self-administered patient histories. Patients react very well to it, and it's been a useful source of information for the surgeon.

Incidentally, in 70% of the patients the primary diagnosis can be made from history alone."

148. F. T. de Dombal et al., "Computer-aided diagnosis of acute abdominal pain." *British Medical Journal* 2 (1972): 9–13.

149. "Computer May Aid Disease Diagnosis," *New York Times*, July 22, 1959.

150. "A Metal Brain for Diagnosis," *New York World Telegram*, July 8, 1959.

151. "Dr. Univac Wanted in Surgery," *New York Post*, Nov. 12, 1959.

152. "Electronic Brain May Some Day Link Doctors over World on Single Case," *Evening Star* (Washington, DC), Nov. 12, 1959. The *Evening Star's* version of the AP article on Ledley and Lusted contains several lines that the *New York Post* version does not. The *Sunday Star* carried an expanded version of the AP article in its Nov. 12, 1959, edition under the title "Electronic Prescriptions." Cautioned the Sunday version of the *Star*, "The sad fact is that the computer system will give out no more than is fed into it. It will turn out no miracle cures unless human brains produce them first."

153. "Computers, Medicine Join Forces," *American Medical Association News* 2, no. 23 (Nov. 16, 1959).

154. "Electronic Computer to Complicate Task of MD, Mathematician Holds," *Scope Weekly*, Aug. 26, 1959.

155. Robert S. Ledley and Lee B. Lusted, "Computers in Medical Data Processing," *Operations Research* 8, no.3 (May–June 1960): 300.

156. Ibid., 310.

157. Ibid.

158. Lusted, "The Proper Province of Automatic Data Processing in Medicine," 855. During the 1960s, H. P. Rome wrote more than a dozen papers advocating the use of computers in psychiatry and related research.

159. Ibid. Pipberger published his findings in: H. V. Pipberger, "Advantages of three lead cardiographic recordings," *Annals of the New York Academy of Science* 126 (1965): 873–81. Most functions of the Veterans Administration were assumed by the Department of Veterans Affairs when it was established in 1989.

160. For a detailed discussion of the development of OR, see Krige, *American Hegemony and the Postwar Reconstruction of Science in Europe.*

2. Building Tomorrow's Biomedicine

1. James Shannon, "Foreword," in *Computers in Biomedical Research*, ed. Ralph W. Stacy and Bruce. D. Waxman (New York: Academic Press, 1965), xi. By using the term "computational technique," Shannon was placing computers into the broader rubric of a mathematized biology he hoped NIH would help to bring about via computerizing the study of life. While Kendrew and Perutz clearly used a digital electronic computer, EDSAC, in their research, Watson and Crick's work was to a substantial degree computational but not dependent on electronic computing equipment.

2. For an extensive account of the growth of the NIH see: Buhm Soon Park, *Health through Science: Biomedical Research Policy at the NIH, 1930–1980* (forthcoming).

3. William F. Raub, "The Life Sciences Computer Resources Program of the National Institutes of Health," *Proceedings of the 1971 26th Annual Conference* (New York: ACM, 1971), 700.

4. In *Calculating a Natural World: Engineers, and Computers During the Rise of U.S. Cold*

War Research (Cambridge, MA: MIT Press, 2007), chaps. 4 and 5, Atsushi Akera demonstrates that significant Air Force sponsorship of research computing extended back to the early 1950s and was a large component of inter-agency struggles over the federal resource allocations and the general direction of the development of computing.

5. Albert W. Hetherington, "Round Table Conference on a Symposium on the Use of Computers in Biology and Medicine" (Washington, DC: National Academy of Sciences–National Research Council, Jan. 18, 1957), transcript, Committee on Uses of Electronic Computers in Biological and Medical Sciences Collection, National Academy of Sciences Archive.

6. Ibid., 4.

7. Ibid., 2.

8. Henry Weinrauch and Albert W. Hetherington, "Computers in Medicine and Biology," *Journal of the American Medical Association* 169 (Jan. 17, 1959): 241.

9. Ibid.

10. Gen. Thomas Sarsfield Power (1905–1970) was neither an expert in medicine nor computing, so it is likely that the impetus to computerize biomedical research came from ARDC researchers. Power is remembered primarily for commanding the Strategic Air Command in the late 1950s, for his outspoken arguments against nuclear weapons test ban treaties, and for leading the first large-scale incendiary raid on Tokyo on Mar. 9–10, 1945.

11. Hetherington, "Round Table Conference on a Symposium on the Use of Computers in Biology and Medicine," 3.

12. Cannan was absent from the round-table discussion itself, and it was instead led by Seymour Jablon, a statistician heavily involved in the Atomic Bomb Casualty Commission. Cannan's absence is the most likely reason the round-table proceedings were recorded and transcribed.

13. R. Keith Cannan, memorandum, Sept. 23, 1957, file: "MED: Committee on Uses of Electronic Computers in Biological and Medical Sciences: Ad hoc (1957–1959)," National Research Council Division of Medical Sciences Collection (1946–1973), National Academy of Sciences Archive.

14. Thomas Haigh, "The Chromium-Plated Tabulator: Institutionalizing an Electronic Revolution: 1954–1958," *IEEE Annals of the History of Computing* 23, no. 4 (2001): 77.

15. E. D. Becker and N. E. Sharpless, "Spectroscopy and Chemical Physics," in *NIH: An Account of Research in Its Laboratories and Clinics*, ed. DeWitt Stetten (New York: Academic Press, 1984), 448.

16. Ralph W. Stacy and Bruce. D. Waxman, "Introduction," in *Computers in Biomedical Research*, eds. Ralph W. Stacy and Bruce. D. Waxman (New York: Academic Press, 1965), 2.

17. Frederick S. Brackett, "Electronic Data Processing and Computing Equipment: The Meaning for NIH," memorandum to James Shannon, Apr. 13, 1956, NIH Electronic Data Processing Collection (RG 443 G2A 64, box 90, file 53), National Archives.

18. Ibid.

19. Ibid.

20. Lee B. Lusted, "Some Roots of Clinical Decision Making," in *A History of Medical Informatics: Proceedings of Association for Computing Machinery Conference on History of Medical Informatics*, eds. Bruce I. Blum and Karen Duncan (New York: ACM Press, 1990), 386.

21. "IBM 650, Introduction 2," IBM Archives, www-03.ibm.com/ibm/history/exhibits/650/650_intro2.html, accessed Dec. 30, 2009.

22. "IBM 650," IBM Archives, www 03.ibm.com/ibm/history/exhibits/650/650_intro.html, accessed Dec, 30, 2009.

23. George H. Leonard, "EDP [Electronic Data Processing] Meeting," Memorandum for the Record, April 20, 1956, NIH Electronic Data Processing Collection (RG 443 G2A 64, box 90, file 53), National Archives. The anti-650 remark was attributed to Alexander Rich.

24. Arnold W. Pratt, "Computers in Biomedical Research," in *NIH: An Account of Research in Its Laboratories and Clinics*, ed. DeWitt Stetten (New York: Academic Press, 1984), 461.

25. Ibid. There were no general-purpose digital electronic computers in Dorn's facility.

26. Harold Dorn, "Purchase Cost of IBM 650 Equipment," memorandum, March 29, 1957, NIH Electronic Data Processing Collection (RG 443 G2A 64, box 90, file 52), National Archives.

27. Ibid.

28. Alexander Rich is best known for his work on the structure of DNA, RNA, and ribosomes. During the mid-1950s he was a core member of Gamow's RNA Tie Club. He has been based at MIT since 1958. For discussion of Rich's interaction with the Cavendish group, see Soraya de Chadarevian, *Designs for Life: Molecular Biology after World War II* (Cambridge, UK: Cambridge University Press, 2002).

29. Leonard, "EDP [Electronic Data Processing] Meeting," Apr. 20, 1956. Leonard's meeting minutes attribute these remarks to Rich.

30. Joseph S. Murtaugh, "Meeting of the EDP and Computing Committee," Memorandum for the Record, June 27, 1956, NIH Electronic Data Processing Collection (RG 443 G2A 64, box 90, file 53), National Archives. Murtaugh attributes the "survey" of cancer researchers to Arnold Pratt.

31. Frederick S. Brackett, Memorandum to James Shannon, "Report of Committee," November 21, 1956, NIH Electronic Data Processing Collection (RG 443 G2A 64, box 90, file 51), National Archives.

32. Ibid.

33. Harold Dorn, "Round Table Conference on a Symposium on the Use of Computers in Biology and Medicine," 39–40.

34. For more on Aiken's approach to using computers in science, see I. Bernard Cohen and Gregory W. Welch, eds., *Makin' Numbers: Howard Aiken and the Computer* (Cambridge, MA: MIT Press, 1999).

35. Howard Aiken, "Round Table Conference on a Symposium on the Use of Computers in Biology and Medicine," inserted page. This insert indicates that the recorder, "HNG," paraphrased some of Aiken's remarks.

36. Pratt, "Computers in Biomedical Research," 461.

37. Ibid., 460–61.

38. Ibid., 461.

39. Belle Waring, "NIDDK Laboratory of Biological Modeling Turns 50," *NIH Record* 41, no. 24 (Nov. 30, 2007).

40. Ibid.

41. Senate Resolution 42, 86th Congress of the United States.

42. Hubert H. Humphrey, "Your Cooperation Invited in Filling in Questionnaire," International Health Study (Pursuant to S. Res. 42, 86th Congress), June 8, 1959, US Senate Record, NIH Electronic Data Processing Collection (RG 443 G2A 64 box 90, file 54), National Archives.

43. Hubert H. Humphrey to John A. McCone, July 12, 1960, Robert S. Ledley Papers, National Biomedical Research Foundation.

44. Hubert H. Humphrey, "Engineers and Information," *Mecheleciv* 7 (Dec. 1959): 30. *Mecheleciv* (*Mech*anical, *el*ectrical, *civ*il engineering) was the monthly student magazine for the George Washington University School of Electrical Engineering, Washington, DC. Michael Mahoney suggests that Humphrey picked up the "information gap" rhetoric from Douglas C. Engelbart.

45. Humphrey, "Engineers and Information," 30.

46. Robert S. Ledley, "Digital Electronic Computers in Biomedical Science," *Science* 130 (Nov. 6, 1959): 1225.

47. Ibid., 1230.

48. Ibid.

49. Lee Lusted, "The Development of National Biomedical Computing Capability," in *Data Acquisition and Processing in Biology and Medicine: Proceedings of the 1961 Rochester Conference*, 4 vols., ed. Kurt Enslein (New York: Pergamon Press, 1962), 6. Lusted quoting C. E. Hopkins and V. B. Berry, "On Mathematical Literacy of Medical Students," *Journal of Medical Education* 36 (1961): 338–41.

50. Ledley, "Digital Electronic Computers in Biomedical Science," 1230–31.

51. Ibid., 1232.

52. Ibid. Ledley's caveat: "I do not intend to give the impression that all computer utilization will have this characteristic, for this is far from true." Ledley did not provide discussion, however, of any other modes of computer use.

53. Ibid.

54. Lee Lusted, "Foreword," Robert S. Ledley, *Report on The Use of Computers in Biology and Medicine*, NAS-NRC document 26,238 (Washington, DC: National Research Council, Division of Medical Science, 1960), vii–viii. This passage reappeared almost verbatim in the introduction to Ledley's 1965 textbook, *Use of Computers in Biology and Medicine*.

55. Frederick L. Stone and J. H. U. Brown, "Technology in Medicine," *BioScience* 15, no. 11 (Nov. 1965), 716.

56. Nelson Y. S. Kiang (Founder, Eaton-Peabody Laboratory of Auditory Physiology), interview with author, Feb. 2004.

57. Joshua Lederberg comments on Joseph November, "Impossible by Any Other Means: Early Advocacy for the Use of Computers in Biology," Joint Atlantic Seminar on the History of Biology, Apr. 2003.

58. Wesley Clark interview with author June 24, 2004.

59. For a detailed examination of the legacy of Feynman's talk, see Chris Toumey, "Reading Feynman into Nanotechnology: A Text for a New Science," *Techné* 13, no. 3 (2008): 133–68.

60. Richard P. Feynman, "There's Plenty of Room at the Bottom: An Invitation to Enter a New Field of Physics," lecture to American Physical Society Annual Meeting, Dec. 29, 1959. Published in *Engineering and Science* 23 (Feb. 1960): 22–36. Emphasis in the original.

61. J. Barkley Rosser, memorandum to Cohen, Cannon, Eisenhart, Lusted, Dec. 12, 1960, file: "Committee to Review Division of Medical Sciences Report on Uses of Computers in Biology and Medicine 1960–1961," National Research Council Division of Medical Sciences Collection (1946–1973), National Academy of Sciences Archive.

62. Ibid.

63. Robert S. Ledley interview with author Feb. 14, 2006.

64. J. S. Barlow and M. A. Brazier, MIT Technical Report 351.

65. John S. Barlow to Robert S. Ledley, Jan. 30, 1961, file: "Com. on Uses of Electronic Computers in Biological and Medical Sciences: Ad hoc. 1960–1961," National Research Council Division of Medical Sciences Collection (1946–1973), National Academy of Sciences Archive.

66. Ledley, "Medical Informatics: A Personal View of Sowing the Seeds," 94.

67. Ledley in Robert S. Ledley and Joseph A. November, "A Lifetime of Biomedical Computing: A Conversation with Robert S. Ledley," Feb. 21, 2008, NIH Public Lecture.

68. Bruce Waxman, "Planting the Seeds: A Panel Discussion," in eds. Bruce I. Blum and Karen Duncan, *A History of Medical Informatics: Proceedings of Association for Computing Machinery Conference on History of Medical Informatics* (New York: ACM Press, 1990), 64. Waxman noted, "We were fortunate enough not to have realized that was the game plan, and we wound up spending 50 or 60 million dollars over five years."

69. Lusted, "Some Roots of Clinical Decision Making," 386. Lusted awards Shannon much credit for the development of biomedical computing: "In my opinion, [Shannon] is responsible, in large part, for stimulating the growth of biomedical computing in the United States, an effort which enabled scientists and clinicians in the 1960s and 1970s to provide worldwide leadership in the development of biomedical computing and computing aids to medical diagnosis, a development that led to medical informatics." Shannon also routed some of the funds to Frederick Brackett, for building space and equipment for his Mathematical Research Branch, and to promote computer use among researchers based at NIH. The MRB still exists today as part of the NIH's Center for Information Technology, specializing in mathematical modeling.

70. Ibid., 388–89.

71. Robert S. Ledley interview with author Dec. 19, 2007. When asked why he focused most of his attention on the NBRF in 1960, rather than lead the NIH effort, Ledley responded, "I was having too much fun!"

72. Lusted, "Some Roots of Clinical Decision Making," 388.

73. Ibid.

74. Ibid., 391.

75. Lee B. Lusted, "Quantification in the Life Sciences," *IRE Transactions on Bio-Medical Electronics* 9 (Jan. 1962): 1.

76. Lee B. Lusted, "The Development of National Biomedical Computing Capability," 3.

77. Lusted, "Quantification in the Life Sciences," 1. Lusted was quoting Ralph. W. Gerard, "Quantification in Biology," *Isis* 52, no. 2 (June 1961): 334–35.

78. Lusted, "Quantification in the Life Sciences," 1. Lusted qtd. in Thomas. S. Kuhn, "The Function of Measurement in Modern Physical Science," *Isis* 52, no. 2 (June 1961): 190.

79. Lusted, "Quantification in the Life Sciences," 1. Lusted qtd. in T. S. Kuhn, "The Function of Measurement in Modern Physical Science," 160.

80. Lusted, "Quantification in the Life Sciences," 2.

81. Ibid., 1.

82. Lusted, "The Development of National Biomedical Computing Capability," 6–7.

83. Ibid., 7. Lusted pointed to Chauncey D. Leake's AAAS talk, "Standards and Nursery Rhymes," as the inspiration for his view that the standards themselves held little value.

84. Ibid., 5.

85. Ibid., 7.

86. Lusted, "Quantification in the Life Sciences," 2.

87. Ibid., 3. Lusted envisioned a network of computers, that could "hardly compare in complexity" to the computer systems at the heart of the control center in the Sky Shield II exercises of October 1961.

88. Raub, "The Life Sciences Computer Resources Program of the National Institutes of Health," 694.

89. Lusted, "The Development of National Biomedical Computing Capability," 5.

90. Lee B. Lusted, "Guidelines for the National Institutes of Health Support of Biomedical Computing: Final Report to the Director, National Institutes of Health, by the Advisory Committee on Computers in Research," Mar. 31, 1964, 14. LINC Collection, MIT Museum. All subsequent references are to this report.

91. Ledley, "Biomedical Computer and Biomathematics Research Center," Application for Research Grant, National Institutes of Health, B-RG-2075 (formerly RG 7323), Nov. 1, 1959, 26. Robert S. Ledley Papers, National Biomedical Research Foundation.

92. Lusted, "The Development of National Biomedical Computing Capability," 4.

93. Fay M. Hemphill and James A. Shannon, "Medical Research Potentials in the Light of Modern Data Processing," *Proceedings of the 3rd IBM Medical Symposium* (Endicott, NY: IBM, 1961): 18.

94. Hemphill and Shannon, "Medical Research Potentials in the Light of Modern Data Processing," 17. Hemphill and Shannon pointed to the following influential figures as "staunch proponents of instrumentation centers": Francis Schmitt, Paul Klopsteg, Stanhope Bayne-Jones, Sidney Farber, Howard Rusk, William Kubicek, Vladimir Zworykin, Boisfeuillet Jones Sr., Senators Lister Hill and Hubert Humphrey, and Representative John Fogarty.

95. "The First Problem . . . When to Use Machines?," *Journal of the American Medical Association*, 196, no. 2 (Apr. 11, 1966): 32.

96. Waxman, "Planting the Seeds: A Panel Discussion," 27.

97. Timothy Lenoir, "Shaping Biomedicine as an Information Science," in *Proceedings of the 1998 Conference on the History and Heritage of Science Information Systems*, ed. Mary Ellen Bowden et al. (Medford, NJ: Information Today, 1999), 28.

98. Maxine Rockoff, obituary of Bruce Waxman, 1998, personal papers of Maxine Rockoff. As George Malindzak put it to Rockoff: "The real impact of [Waxman's] program was that within each of our laboratories and research institutions, we spawned a whole generation of young scientists and colleagues who began looking at science in a completely different way. The computer was now more friendly and approachable, and the LINC's analog-to-digital conversion feature permitted the first realistic on-line digital processing of analog biological data in biomedical research facilities outside the MIT area."

99. Homer R. Warner, "History of Medical Informatics at Utah," in *A History of*

Medical Informatics: Proceedings of Association for Computing Machinery Conference on History of Medical Informatics, eds. Bruce I. Blum and Karen Duncan (New York: ACM Press, 1990), 361. Warner made this comment in Nov. 1987, during the heyday of North's cultural notoriety.

100. Wesley Clark, "The LINC Was Early and Small," in *A History of Personal Workstations*, ed. Adele Goldberg (New York: ACM Press, 1988), 370.

101. Paul Castleman, "Medical Application of Computers at BBN," *IEEE Annals of the History of Computing* 28, no. 1 (2006): 9.

102. Hunter Crowther-Heyck, *Herbert Simon: The Bounds of Reason in Modern America* (Baltimore: Johns Hopkins University Press, 2005), 260. Crowther-Heyck contends that with the NIH money Simon and Newell grew more bold, envisioning the computerization of a broad swath of Carnegie psychology research. Simon, for instance, claimed that " 'information processing models tend to be models of an individual' and that therefore 'a common bond of concern with the individual ties clinical work and simulation together.' " Crowther-Heyck acknowledges that Simon's claim was to a degree "grant-swinging rhetoric," but he argues that "Simon and Newell had repeatedly found in their work [that] computer simulation techniques had strong implications for experimental design."

103. One applicant for NIH support, R. Wade Cole of Stanford University, summed up what he believed were the NIH's five criteria for selecting a computing project to fund: "1) High-quality institution; 2) Large volume of good research output; 3) More research, less clinical practice; 4) More than one field of interest must be involved; 5) Within applying institution, investigations must be super-departmental." These criteria were indeed roughly consistent with the ACCR's preferences, which were not documented. R. Wade Cole, memorandum, "NIH News," 23 January 1963, file 2, box 1, ACME Collection (SC 236), Stanford University Archives.

104. Martin H. Weik, *A Fourth Survey of Domestic Electronic Digital Computing Systems*, Ballistic Research Laboratories Report No. 1227 (Aberdeen, MD: BRL,1964), 162. Ed Thelen, "IBM 7040," http://ed-thelen.org/comp-hist/BRL64-i.html, accessed Dec. 20, 2010.

105. IBM, "7090 Data Processing System," technical fact sheet distributed on Oct. 4, 1960, IBM Archives, www-03.ibm.com/ibm/history/exhibits/mainframe/mainframe_PP7090.html, accessed Jan. 18, 2010.

106. Ceruzzi, *A History of Modern Computing* (Cambridge, MA: MIT Press, 2003), 71.

107. Ledley, "Biomedical Computer and Biomathematics Research Center," 29.

108. Martin H. Weik, *A Third Survey of Domestic Electronic Digital Computing Systems*, Ballistic Research Laboratories Report No. 1115 (Aberdeen, MD: BRL, 1961), 527–29. Ed Thelen, "IBM 1401 Data Processing System," http://ed-thelen.org/comp-hist/BRL61-ibm1401.html, accessed Jan. 18, 2010.

109. Robert Ledley, "Planting the Seeds: A Panel Discussion," in *A History of Medical Informatics: Proceedings of Association for Computing Machinery Conference on History of Medical Informatics*, ed. Bruce I. Blum and Karen Duncan (New York: ACM Press, 1990), 61.

110. Wilfrid J. Dixon and Patricia M. Britt, "Health Sciences Computing Facility, University of California, Los Angeles, 1959–1979," in *A History of Medical Informatics: Proceedings of Association for Computing Machinery Conference on History of Medical Informatics*, ed. Bruce I. Blum and Karen Duncan (New York: ACM Press, 1990), 78.

111. Ibid., 76.

112. Wilfrid Dixon, "Planting the Seeds: A Panel Discussion," in eds. Bruce I. Blum and Karen Duncan, *A History of Medical Informatics: Proceedings of Association for Computing Machinery Conference on History of Medical Informatics* (New York: ACM Press, 1990), 55. Today, the package has been renamed as Statistical Product and Service Solutions in order to appeal to a broader market. Generally, however, it is referred to simply as SPSS.

113. Thelma Estrin, "The UCLA Brain Research Institute Data Processing Laboratory," in *A History of Medical Informatics: Proceedings of Association for Computing Machinery Conference on History of Medical Informatics*, ed. Bruce I. Blum and Karen Duncan (New York: ACM Press, 1990), 158. Adey studied how organisms reacted to electromagnetic radiation, and is today known for recently leading a campaign to raise public awareness of what he believes are the health risks of using cell phones. His earlier work on "mind-altering radio waves" and "electromagnetic behavior control" has frequently been cited by elements of the counterculture.

114. Ibid., 158–59.

115. Estrin herself has a history worthy of further study. As one of the very few female electrical engineers trained in the late 1940s, she found entry into the traditionally exclusively male domain difficult, and wound up supporting her husband's (Gerald Estrin) computer work at the Institute for Advanced Study, in Princeton, NJ. There she helped build the Johnniac and became interested in neurophysiology. During the early 1950s she befriended John von Neumann, who "always queried me about the status of my EEG research. Johnny's interest in the brain stemmed from his interest in automata" ("The UCLA Brain Research Institute Data Processing Laboratory," 157). In 1954, she went to Israel's Weizmann Institute of Science, where she built another Johnniac. Still unable to find employment in the United States despite her exceptional qualifications, she followed her husband to UCLA, eventually working for Brazier at the BRI.

116. Ibid., 159.

117. Ibid., 160.

118. This project was also supported by NASA and the USAF.

119. Mary A. B. Brazier, "The Electrical Activity of the Nervous System," *Science* 146 (Dec. 11, 1964): 1423.

120. Ibid., 1428.

121. Dixon, "Planting the Seeds: A Panel Discussion," 54.

122. Max A. Woodbury, "The Impact of Biological Computing," in *Data Acquisition and Processing in Biology and Medicine: Proceedings of the 1963 Rochester Conference*, ed. Kurt Enslein (New York: Pergamon Press, 1964), 9.

123. Weik, *A Third Survey of Domestic Electronic Digital Computing Systems*, 536–37.

124. Ibid.

125. Control Data Corporation, "Control Data 160-A Computer" sales brochure (Minneapolis, MN: CDC, 1963), Computer History Museum Archive, http://archive .computerhistory.org/resources/text/CDC/CDC.160A.1962.102646114.pdf, accessed Dec. 20, 2010.

126. Wesley A. Clark, "Data Processing Aspects of Biomedical Computing Centers," Lincoln Laboratory Report C.13.3, Nov. 22, 1961. Wesley Clark, Personal Collection.

127. Bonnie Kaplan, "The Computer Prescription: Medical Computing, Public Policy, and Views of History," *Science, Technology, & Human Values* 20, no. 1 (Winter 1995): 30.

128. Homer R. Warner et al., "A mathematical approach to medical diagnosis. Appli-

cation to congenital heart disease." *Journal of the American Medical Association*, 177 (1961): 183.

129. Edward A. Feigenbaum interview with author June 20, 2004.

130. Peter Wortsman, "Donald A. B. Lindberg: A Digital Pioneer at the National Library of Medicine," *Journal of the College of Physicians and Surgeons of Columbia University* 18, no. 3 (Fall 1998), www.cumc.columbia.edu/news/journal/journal-o/archives/jour_v18no3/profile.html, accessed Dec. 20, 2009.

131. Helen H. Gee, "Organization and Influence in Biomedical Computing," Proceedings of Journées d'Informatique Médicale / Days for Medical Information (Rocquencourt, 1970), 440.

132. Ibid., 439.

133. Helen Hofer Gee, "Session I—Computer Applications I: Rapporteur's Summary," *Computers in Life Science Research*, eds. William Siler and Donald A. B. Lindberg (Bethesda, MD: FASEB, 1975), 43.

134. Raub, "The Life Sciences Computer Resources Program of the National Institutes of Health," 694.

135. "The First Problem . . . When to Use Machines?," *Journal of the American Medical Association*, 32.

136. Raub, "The Life Sciences Computer Resources Program of the National Institutes of Health," 694. Emphasis in original.

137. Division of Research Facilities and Resources (DRFR), *Special Research Resources for the Biomedical Sciences* (Bethesda, MD: NIH, 1965), 9, ACME Collection (SC 236 box 1, file 9), Stanford University. The DRFR stated, "The principal goal of the special research resources program . . . is to provide grants for such large-scale, specialized or unusual resources." Subsequent references are to this report.

138. William Yamamoto, "Planting the Seeds: A Panel Discussion," in eds. Bruce I. Blum and Karen Duncan, *A History of Medical Informatics: Proceedings of Association for Computing Machinery Conference on History of Medical Informatics* (New York: ACM Press, 1990), 66.

139. Castleman et al., "The implementation of the PROPHET system," *Proceedings of the May 6–10, 1974 National Computer Conference and Exposition* (New York: AFIPS/ACM, 1974), 457. By the mid-1970s, PROPHET had evolved to what historian Eric Francoeur describes as "a time-shared, interactive, graphics-oriented database-management system for laboratory and clinical scientists studying the relationship between molecular structure and biological function." (Eric Francoeur, "Cyrus Levinthal, the Kluge and the origins of interactive molecular graphics," *Endeavour* 26, no. 4 (Dec. 2002): 130.

140. Raub, "The Life Sciences Computer Resources Program of the National Institutes of Health," 699.

141. Morris Frank Collen, *A History of Medical Informatics in the United States* (Bethesda, MD: American Medical Informatics Association, 1995), 59.

142. Gee, "Organization and Influence in Biomedical Computing," 446.

143. Ibid. In more recent and prosperous decades, the DRFR's successor, the NCRR, has spent hundreds of millions of dollars establishing informatics centers for biomedical research.

144. Waxman, "Planting the Seeds: A Panel Discussion," 66.

145. Ibid., 64. By way of example, Waxman cited (among others) many of the projects discussed in this book: Dixon's statistical software packages, the development of the

LINC, Robert Ledley's and Jerome Cox's imaging work, computerized hospital management and medical diagnosis, and Hubert Pipberger and Caesar Cacerces's work on processing EKG signals.

146. Bruce D. Waxman, *The Venusian Conundrum* (Huntington, WV: University Editions, 1997), 98. The novel is set in the late 1990s and is ostensibly about former President Jimmy Carter's efforts to organize a Manhattan Project–like response to the imminent destruction of civilization by several large asteroids.

147. Bruce D. Waxman, "Planting the Seeds: Personal Observations," in eds. Bruce I. Blum and Karen Duncan, *A History of Medical Informatics: Proceedings of Association for Computing Machinery Conference on History of Medical Informatics* (New York: ACM Press, 1990), 115.

148. Waxman, *The Venusian Conundrum*, 97. To this, Waxman's protagonist adds, "I'm mad as hell that our medical-heath care system is so greed-ridden and our national biomedical research establishment so unaccomplished and undirected as to have produced little of significance despite the expenditures of over $100 billion in the last three decades."

149. Ibid., 99. Waxman via his *Venusian Conundrum* protagonist described the fruit of NIH's traditional, serendipity-oriented approach to applied research as "pathetic": "The list of such largely uncontrolled diseases is well known: cancer, diabetes, sickle-cell anemia, AIDS, Alzheimer's disease, schizophrenia, heart disease. It is agonizing that so little has been accomplished despite the vast amounts of money spent by the NIH over the last three decades. If challenged, the NIH will bring out its short success list and talk about the overwhelming theoretical obstacles needed to overcome AIDS, cancer, and most other serious diseases. They will demonstrate the Alpha Helix, the description of the HIV virus and advances in the survival of some types of leukemia. An objective look at the achievements relative to the time and expenditures involved is, by any objective standard, pathetic."

150. Ibid., 97–98.

151. Ibid., 99.

152. Helen Hofer Gee, "Session I—Computer Applications I: Rapporteur's Summary," 43–44. She qualified the $100 million figure, noting, "Although this figure represents the total costs of the identified research, not just the computer costs, it commands attention."

3. The LINC Revolution

1. A concise account of these events can be found in Joe November, "LINC: Biology's Revolutionary Little Computer," *Endeavour* 28, no. 3 (2004): 125–31.

2. Jeffrey S. Young hailed Clark as "the most brilliant computer designer of his generation." Jeffrey S. Young, *Forbes Greatest Technology Stories: Inspiring Tales of the Entrepreneurs and Inventors who Revolutionized Modern Business* (New York: John Wiley & Sons, 1998), 318. In an interview with the author on June 26, 2004, Clark qualified Young's description by remarking that "generations are very short."

3. Wesley A. Clark, "The LINC Was Early and Small," in *A History of Personal Workstations*, ed. Adele Goldberg (New York: ACM Press, 1988), 350.

4. Wesley Clark interview with author June 26, 2004.

5. For a general description of Simon see Edmund C. Berkeley, *Giant Brains, or Machines That Think* (New York: John Wiley & Sons, 1949).

6. Clark, "The LINC Was Early and Small," 350. Clark meant not that the possibilities were fewer or of less importance, but that there were great possibilities in small-scale computing.

7. Wesley Clark correspondence to Personnel Director, Digital Computer Laboratory, Lincoln Laboratory Application, Oct. 31, 1951. Wesley Clark, Personal Collection.

8. Wesley Clark interview with author June 26, 2004.

9. Clark, "The LINC Was Early and Small," 350.

10. "Batch processing" is anachronistic in this case. The term originated in the 1950s when users entered programs on punch cards. Users would give a "batch" of these programmed cards to the system operator, who would input them into the computer.

11. Young, *Forbes Greatest Technology Stories*, 318.

12. Charles E. Molnar, Charles E. and Wesley A. Clark, "Development of the LINC," in *A History of Medical Informatics: Proceedings of Association for Computing Machinery Conference on History of Medical Informatics*, ed. Bruce I. Blum and Karen Duncan (New York: ACM Press, 1990), 122.

13. Young, *Forbes Greatest Technology Stories*, 93. Young notes that Whirlwind was referred to as "Forrester's Folly" and "Forrester's Private Pyramid" by those who saw it as an extravagance.

14. The common wire provided half the charge while the individual wires provided the remaining charge necessary to change the direction in which the core was magnetized.

15. Clark, "The LINC Was Early and Small," 350. Clark called the programming "a primitive affair carried out with the aid of heavily ruled coding forms on which to write out absolute-address instructions and octal instructions."

16. Wesley Clark correspondence to Personnel Director, Digital Computer Laboratory, Lincoln Laboratory Application, Oct. 31, 1951. Wesley Clark, Personal Collection.

17. Atsushi Akera, *Calculating a Natural World: Engineers, and Computers During the Rise of U.S. Cold War Research* (Cambridge, MA: MIT Press, 2007), 192.

18. The time slots were fifteen minutes because Whirlwind's storage tubes could not hold onto information for more than fifteen minutes.

19. Young, *Forbes Greatest Technology Stories*, 98.

20. Mitchell Waldrop compares using Whirlwind to using a late 1970s TRS-80 microcomputer.

21. Clark recalls that the MTC, while drastically miniaturized relative to Whirlwind, still had enough electricity flowing through it that it interfered with local radio reception while in operation: "In those pre-regulation days you could tune a radio to frequencies being broadcast by the MTC's open-wire bus and hear the test program running—or trying to run—from several city blocks away. Sometimes when approaching by automobile for an extra-long simulation run in the dead of night the signal was clear enough for a decision to turn back home if things weren't going well" ("The LINC Was Early and Small," 354).

22. Akera, *Calculating a Natural World*, 192. Akera points to Vannevar Bush and the Servomechanisms Lab as the originators of Lincoln's encouragement of interdisciplinary collaboration.

23. The Communications Biophysics Group was known by the abbreviation CBL because everybody referred to it as a "laboratory."

24. Clark, "The LINC Was Early and Small," 350.

25. Molnar in Molnar and Clark, "Development of the LINC," 120. Lily E. Kay cast McCulloch's work as an effort to reduce the "mind" to a phenomenon of interacting binary signals: "From McCulloch's 'experimental epistemology,' the mind—purposes and ideas—emerged out of the regularities of neuronal interactions, or nets. That science of the mind thus became a science of signals based on binary logic with clearly defined units of perception and precise rules of formation and transformation for representing mental states." Unifying physical and mental were neural nets—as Kay put it, "aimed at bridging the gulch between body and mind (matter and form) and the technical gulf between things man-made and things begotten, neural nets also laid the foundation for the field of artificial intelligence." Lily E. Kay, "From logical neurons to poetic embodiments of mind: Warren S. McCulloch's project in neuroscience," *Science in Context* 14, no. 4 (2001): 591.

26. John S. Barlow, "The Early History of EEG Data-Processing at the Massachusetts Institute of Technology and the Massachusetts General Hospital," *International Journal of Psychophysiology* 26 (1997): 447.

27. Molnar in Molnar and Clark, "Development of the LINC," 120.

28. Barlow, "The Early History of EEG Data-Processing," 444.

29. Y. W. Lee et al., "Application of Correlation Analysis to the Detection of Periodic Signals in Noise," *Proceedings of the IRE* 38 (1950): 1166.

30. Barlow, "The Early History of EEG Data-Processing," 449.

31. Ibid., 450.

32. John Barlow, Nelson Y.S. Kiang, Ishmael Stefanov-Wagner, and David Steffens interview with author Feb. 5, 2004. Barlow noted in the interview that CBL was not supposed to know anything about Whirlwind or MTC, which were both classified, but went on to state, "People at Lincoln bragged to RLE people who bragged to us."

33. For a detailed introduction to MCP neurons, see the website hosted by The Mind Project (Illinois State University), www.mind.ilstu.edu/curriculum/modOverview .php?modGUI=212, accessed July 25, 2011.

34. Nelson Kiang interview with author Feb. 5, 2004. Clark confirmed his enthusiasm for Kiang's scheme in the June 20, 2004, interview with the author.

35. Belmont G. Farley and Wesley A. Clark, "Simulation of self-organizing systems by digital computer," *I.R.E. Transactions on Information Theory* 4 (1954): 76.

36. According to Clark (conversation with author Apr. 9, 2008), Farley was inspired by the writing and lectures of Canadian psychologist Donald Olding Hebb (1904–1985).

37. Clark, "The LINC Was Early and Small," 354.

38. Wesley A. Clark, "Design Considerations for an Experimental Computer," Lincoln Lab memo 6M-3536, 1955. Wesley Clark, Personal Collection.

39. Clark and Olsen used Motorola hearing-aid transistors (eighty dollars apiece) in their design. It should be noted that in the TX series of computers the transistors and circuits were not integrated as they are in laptop and desktop computers today.

40. Sixteen bits were required for address information, leaving only 2 bits for instructions, which raises the question: "How do you build a sensible machine code with just two bits?" Jack Dennis, who worked for Clark and who went on to become a founder of the MULTICS project, supplied the answer: (1) You must be able to store information into memory locations; (2) You must be able to get information out of the memory, so one can operate on it in the central processing unit. The TX-0 does not have an instruction

code "load." In the TX-0, one got information into the accumulator by clearing the accumulator and then executing an "add" instruction; (3) The third instruction of the TX-0 was transfer negative: transfer control to the location specified by the address; (4) The operate instruction was next. Anything not done by the other three kinds of instructions was done by operate instructions. The remaining 16 bits instead of referring to a memory location were simply a micro-coded extension of the operation code. One combination would cause a point to be displayed on the cathode ray tube (CRT) whose coordinates were the right half of the accumulator and the left half of the accumulator. In the same instruction you could transform the contents of the accumulator so that it would cause (on the next repetition of instruction) a different point to be plotted on the CRT. Jack Dennis, "The TX-0 at MIT," *The Computer Museum Report* 8 (1984), www.bitsavers.org/pdf/mit/tx-0/TX-0_history_1984.txt, accessed July 25, 2011.

41. Gwen Bell, "The TX-0 at the Lincoln Labs," *The Computer Museum Report* 8 (Spring 1984), http://ed-thelen.org/comp-hist/TheCompMusRep/TCMR-V08.html#Past, accessed Jan. 19, 2010. Bell quoted Gilmore directly. Clark noted that Hark was named for a character in James Thurber's children's fantasy novel *The 13 Clocks* (1950).

42. Clark, "The LINC Was Early and Small," 357.

43. John T. Gilmore, "Retrospectives II, The Early Years in Computer Graphics at MIT, Lincoln Lab, and Harvard," International Conference on Computer Graphics and Interactive Techniques, Boston, July 31–Aug. 4, 1989. Reprinted in *ACM SIGGRAPH '89 Panel Proceedings* 336 (New York: ACM Press, 1989), 44.

44. Belmont G. Farley et al. "Computer Techniques for the Study of Patterns in the Electroencephalogram," Lincoln Laboratory Technical Report No. 165 (Nov. 6, 1957), 2–4.

45. John T. Gilmore, "Retrospectives II," 44. The original paper describing the "Moving Window Display Program" is: B. G. Farley et al., Group 63 Report #165, N 6 Nov. 1957.

46. Gilmore, "Retrospectives II," 43–44.

47. Ivan Sutherland, who was then an electrical engineering graduate student at MIT, was particularly captivated by the interactive aspect of the TX-2's CRT display, and dedicated several years to developing Sketchpad, a system that displayed drawings that the user could stretch, bend, and otherwise manipulate in real time. Sketchpad inspired much of Douglas Engelbart's work with computer graphics in the 1960s, and was the basis for many of the graphical programs that became important to the development of GUIs in the 1970s as well as the CAD (Computer-Aided Design) programs that appeared in more recent decades.

48. Severo M. Ornstein, *Computing in the Middle Ages: A View from the Trenches 1955–1983* (Bloomington, IN: 1st books Library, 2002), 82. Severo Ornstein is the son of "ultra-modernist" composer Leo Ornstein (1892–2002). He is also a son-in-law of mathematician Derrick Henry Lehmer (1905–1991).

49. Ibid. Ornstein recalls believing Clark had "gone too far" in one late 1950s Lincoln Lab lecture, during which Clark envisioned a computer as "something that would one day perhaps just be painted onto any handy surface."

50. M. Mitchell Waldrop, *The Dream Machine: J. C. R. Licklider and the Revolution That Made Computing Personal* (New York: Viking, 2001), 141. There is a popular misunderstanding that Wesley Clark and J. C. R. Licklider collaborated extensively on research

in the late 1950s. At the time, Licklider coauthored papers with Weldon Clark, not Wesley Clark.

51. Ibid., 147. Emphasis in original.

52. Ibid., 148.

53. J. C. R. Licklider, "Man-Computer Symbiosis," *IRE Transactions on Human Factors in Electronics* HFE-1 (Mar. 1960): 6–7. Clark remarked during a 2008 conversation with the author that Licklider, a trained psychologist, should have been aware of the importance of images to thinking. Clark also wondered why Licklider shunned graphical computers.

54. Waldrop, *The Dream Machine*, 149.

55. Molnar in Molnar and Clark, "Development of the LINC," 119. Molnar recalled in 1990 that his notion was reinforced in 1956 when he read Norbert Wiener's book, *Cybernetics: Or Control and Communication in the Animal and the Machine*.

56. Ibid. Molnar noted, "Wes Clark . . . frustrated me severely by refusing to tell me what to do. It took me all summer to get the message; I painfully began to acquire the habit of deciding for myself."

57. Clark, "The LINC Was Early and Small," 357.

58. Nelson Kiang interview with author Feb. 5, 2004. Kiang came up with the name ARC.

59. W. A. Clark et al., "The Average Response Computer (ARC): A Digital Device for Computing Average and Amplitude and Time Histograms of Electrophysiological Response," *IRE Transactions on Bio-Medical Electronics* 35 (1961): 46–47.

60. Clark, "The LINC Was Early and Small," 359. An inspection of the ARC by MIT Museum Curator Deborah Douglas reveals that while it was not aesthetically pleasing the ARC's case was professionally crafted out of the best available material and that considerable care had gone into ensuring that the machine looked more like a laboratory appliance than computer cobbled together for the CBL. Douglas pointed to the attention given to rounding edges and corners, and the stylish, embedded handles on the machine's panel doors. Clark's other machines lacked this degree of polish.

61. W. A. Clark et al., "The Average Response Computer," 49.

62. Clark, "The LINC Was Early and Small," 359.

63. W.A. Clark, "Digital Techniques in Neuro-electric Data Processing," In *Computer Techniques in EEG Analysis*, ed. Mary A.B. Brazier, *EEG J.* supplement 20 (Elsevier, 1961), n.p.

64. Ibid.

65. Donna Molnar interview with author June 10, 2004.

66. Ornstein, *Computing in the Middle Ages*, 93.

67. John McCarthy, "Reminiscences on the History of Time Sharing," 1983, www-formal.stanford.edu/jmc/history/timesharing/timesharing.html, accessed Dec. 22, 2010. McCarthy noted: "The major technical error of my 1959 ideas was an underestimation of the computer capacity required for time-sharing. I still don't understand where all the computer time goes in time-sharing installations, and neither does anyone else."

68. When Minsky was asked, MAC stood for "Machine Aided Cognition." Others contend that MAC stands for "Multiple Access Computer" or "Man And Computer."

69. Ronda Hauben, "Cybernetics, Time-sharing, Human-Computer Symbiosis and On-line Communities: Creating a Supercommunity of On-line Communities," in *Netizens: An Anthology*, eds. Michael Hauben and Ronda Hauben (New York: Columbia Uni-

versity, 1996), www.columbia.edu/~rh120/ch106.x06/, accessed July 25, 2011. Hauben adds: "Corbato describes how CTSS (Compatible Time-Sharing System), as the time-sharing system he was working on was called, couldn't go into operation until the transistorized IBM 7090 hardware had arrived and could be used in early spring of 1962. Only then could they begin to deal with the real problems to make a working system."

70. Clark, "The LINC Was Early and Small," 358. Clark maintains his opposition to time-sharing but acknowledges that it has "resulted in a huge and productive impetus to computer science at a critical time."

71. Thierry Bardini, *Bootstrapping: Douglas Engelbart, Coevolution, and the Origins of Personal Computing* (Stanford: Stanford University Press, 2000), 31. Throughout the 1960s Engelbart was marginalized for his opposition to timesharing.

72. Hauben, "Cybernetics, Time-sharing, Human-Computer Symbiosis and On-line Communities," www.columbia.edu/~rh120/ch106.x06, accessed July 25, 2011.

73. Clark recalled in an April 9, 2008, conversation with the author that Teager also objected to the committee's decision, but on the grounds that they were not implementing time-sharing rapidly or extensively enough.

74. Clark, panel discussion comments on "The LINC Was Early and Small," as quoted in Goldberg, ed., *A History of the Personal Workstation*, 402.

75. Clark, "The LINC Was Early and Small," 358.

76. Wesley Clark interview with Judy O'Neill May 3, 1990, Charles Babbage Institute, University of Minnesota. Thierry Bardini notes that Douglas Engelbart objected to time-sharing for many of the same reasons as Clark. Clark's position, Bardini claims, "is very close to Engelbart's criticism of the way people become subservient to a big technological system like a steamship or locomotive, instead of being given their autonomy." Engelbart, now best known for inventing the computer mouse, received only grudgingly-given funding from Licklider, and was marginalized during the 1960s because of his objections to timesharing. (*Bootstrapping*, 31.)

77. Clark, "The LINC Was Early and Small," 358.

78. Clark remarked to the author in June 2004 that there was no personal animosity between the two men.

79. J. C. R. Licklider, "Man-Computer Symbiosis," 8.

80. Ibid.

81. J. C. R. Licklider, "Some Reflections on Early History," in ed. Adele Goldberg, *A History of the Personal Workstation*, 118.

82. Waldrop, *The Dream Machine*, 203.

83. Wesley A. Clark, "Data Processing Aspects of Biomedical Computing Centers," Lincoln Laboratory Report C.13.3, Nov. 22, 1961. In author's possession. All subsequent references are to this report.

84. Clark's understanding of computer use at MIT was based on MIT Semi Annual Report No. 8 (Jan. 1961).

85. Lusted, "Guidelines for the National Institutes of Health Support of Biomedical Computing : Final Report to the Director, National Institutes of Health, by the Advisory Committee on Computers in Research," Mar. 31, 1964, 16. LINC Collection, MIT Museum.

86. Max A. Woodbury, "The Impact of Biological Computing," in *Data Acquisition and Processing in Biology and Medicine: Proceedings of the 1963 Rochester Conference*, ed. Kurt Enslein (New York: Pergamon Press, 1964), 7.

87. Ornstein, *Computing in the Middle Ages*, 97.

88. Wesley A. Clark and Charles E. Molnar, "A Description of the LINC," in *Computers in Biomedical Research*, ed. Ralph W. Stacy and Bruce D. Waxman (New York: Academic Press, 1965), 2:38.

89. Ibid. All five points have been quoted in the order in which they originally appeared.

90. Clark, "The LINC Was Early and Small," 360.

91. Ibid., 361.

92. Clark and Molnar, "A Description of the LINC," 38.

93. Molnar in Molnar and Clark, "Development of the LINC," 136.

94. Clark and Molnar, "A Description of the LINC," 47.

95. Clark, "The LINC Was Early and Small," 363.

96. This was inspired by Clark's use of a radio to listen in on the MTC.

97. Clark and Molnar, "A Description of the LINC," 51–53.

98. Ornstein, *Computing in the Middle Ages*, 112.

99. Waldrop, *The Dream Machine*, 262.

100. Clark, "The LINC Was Early and Small," 367. Clark notes that at the question-and-answer session immediately following his and Molnar's presentation of the Linc, the enthusiasm among audience members was not apparent. The only question they received pertained to the durability of wiring insulation.

101. Samuel A. Rosenfeld, "Laboratory Instrument Computer (LINC): The Genesis of a Technological Revolution," Seminar in Celebration of the Twentieth Anniversary of the LINC Computer (Bethesda: National Institutes of Health, 1983), 4, http://history.nih.gov/exhibits/linc/index.html, accessed Dec. 22, 2010. Several interviews revealed that Clark's ashtray demonstration appealed to the many biomedical researchers who, despite the known dangers, nevertheless smoked regularly. Some of the LINCs built by DEC in the mid 1960s indeed came with ashtrays installed.

102. Nelson Yuan-Sheng Kiang, *Discharge Patterns of Single Fibers in the Cat's Auditory Nerve* (Cambridge, MA: MIT Press, 1965), 3–6.

103. Charles Molnar, personal notebook, duplication in author's possession. This notebook was partially copied in an appendix to Molnar and Clark, "Development of the LINC." Donna Molnar loaned me the original in June 2004.

104. Rosenfeld, "Laboratory Instrument Computer (LINC): The Genesis of a Technological Revolution," 4.

105. Years later, Bill Simon wrote a program to find signals in exponentially decomposing systems. Clark, "The LINC Was Early and Small," 368.

106. Wesley Clark interview with author June 26, 2004.

107. Waldrop, *The Dream Machine*, 189.

108. Ornstein, *Computing in the Middle Ages*, 102.

109. Ibid., 114.

110. Waldrop, *The Dream Machine*, 190. As Waldrop colorfully put it: "So as the summer of 1962 turned into fall, Clark and his handful of visionaries were still figuratively wandering in the wilderness, looking for their promised land."

111. Waldrop casts this differently: "Lick immediately tried to snap them [the Linc group] up for BBN, of course, but without success: Clark an academic to his soul, was uncomfortable with the idea of working for a commercial firm" (*The Dream Machine*, 190).

112. Clark, "The LINC Was Early and Small," 370.

113. Ibid., Rosenfeld explains how the support was divided: "Bruce Waxman was able to get about $400,000 from Fred Stone of the NIH Division of Research Facilities and Resources and had to turn elsewhere for the remainder. Since LINC was so obviously useful for neuroscientific applications, Waxman asked Philip Sapir and Louis Wienck-owski, who were administering the NIMH extramural research program, to help support an evaluation of LINC's utility in the lab. Sapir, who had a history of supporting successful innovations, was enthusiastic about LINC's prospects and came up with another $300,000. Still quite a bit short, Clark suggested that Waxman contact Orr Reynolds at NASA, who had once been at the Office of Naval Research, which had supported computer development at Lincoln Lab since the days of Whirlwind, the first large defense oriented computer. Reynolds, newly appointed as director of bioscience programs at NASA, was interested in an automated biological laboratory to search for extraterrestrial life, especially on the planet Mars. He saw LINC as an opportunity to support NASA's mission. So, NASA pitched in another $700,000. The project was 'go.'" "Laboratory Instrument Computer (LINC): The Genesis of a Technological Revolution," 8.

114. "New Computing Center for MIT," *NIH Record* (Jan. 1963).

115. Four other "phantom" LINCs were built. Two were used by the LINC team for development. The third was given to Keith Killam at Stanford University in what seems to have been an effort to keep Stanford involved in biomedical computing after his and George Forsythe's grant application fell through (see chap. 5). The fourth LINC was given to Nelson Kiang at the Eaton-Peabody Laboratory of Auditory Physiology as a reward for his earlier work with Clark. Kiang's LINC ended up becoming the longest-running fully operational classic LINC—it was used continuously between 1963 and 1990. It is now part of the MIT Museum's collection.

116. Rosenfeld, "Laboratory Instrument Computer (LINC): The Genesis of a Technological Revolution," 6.

117. Ornstein, *Computing in the Middle Ages*, 118.

118. Rosenfeld, "Laboratory Instrument Computer (LINC): The Genesis of a Technological Revolution," 6.

119. Wesley Clark interview with author June 26, 2004.

120. Ornstein, *Computing in the Middle Ages*, 119.

121. By 1965, Clark brought the price of the "classic LINC" down to about $32,000.

122. Ledley, "Digital Electronic Computers in Biomedical Science," *Science* 130 (Nov. 6, 1959): 1225–34.

123. Clark in Molnar and Clark, "Development of the LINC," 130.

124. Clark, "The LINC Was Early and Small," 370. From the biologists' perspective, bringing golf clubs to the LINC Summer may not have indicated a lack of seriousness about the endeavor of learning to use computers. As Philip J. Pauly notes, biologists maintained a tradition of mixing research and recreation during summer months. In the case of the Woods Hole resort on Cape Cod, this mixture was quite productive: "Scientists associated with the Woods Hole summer colony produced research of major significance. The cell lineage studies of the 1890s formed one of the first instances of an independent and conceptually fruitful tradition of American laboratory science. Interest in experimental embryology led by the end of the century to Jacques Loeb's spectacular invention of artificial parthenogenesis, and, in the years prior to World War I, to Frank Lillie's creation of the foundations for modern understanding of sexual reproduction.

Cytologists such as E. B. Wilson and Nettie Stevens linked chromosomal mechanics to the phenomena of Mendelian heredity; T. H. Morgan's interactions with these colleagues formed the background for his work on Drosophila genetics, which earned him a Nobel Prize. Biologists associated with Woods Hole were the first group of American laboratory scientists to become international research leaders, both experimentally and theoretically; this new status became evident after 1900 as the flow of American biology students to Germany ended, and Europeans began to come to the United States for postgraduate study." Philip J. Pauly, "Summer Resort and Scientific Discipline: Woods Hole and the Structure of American Biology, 1882–1925," in *The American Development of Biology*, ed. Ronald Rainger et al. (Philadelphia: University of Pennsylvania Press, 1988), 136.

125. Clark, "The LINC Was Early and Small," 350.

126. C. Alan Boneau, "Final Report to the LINC Evaluation Program," in *Proceedings of the Final LINC Evaluation Program Meeting* (St. Louis: Computer Research Laboratory, Washington University, St. Louis, 1965), 5–9.

127. The biologists did, though, prove adept at the complex and onerous task of wiring the LINC back panels, using surgical ties to organize bundles of loose wires (Molnar and Clark, "Development of the LINC,"134).

128. Clark, "The LINC Was Early and Small," 380.

129. Molnar in Molnar and Clark, "Development of the LINC," 135.

130. Ornstein, *Computing in the Middle Ages*, 132.

131. Wesley Clark interview June 26, 2004.

132. Ornstein, *Computing in the Middle Ages*, 132.

133. Pake's research in the 1940s on nuclear magnetic resonance provided the basis for the later development of magnetic resonance imaging (MRI).

134. Ornstein, *Computing in the Middle Ages*, 132.

135. Jerome R. Cox, "Recollections on the Processing of Biomedical Signals," in eds. Bruce I. Blum and Karen Duncan, *A History of Medical Informatics* (New York: ACM Press, 1990), 98.

136. Cox explains how HAVOC led him to general-purpose computers: "I could see after building HAVOC there was an important role for computers in physiology lab. Special-purpose computers weren't going to cut it." Cox remains proud of HAVOC and points to its success as a factor in the emergence of evoked response audiology for infants—the tests that HAVOC performed are now mandatory for infants in 40 states. (Jerome Cox interview with author July 7, 2004.)

137. Ibid.

138. Ibid.

139. Ornstein, *Computing in the Middle Ages*, 135.

140. Ibid.

141. Mort Ruderman, DEC Interoffice Memorandum, July 15, 1964, LINC-8 file, DEC Collection, Computer History Museum Archive, Mountain View, CA. The advent of inexpensive integrated circuits allowed DEC to shrink the LINC-8, both physically and in terms of cost. It sold for about $27,000.

142. Spear Microelectronics advertisement pamphlet, DEC Collection, Computer History Museum Archive, Mountain View, CA.

143. Ibid.

144. Gordon Bell, transcribed comment in Adele Goldberg, ed., *A History of the Personal Workstation*, 9–10.

145. Alan C. Kay, "How to Predict the Future," Feb. 1, 1985, D-9. Transcript in author's possession.

146. Alan C. Kay, "The Early History of Small Talk," *ACM SIGPLAN Notices* 28, no. 3 (Mar. 1993): 72. There is a consensus among the LINC users interviewed by the author that they were the earliest users of personal computers. Clark, however, never regarded the LINC as a commodity, and he did not envision a significant market for these machines beyond scientific settings.

147. Alan Kay and Adele Goldberg, "Personal Dynamic Media," *Computer* 10, no. 3 (Mar. 1977): 31.

148. Ibid., 32.

149. Wesley Clark quoted in Severo Ornstein, "The LINC: A Paradigm Shift," address to Vintage Computer Festival 10.0, Nov. 3, 2007, Digibarn Computer Museum, Boulder Creek, CA, www.digibarn.com/history/07-11-04-VCF10-LINC/index.html, accessed July 25, 2011.

4. A New Way of Life

1. G. Octo Barnett and Robert A. Greenes, "Interface Aspects of a Hospital Information System," *Annals of the New York Academy of Sciences* 161 (1969): 756.

2. David E. Clark, "Computers in Medicine," *British Medical Journal* 4, no. 5729 (Oct. 24, 1970): 241.

3. Pointing to the prevalence of the term "impact" at the NIH, Max Woodbury joked, "The most piercing twinge comes from recollection of a 'computernik' colleague speaking of 'impacting (an area) with a computer' and picturing someone with borrowed dentist's forceps having to extract the 'impacted computer' like a buried wisdom tooth so normal development could take place." Max A. Woodbury, "The Impact of Biological Computing," in *Data Acquisition and Processing in Biology and Medicine: Proceedings of the 1963 Rochester Conference*, ed. Kurt Enslein (New York: Pergamon Press, 1964), 7.

4. Ibid., 8.

5. Ibid.

6. NIH approved all but one request to keep the LINC. The exception was John C. Lilly's group at the Communication Research Institute (US Virgin Islands), which was using the computer to create a language that would allow humans and dolphins to communicate. At the time Lilly was using the LINC, he was also experimenting with psychedelic drugs and sensory deprivation tanks (which he developed), as well as drifting away more generally from mainstream science. By the late 1960s Lilly had become a major figure in countercultural circles. When the NIH reclaimed its LINC in 1966, the machine had been heavily damaged by humidity and direct contact with water (sprayed by the dolphins). In the 1980s, Lilly attempted again to synthesize a human-dolphin common language, this time using microcomputers.

7. M. Mitchell Waldop, *The Dream Machine: J. C. R. Licklider and the Revolution That Made Computing Personal* (New York: Viking, 2001), 262.

8. Jerome Cox interview with author July 7, 2004.

9. "Resolution," in *Proceedings of the Final LINC Evaluation Program Meeting* (St. Louis: Computer Research Laboratory, Washington University, 1965), 1.

10. Users of the four "phantom" LINCs were not present. This includes Nelson

Kiang et al., at the Massachusetts Eye and Ear Infirmary's Eaton-Peabody Laboratory of Auditory Physiology, as well as Keith Killam et al. at Stanford.

11. George S. Malindzak Jr. and Frederick L. Thurstone, "Studies Related to the Hydrodynamics and the Transmission Characteristics of the Arterial System," in *Proceedings of the Final LINC Evaluation Program Meeting* (St. Louis: Computer Research Laboratory, Washington University, 1965), chap. 2, 11.

12. Ibid. Specifically, Malindzak and Thurstone were trying to calculate "incident and reflected wave parameters from time and space pressure pulse data measure along the axis of the vessel."

13. Ibid., chap. 2, 10.

14. Ibid. A subroutine is a set of instructions designed to be stored in a computer's memory so that larger programs can make use of it repeatedly without its being written into the program each time it is used.

15. Ibid., chap. 2, 13.

16. Molnar in Charles E. Molnar and Wesley A. Clark, "Development of the LINC," in *A History of Medical Informatics: Proceedings of Association for Computing Machinery Conference on History of Medical Informatics*, eds. Bruce I. Blum and Karen Duncan (New York: ACM Press, 1990), 137.

17. Malindzak and Thurstone, "Studies Related to the Hydrodynamics," chap. 2, 13.

18. Ibid., chap. 2, 15.

19. Ibid., chap. 2, 15–16.

20. Ibid., chap. 3, 19–20. The third psychologist to employ an original LINC, John C. Lilly, the director of the Communication Research Institute in Miami, Florida, used the computer in a vastly different capacity: to facilitate his effort to study "the dolphin's ability to solve problems using [a] newly developed primitive language . . . [based on] a simple five-element code." (John C. Lilly, "An Experimental Investigation of the Dolphin's Communication Abilities by Means of a Dolphin Machine Code," in *Proceedings of the Final LINC Evaluation Program Meeting* (St. Louis: Computer Research Laboratory, Washington University, 1965), chap. 4, 1

21. C. George Boeree, "B.F. Skinner, 1904-1990," *Personality Theories*, http://web space.ship.edu/cgboer/skinner.html, accessed July 27, 2011.

22. Donald S. Blough and Lloyd Marlowe, "Report on Use of LINC Computer Through February, 1965, and Proposal for Its Continued Use," in *Proceedings of the Final LINC Evaluation Program Meeting* (St. Louis: Computer Research Laboratory, Washington University, 1965), chap. 3, 2.

23. Donald S. Blough, "Reinforcement of Least-frequent Inter-response Times," in *Proceedings of the Final LINC Evaluation Program Meeting* (St. Louis: Computer Research Laboratory, Washington University, 1965), chap. 3-B, 15.

24. Ibid., chap. 3-B, 14.

25. Charles P. Shimp, "Synthetic Variable-Interval Schedules of Reinforcement," *Journal of the Experimental Analysis of Behavior* 19, no. 2 (Mar. 1973): 311.

26. Blough and Marlowe, "Report on Use of LINC Computer," chap. 3, 2.

27. Ibid., chap. 3, 5.

28. Ibid.

29. Marlowe died in the late 1960s, just after receiving his psychology doctorate from Brown.

30. Blough and Marlowe, "Report on Use of LINC Computer," chap. 3, 6. In

Blough's opinion, "The arduous and no doubt uninteresting work of preparing such material might in the end be of more service than equal effort on technical matters."

31. Outline adapted from Alan C. Boneau, "Final Report to the LINC Evaluation Program," in *Proceedings of the Final LINC Evaluation Program Meeting* (St. Louis: Computer Research Laboratory, Washington University, 1965), chap. 5, 2–3.

32. Ibid., chap. 5, 3.

33. Ibid., chap. 5, 2. Once the LINC was running, the laboratory's "day" expanded to twenty-four hours.

34. Ibid., chap. 5, 10.

35. Ibid., chap. 5, 6–7.

36. Ibid., chap. 5, 8. Boneau also wanted to employ the LINC to test the "fatigue" hypothesis by pacing the pigeons: "We also intend to train pigeons to respond with different mean latency distributions to determine whether we might increase discrimination performance by forcing them to wait longer." Boneau published this finding in C. Alan Boneau, "Decision Theory, the Pigeon, and the Psychophysical Function," *Psychological Review* 74 (Mar. 1967): 123–35. In a September 1965 *Science* letter, "Color-Discrimination Performance of Pigeons: Effects of Reward," Boneau and his colleagues reported that their trials gave rise to yet more questions. They observed: "After a reward the probability that the birds would respond to light stimuli that were never rewarded was higher than before the reward was given, but paradoxically the birds showed no general decline in their ability to differentiate stimuli at wavelengths 1 millimicron [1 nanometer] apart." C. Alan Boneau et al., *Science* 149 (Sept. 1965): 1113.

37. Boneau, "Final Report to the LINC Evaluation Program," chap. 5, 7.

38. Ibid.

39. Ibid., chap. 5, 9.

40. Ibid., chap. 5, 10.

41. E. O. Attinger and A. Anne, "LINC Evaluation Program, Final Report," *Proceedings of the Final LINC Evaluation Program Meeting* (St. Louis, Computer Research Laboratory, Washington University, 1965), chap. 9, 16.

42. Joshua Lederberg and Lee Hundley, "Final Report: LINC Evaluation Program," *Proceedings of the Final LINC Evaluation Program Meeting* (St. Louis, Computer Research Laboratory, Washington University, 1965), chap. 13, 8.

43. Bernard Weiss, "LINC Evaluation Report," *Proceedings of the Final LINC Evaluation Program Meeting* (St. Louis, Computer Research Laboratory, Washington University, 1965), chap. 7, 16.

44. Fred S. Grodins and James E. Randall, "LINC Computer Evaluation for Grant FR 00146-01," *Proceedings of the Final LINC Evaluation Program Meeting* (St. Louis: Computer Research Laboratory, Washington University, 1965), chap. 8, 1.

45. Joseph E. Hind and Chris D. Geisler, "Final Report on LINC Computer Evaluation," NIH Grant MH0835401 *Proceedings of the Final LINC Evaluation Program Meeting* (St. Louis, Computer Research Laboratory, Washington University, 1965), chap. 12, 8.

46. Ibid.

47. Ibid.

48. Attinger and Anne, "LINC Evaluation Program, Final Report," chap. 9, 15.

49. Ibid., chap. 9, 16.

50. Ibid., chap. 9, 30. Anne stayed in Philadelphia until 1966, when he was recruited by Clark and Molnar to join the LINC team at Washington University.

51. Nelson Y. S. Kiang interview with author Feb. 5, 2004.

52. John F. Cook, "Lights out for the Last LINC," *RLE Currents* 6, no. 1 (Fall 1992): 24.

53. Mountcastle stated to the author in a Mar. 10, 2008, interview that "Talbot could make the computer sing."

54. Molnar in Molnar and Clark, "Development of the LINC," 136.

55. Lederberg and Lee Hundley, "Final Report: LINC Evaluation Program," chap. 13, 9.

56. "Now, what would I want with a computer in my laboratory?," DEC memorandum, 1966, LINC-8 files, DEC collection, Computer History Museum Archive, Mountain View, CA, 1. To a lesser extent, IBM also marketed computers to researchers in the life science in the mid-1960s. All subsequent references are to this memorandum.

57. DEC would offer two-week programming courses for neophyte users.

58. Spear Microelectronics advertisement pamphlet, LINC-8 files, DEC collection, Computer History Museum Archive, Mountain View, CA.

59. Ibid.

60. Morris Frank Collen, *A History of Medical Informatics in the United States* (Bethesda, MD: American Medical Informatics Association, 1995), 149–51.

61. Ibid., 164.

62. Lee B. Lusted and Robert W. Coffin, "PRIME: An Operational Model for a Hospital Automated Information System," *Proceedings of the IEEE* 57, no. 11 (Nov. 1969): 1961–73.

63. Homer Warner of the NIH's CRSS did visit Collen's screening facility in Oakland and later recommended funding, but it appears that most of the cost was borne by KP. W. Edward Hammon, "Presentation of the Morris F. Collen M.D. Medal to Dr. Morris F. Collen," *Journal of the American Medical Informatics Association* 1, no. 2 (Mar.–Apr. 1994): 202.

64. Jochen R. Moehr, "To Morris F. Collen: Happy Ninetieth!" *Journal of the American Medical Informatics Association* 10, no. 6 (Nov.–Dec. 2003): 613

65. "Enter the Robot M.D.," *Newsweek*, Oct. 3, 1966, 92.

66. Moehr, "To Morris F. Collen: Happy Ninetieth!," 613.

67. "Enter the Robot M.D.," 92.

68. Moehr, "To Morris F. Collen: Happy Ninetieth!," 614.

69. Early objections among physicians and patients to multiphasic screening are documented in Paul von Oeyen, "Opinions of Rhode Island Physicians on Automated Multiphasic Screening," *Health Service Reports* 87, no. 4 (Apr. 1972): 366–74.

70. Moehr, "To Morris F. Collen: Happy Ninetieth!," 615.

71. David E. Clark, "Computing Requirements of the Hospital and Medical School," Jan. 23, 1967, report to Medical Computing Unit, University of Manchester, box 1, folder 9, ACME Collection (SC 236) Stanford University Archives. All subsequent references are to this report. The UK was long interested in US biomedical computing; the Ministry of Health sent a team to America in Autumn 1963, but according to Clark their results were never published.

72. By Clark's reckoning, as of June 30, 1965, the NIH supported fifty-three centralized research resources; thirty-nine were computer centers. The UK trailed far behind: the only major computing unit in Britain dedicated to medical work at the time was implemented to automate hospital payroll (9).

73. Chuck Appleby, "IT Visionary: G. Octo Barnett, M.D.," *Healthcare's Most Wired Magazine*, Mar. 26, 2008.

74. G. Octo Barnett, "History of the Development of Medical Information Systems at the Laboratory of Computer Science at Massachusetts General Hospital," in *A History of Medical Informatics: Proceedings of Association for Computing Machinery Conference on History of Medical Informatics*, eds. Bruce I. Blum and Karen Duncan (New York: ACM Press, 1990), 143.

75. Robert A. Greenes, "Presentation of the Morris F. Collen Award to G. Octo Barnett, MD," *Journal of the American Medical Informatics Association* 4, no. 2 (Mar.–Apr. 1997): 155.

76. G. Octo Barnett, "Computer Applications in Medical Communication and Information Retrieval Systems as Related to the Improvement of Patient Care and the Medical Record," report to the NIH Computer Research Study Section, Division of Research Grants, Sept. 26, 1966, 4. All subsequent references are to this report.

77. Barnett, "History of the Development of Medical Information Systems," 145.

78. One example of such incompatibility could be found during the development of Lockheed's Technicon Medical Information System (TMIS) at El Camino Hospital in Mountain View, California. There, as Rachel Plotnick shows, the IBM 370 in which the system was based had to be reconfigured to allow multiple hospital staff to access and modify records in real time. Implementing this change meant (at first) removing long-term archiving functions, which were a standard part of the computer's operations in almost all other settings. Rachel Plotnick, "Computers, Systems Theory, and the Making of a Wired Hospital: A History of Technicon Medical Information System, 1964–1987," *Journal of the American Society for Information Science and Technology* 61, no. 6 (June 2010): 1285.

79. Donald A..B. Lindberg, "Commentary on G. Octo Barnett's Report to the Computer Research Study Section," *Journal of the American Medical Informatics Association* 13, no. 2 (Mar.–Apr. 2006): 137.

80. G. O. Barnett et al., "MUMPS: A Support for Medical Information Systems," *Medical Informatics* 1 (1976): 183.

81. R. A. Greenes et al., "Design and Implementation of a Clinical Data Management System," *Computers in Biomedical Research* 2 (1969): 477.

82. Collen, *A History of Medical Informatics*, 15.

83. Robert Ledley, "Preface" to National Biomedical Research Foundation, *NBR Research Accomplishments 1960–1970* (Washington, DC: NBRF, 1973), xv.

84. Helen Hofer Gee, "Session I—Computer Applications I: Rapporteur's Summary," in *Computers in Life Science Research*, ed. William Siler and Donald A. B. Lindberg (Bethesda, MD: FASEB, 1974), 43–44.

85. National Biomedical Research Foundation, *NBR Research Accomplishments 1960–1970* (Washington, DC: NBRF, 1973), 7.

86. Robert S. Ledley, "Automatic Pattern Recognition for Clinical Medicine," *Proceedings of the IEEE* 56, no. 11 (1968): 2018.

87. Ibid.

88. National Biomedical Research Foundation, *NBR Research Accomplishments 1960–1970*, 5.

89. Ledley, "Planting the Seeds: A Panel Discussion," in *A History of Medical Infor-*

matics: Proceedings of Association for Computing Machinery Conference on History of Medical Informatics, eds. Bruce I. Blum and Karen Duncan (New York: ACM Press, 1990), 94.

90. Ibid., 98.

91. Examples drawn from *Pattern Recognition* 43, no. 6 (June 2010).

92. Ledley, "Planting the Seeds: A Panel Discussion," 94.

93. Dean F. Sittig et al., "The Story Behind the Development of the First Whole-body Computerized Tomography Scanner as Told by Robert S. Ledley," *Journal of the American Medical Informatics Association* 13, no. 5 (Sept.–Oct. 2006): 467–68). Ledley recalled in 2006: "I was going to use convolution. How did I know that? Well, *Science* magazine began putting pictures on their covers in the late '60s, I think. And they had a picture of a virus. They made the picture of the cross-section of a virus, and it looked kind of interesting. They took an electron microscope, and they scanned the virus right across. And then they couldn't really rotate it, so they said it's circularly symmetric, and they did what Cormack had done . . . what they did use was [convolution]. Great! People were talking about [convolutions] because you could take scratches out of pictures and things like that. So I figured, 'That's it!' " Sittig et al., "The Story Behind the Development of the First Whole-body Computerized Tomography Scanner," 468.

94. Ibid., 467–68.

95. Bettyann H. Kevles, *Naked To The Bone: Medical Imaging in the Twentieth Century* (New York: Basic Books, 1998), 162. Oldendorf and Hounsfield shared the Albert and Mary Lasker Award in 1975, and Cormack and Hounsfield shared a Nobel Prize in 1979. In both cases the prizes were awarded to the men for independently arriving at the concepts upon which CT scanners are built.

96. Sittig et al., "The Story Behind the Development of the First Whole-body Computerized Tomography Scanner," 465.

97. Stuart S. Blume, *Insight and Industry: On the Dynamics of Technological Change in Medicine* (Cambridge, MA: MIT Press, 1992), 183, 187.

98. Margaret O. Dayhoff et al., *Atlas of Protein Sequence and Structure* (Silver Spring, MD: National Biomedical Research Foundation, 1965).

99. Margaret O. Dayhoff and George E. Kimball, "Punched Card Calculation of Resonance Energies," *Journal of Chemical Physics* 17 (1949): 706–17.

100. Margaret Dayhoff, "Molecular Resonance Energies of Organic Molecules (Computer Calculation)," Ph.D. thesis, Columbia University, 1949, www.dayhoff.cc/MODayhoff_Thesis.html, accessed July 27, 2011.

101. Ledley, "Preface" to *NBR Research Accomplishments 1960–1970*, xviii.

102. Richard V. Eck and Margaret O. Dayhoff, "Evolution of the Structure of Ferredoxin Based on Living Relics of Primitive Amino Acid Sequences," *Science* 152, no. 3720 (Apr. 15, 1966): 363.

103. Helen Hofer Gee, "Session I—Computer Applications I: Rapporteur's Summary," 43–44.

104. Bruno J. Strasser, "Collecting, Comparing, and Computing Sequences: The Making of Margaret O. Dayhoff's *Atlas of Protein Sequence and Structure*, 1954–1965," *Journal of the History of Biology* 43, no. 4 (Dec. 2010): 643.

105. To raise the profile of the *Atlas*, Ledley distributed free copies to prominent researchers in biology and medicine. (Ledley and November, "A Lifetime of Biomedical Computing: A Conversation With Robert S. Ledley," NIH Public Science Lecture, Feb. 21, 2008.)

106. Strasser, "Collecting, Comparing, and Computing Sequences," 623.

107. Bruno J. Strasser, "Genbank: Natural History in the 21st Century?" *Science* 322 (2008): 537–38.

108. Bruno J. Strasser, "The Experimenter's Museum: GenBank, Natural History, and the Moral Economies of Biomedicine," *Isis* 102, no. 1 (Mar. 2011): 82–84.

109. Strasser, "Collecting, Comparing, and Computing Sequences," 653.

110. David G. George et al., "The Protein Identification Resource (PIR)," *Nucleic Acids Research* 14, no. 1 (1986): 11–15.

5. Martians, Experts, and *Universitas*

1. UCLA and NYU both had programs in the early 1960s that enabled physiologists to store and analyze data on campus mainframes.

2. For more on Stanford during the 1940s and 1950s, see Rebecca S. Lowen, *Creating the Cold War University: The Transformation of Stanford* (Berkeley: University of California Press, 1997).

3. Eric J. Vettel, "The Protean Nature of Stanford University's Biological Sciences 1946–1972," *Historical Studies in the Physical and Biological Sciences* 35, no.1 (2004): 95–113. C. Stewart Gillmor, *Fred Terman at Stanford: Building a Discipline, a University, and Silicon Valley* (Stanford: Stanford University Press, 2004). Timothy Lenoir, "Biochemistry at Stanford: A Case Study in the Formation of an Entrepreneurial Culture," Lenoir Second Quarter Progress Report, Apr. 21, 2002, www.stanford.edu/dept/HPS/TimLenoir/Startup/QuarterlyRpts/Lenoir–StartupRptApr02.pdf, accessed Apr. 12, 2004. Timothy Lenoir, "Myths about Stanford's Interaction with Industry," http://iis-db.stanford.edu/evnts/4097/TLenoir_Myths_about_Stanford.pdf, accessed Dec. 21, 2010. Robert Kargon and W. Stuart Leslie, "Imagined Geographies: Princeton, Stanford and the Boundaries of Useful Knowledge in Postwar America," *Minerva* 32 (Summer 1994): 121–43.

4. Frederick Terman's father was Stanford cognitive psychologist Lewis Madison Terman (1877–1956). The elder Terman developed the "Terman Test" and vigorously promoted the use of the IQ test in the United States. He notably conducted several experiments pertaining to the education of gifted children. Politically, L. M. Terman was a progressive, one who fervently supported both Roosevelts.

5. Vettel, "The Protean Nature of Stanford University's Biological Sciences," 96.

6. In "Choosing the Future: The US Research Community, 1944–1946," *Historical Studies in the Physical and Biological Sciences* 25, no. 2 (1995): 301–28, Nathan Reingold shows that Vannevar Bush and Warren Weaver were in part motivated by this circumstance in their efforts to consolidate and coordinate research.

7. Vettel, "The Protean Nature of Stanford University's Biological Sciences," 96.

8. Ibid., 98–99.

9. Ibid. In "Selling Pure Science in Wartime: The Biochemical Genetics of G.W. Beadle," *Journal of the History of Biology* 22, no. 1 (1989): 73–101, Lily E. Kay points out that during the war Beadle secured federal support for his "pure" *Neurospora* research by convincing funding bodies that it had wartime applications.

10. Committee on Curriculum, Medical Council of Stanford University, "A Program of Education for Medicine at Stanford University," July 1956, 4. According to John Long Wilson, an Associate Dean at the Stanford School of Medicine from 1968 to 1984, "This Program [was] the crucial planning document of the School. . . . The Program was origi-

nally approved by the Medical Council in 1956 and subsequently modified and endorsed by President Sterling and the Board of Trustees." (Wilson, *Stanford University School of Medicine and the Predecessor Schools*, chap. 37).

11. Vettel, "The Protean Nature of Stanford University's Biological Sciences," 96.

12. Gillmor, *Fred Terman at Stanford*, 349.

13. Tim Lenoir, "Biochemistry at Stanford: A Case Study in the Formation of an Entrepreneurial Culture," *Lenoir Second Quarter Progress Report*, Apr. 21, 2002, 1, www .stanford.edu/dept/HPS/TimLenoir/Startup/QuarterlyRpts/Lenoir-StartupRptApr02 .pdf, accessed Apr. 3, 2004.

14. Ibid. Also shaping Sterling's decision to reorient the Medical School toward research was lobbying by the "Clay Street Marching and Chowder Society," an informal but exclusive group of friends of the Medical School (Kaplan was a member) who saw research as more important to the advancement of medicine than patient care per se. (See Gillmor, 353–55.)

15. Committee on Curriculum, Medical Council of Stanford University, "A Program of Education for Medicine at Stanford University," 5–6.

16. Ibid., 6.

17. AnnaLee Saxenian, "Creating a Twentieth Century Technical Community: Frederick Terman's Silicon Valley," The Inventor and the Innovative Society: The Lemelson Center for the Study of Invention and Innovation, National Museum of American History, Smithsonian Institution, Nov. 10–11, 1995, http://people.ischool.berkeley .edu/~anno/Papers/terman.html, accessed July 29, 2011.

18. Lenoir, "Biochemistry at Stanford," 2.

19. Committee on Curriculum, Medical Council of Stanford University, "A Program of Education for Medicine at Stanford University," 6.

20. Gillmor, *Fred Terman at Stanford*, 355. Gillmor took this quote from a booklet that was published for the dedication of the newly relocated Medical School.

21. Ibid., 1.

22. Robert Kargon and Stuart Leslie, "Imagined Geographies: Princeton, Stanford and the Boundaries of Useful Knowledge in Postwar America," *Minerva* 32 (Summer 1994): 121.

23. Committee on Curriculum, Medical Council of Stanford University, "A Program of Education for Medicine at Stanford University," 6.

24. Gillmor, *Fred Terman at Stanford*, 350.

25. Lenoir notes in "Biochemistry at Stanford" that much of the cost of the initial move was defrayed by a large grant from the Ford Foundation.

26. John Long Wilson, *Stanford University School of Medicine and the Predecessor Schools: An Historical Perspective* (Stanford: Lane Medical Library, 1999), chap. 37. Kaplan stayed because his approach to medicine was compatible with the Sterling-Terman vision for Stanford biomedical research. His project "Clinac," built primarily by Edward Ginzton of the Stanford Microwave Laboratory, a 6-million-volt linear electron accelerator, could shoot X-rays into even the deepest cancerous tissue and served as the centerpiece of a large anti-cancer program that ran at Stanford from 1956 to 1958. The program encompassed twenty-eight projects, drew funding from five federal agencies, and encouraged collaboration between medical researchers and engineers. Clinac was later developed for commercial use by Varian Associates.

27. Ibid. According to J. L. Wilson, Alway, an Associate Dean of the School of Medi-

cine from 1968 to 1984, took to heart Stanford Trustee Herbert Hoover's advice "to appoint illustrious men."

28. Doogab Yi notes that Kornberg chose only to bring over some of his departmental faculty, carefully choosing who would come to Stanford with him. Doogab Yi, "The Coming of Reversibility: The Discovery of DNA Repair between the Atomic Age and the Information Age," *Historical Studies in the Physical and Biological Sciences* 37 Supplement (2007): 35–72.

29. Committee on Curriculum, Medical Council of Stanford University, "A Program of Education for Medicine at Stanford University," 4.

30. Joseph November, "George Elmer Forsythe," in *The New Dictionary of Scientific Biography* (New York: Charles Scribner's Sons, 2007).

31. Donald E. Knuth, "George Forsythe and the Development of Computer Science," *Communications of the ACM* 15, no. 8 (Aug. 1972): 721.

32. Ibid., 723.

33. David Salisbury and Gio Wiederhold, "George Forsythe, His Vision and Its Effects," *Stanford News Service*, Nov. 26, 1997, www-db.stanford.edu/pub/voy/museum/ ForsytheNews.html, accessed Dec. 21, 2010.

34. George E. Forsythe, "Educational Implications of the Computer Revolution," in *Applications of Digital Computers*, ed. W. F. Freiberger and William Prager (Boston: Ginn, 1963), 171.

35. George.E. Forsythe and Keith Killam, "Medical Data Processing," grant application prepared for the National Institutes of Health, June 5, 1962, file 2, box 1, ACME Collection (SC 236), Stanford University Archives, 5. Subsequent references are to this document.

36. R. Wade Cole, correspondence to JHU Brown (NIH), Jan. 25, 1963, file 2, box 1, ACME Collection (SC 236), Stanford University Archives. Like Forsythe, Cole was trained as a numerical analyst before devoting his career to electronic computers.

37. George E. Forsythe and Keith Killam, "Medical Data Processing," grant application prepared for the NIH, June 5, 1962, file 2, box 1, ACME Collection (SC 236), Stanford University Archives, 5.

38. Knuth, "George Forsythe and the Development of Computer Science," 722.

39. They added, "It is expected that such an environment would be conducive to future multivariant research exploring the full power of computational techniques as applied to medicine."

40. R. Wade Cole, correspondence to George E. Forsythe, Dec. 11, 1962, file 2, box 1, ACME Collection (SC 236), Stanford University Archives.

41. Ibid.

42. George E. Forsythe, "Suggested Outline for Proposal," memorandum, Nov. 1962, file 2, box 1, ACME Collection (SC 236), Stanford University Archives, 4. Forsythe and Killam prepared this proposal for the NIH in the late summer of 1962. It was turned down along with their original attempt.

43. Ibid.

44. Ibid., 5.

45. Ibid., 6. Forsythe goes on to lament biology's sluggishness in adopting computer technology: "Biology generally lags behind in assimilating advances in the physical sciences into its armamentarium." "It is not surprising then, that modern statistical techniques and computer technology in general have made little impact to date in biology."

46. Ibid., 6–7. In terms of practice, they hoped to enable testing of new types of models beyond contemporary concepts of nervous system, which relied on a linear deterministic model. There is no evidence that this expressed hope ever materialized into a specific research agenda. Though it has a prominent place at the conclusion of Forsythe's proposal outline, it is unclear whether it was crafted for the purpose of strengthening the revised grant proposal or if it represented a glimpse into a substantial volume of thought about how computers would transform the epistemology of modeling the nervous system.

47. George E. Forsythe, "NIH Grant," Nov. 29, 1962, file 2, box 1, ACME Collection (SC 236), Stanford University Archives.

48. Ibid.

49. Ibid.

50. R. Wade Cole correspondence to Thomas J. Kennedy, Jr. (NIH), 5 December 1962, file 2, box 1, ACME Collection (SC 236), Stanford University Archives. Proselytization metaphors abounded in the correspondence of the Forsythe group. In the same letter, Cole remarked: "All of our staff members, the Director and Associate Director included, act both formally and informally as computing missionaries around the campus. Much of this missionary work is accomplished through personal contact."

51. R. Wade Cole correspondence to J. H. U. Brown (NIH), Jan. 25, 1963, file 2, box 1, ACME Collection (SC 236), Stanford University Archives.

52. This hope was articulated in George E. Forsythe memorandum, "One More Pass at NIH," Apr. 30, 1963, box 1, folder 2, ACME Collection (SC 236), Stanford University Archives. This final proposal was never formally submitted to the NIH.

53. George E. Forsythe, "NIH," memorandum, Dec. 4, 1962, file 2, box 1, ACME Collection (SC 236), Stanford University Archives.

54. Ibid.

55. R. Wade Cole correspondence to J. H. U. Brown (NIH), Jan. 25, 1963, file 2, box 1, ACME Collection (SC 236), Stanford University Archives. Forsythe's emphasis on centralized computing ran counter to coalescing preferences among members of the ACCR to give biomedical researchers small machines (such as the LINC) whose operation they could control directly and completely. He likely was not aware of the ACCR's disappointment in the centralized facilities it had already sponsored.

56. Forsythe, "NIH."

57. George E. Forsythe, "More NIH News," memorandum, Dec. 6, 1962. file 2, box 1, ACME Collection (SC 236), Stanford University Archives.

58. Thomas J. Kennedy Jr., correspondence to R. Wade Cole, Dec. 18, 1962, file 2, box 1, ACME Collection (SC 236), Stanford University Archives.

59. Forsythe, "More NIH News."

60. Ibid.

61. Ibid.

62. John G. Harriot, "In Memory of George E. Forsythe," *Communications of the ACM* 15, no. 8 (Aug. 1972): 719–20.

63. National Institutes of Health, "Special Research Resource Annual Report, FY 1967," BBGGYW, Joshua Lederberg Papers, National Library of Medicine. Wade Cole left the Stanford biomedical computing "crusade" altogether, accepting a position at IBM.

64. Lederberg seems to have viewed the discovery of extraterrestrial life as a much more significant contribution to the study of life than the development of molecular biol-

ogy in the 1940s and 1950s. In 1963, he wrote in an essay draft: "A decade ago, we knew the big problems: genes, viruses, proteins, the chemical basis of life. In the large, these molecular problems have now been answered. An immense amount of filling-in needs doing, and there are bound to be many reversals and surprises. In skeletal perspective, the theoretical basis of contemporary molecular biology was already laid by the iconoclastic patriarchs: evolution (Darwin); particulate heredity (Mendel and Morgan); biomolecular architecture (Pasteur, Ehrlich, Landsteiner) — concurrently with the flowering of chemistry and physics. What next in such a perspective? I can formulate only one fundamental possibility: the generalization of terrestrial life, either by artificial synthesis, or by the discovery of life beyond the earth (either through the exploration of Mars and Jupiter or intelligent communication over larger distances)." Joshua Lederberg, "1984—Biology," Sept. 17, 1963, BBGNDT, Joshua Lederberg Papers, National Library of Medicine.

65. Joshua Lederberg, "How DENDRAL Was Conceived and Born," 4. Working Draft, Edward A. Feigenbaum Papers, box 11, folder 2. This is an annotated early version of the essay of the same name that appears in *A History of Medical Informatics: Proceeding of Association for Computing Machinery Conference on History of Medical Informatics*, ed. B. Blum (New York: ACM Press, 1990).

66. Vettel states ("The Protean Nature of Stanford University's Biological Sciences," 103) that Lederberg initially wanted to pursue this agenda by integrating what would be his genetics department and Kornberg's new biochemistry department. Kornberg rejected this proposal on the grounds that he believed Lederberg's work with bacteria "intersected too energetically applied agriculture work." This is strange, especially given that Lederberg was trying to leave Madison for the express purpose of getting away from the agriculture work. It is also very curious that Lederberg, who discovered transduction, had little to do with the Kornberg group's extensive work with transduction in eukaryotes.

67. Angela Creager noted in a conversation with the author that Roger Stanier adopted the term "comparative biochemistry" from van Niel and helped established its popularity among biochemically-oriented microbiologists.

68. Lederberg has since come to regard his concentration on exobiology as an indulgence, noting that his early Nobel Prize had given him the professional stability required "to stay in a non-reputable game. Not disreputable, mind you, but non-reputable. It might have been very, very difficult otherwise and it would [have been] very hard for a capable young scientist who's had a lot of risks to take in his career to hitch it to something as uncertain as exobiology." Lederberg interview by Edward C. Ezell, Aug. 23, 1977, qtd. in Edward Clinton Ezell and Linda Neuman Ezell, *On Mars: Exploration of the Red Planet 1958–1978* (Washington, DC: NASA History Office, 1984), chap. 3, http://history.nasa.gov/SP-4212/ch3.html, accessed July 29, 2011.

69. Audra J. Wolfe, "Germs in Space: Joshua Lederberg, Exobiology, and the Public Imagination, 1958–1964," *Isis* 93 (2002): 189–90.

70. Ibid.

71. Joshua Lederberg, "Exobiology: Approaches to Life Beyond Earth," *Science* 132 (1960): 396.

72. Ibid.

73. Stanley Miller and Harold C. Urey, "Organic Compound Synthesis on the Primitive Earth," *Science* 130 (July 31, 1959): 251.

74. Lederberg, "Exobiology: Approaches to Life Beyond Earth," 398.

75. Wolfe, "Germs in Space," 194.

76. Ibid.

77. A broad (and also deep) history of NASA's involvement in efforts to study extraterrestrial life can be found in Steven J. Dick and James E. Strick, *The Living Universe: NASA and the Development of Astrobiology* (New Brunswick: Rutgers University Press, 2005). This book shows the many of the effects the early dreams of finding life beyond Earth had on American space missions of the 1970s through the early 2000s.

78. William N. Sinton, "Further Evidence of Vegetation on Mars," *Science* 130 (1959): 1234–37. Reacting to Sinton's observations, Lederberg wrote in 1960 that "these studies give little encouragement for the development of a Martian life as rich as Earth's, but they do not rule out a marginal biology whose urgent need is the finding and retention of water." (Joshua Lederberg, "Life in Space," 1960, unpublished draft, BBGNCX, Joshua Lederberg Papers, National Library of Medicine.)

79. Robert S. Ledley, "Digital Electronic Computers in Biomedical Science," *Science* 130 (Nov. 6, 1959): 1225–34. Lederberg seems to have been a great admirer of Ledley's ideas and work, which he followed closely during the subsequent decades. During a 2007 conversation with the author, Ledley recalled that Lederberg had repeatedly urged him to write an autobiography.

80. Joshua Lederberg comments on Joseph November, "Impossible by Any Other Means: Early Advocacy for the Use of Computers in Biology," Joint Atlantic Seminar on the History of Biology, Apr. 5, 2003.

81. See chap. 6 for a discussion of biomedical computing at Stanford and Lederberg's priorities for the Department of Genetics.

82. Edward A. Feigenbaum interview with the author June 20, 2004.

83. Lederberg, "How DENDRAL Was Conceived and Born," 4.

84. Ibid.

85. The day-to-day research and development activities of the IRL were directed by Elliott C. Levinthal (not to be confused with molecular biologist Cyrus Levinthal).

86. Ibid., 1–2.

87. Joshua Lederberg interview with author Mar. 28, 2005.

88. Joshua Lederberg, "An Instrumentation Crisis in Biology," application for NIH grant, May 1963, BBGCVS, Joshua Lederberg Papers, National Library of Medicine, 1.

89. Ibid.

90. Ibid., 2.

91. Joshua Lederberg interview with author Mar. 28, 2005.

92. Lederberg, "An Instrumentation Crisis in Biology," 9–10.

93. Ibid., 9.

94. Ibid.

95. Ibid., 3.

96. Eugene Garfield established the Institute for Scientific Information (ISI) in 1960; it is today known as Thomson ISI and hosts widely used tools like the Scientific Citation Index. An overview of Garfield's efforts to create a computerized, multi-disciplinary citation index can be found in Blaise Cronin and Helen Barsky Atkins, ed., *The Web of Knowledge: A Festschrift in Honor of Eugene Garfield* (Medford, NJ: Information Today, 2000).

97. Ibid., 4–5. McCarthy also reintroduced Lederberg to Minsky's AI work.

98. For a historically thorough and technically sound examination of Djerassi's development of mass spectrometry techniques in the context of the technological, methodolog-

ical, institutional, and social transformations of chemistry in the mid-twentieth century, see Carsten Reinhardt, *Shifting and Rearranging—Physical Methods and the Transformation of Modern Chemistry* (Sagamore Beach, MA: Science History Publications, 2006).

99. Joshua Lederberg, "An Instrumentation Crisis in Biology."

100. Feigenbaum, E. A., and R. Watson, "An initial problem statement for a machine induction research project," *Stanford AI Memo* 40 (1965).

101. Joshua Lederberg and Edward Feigenbaum, "Mechanization of Inductive Inference in Organic Chemistry," *Stanford AI Memo* 54 (Aug. 2, 1967): 5.

102. Joshua Lederberg, "How DENDRAL Was Conceived and Born," 6.

103. Joshua Lederberg, "Topological mapping of organic molecules," *Proceedings of the National Academy of Sciences* 53 (1965): 134.

104. Ibid., for further examples.

105. Lederberg ran this program on the LINC, the small, programmable, general-purpose digital computer designed specifically for biologists. Lederberg won one of the coveted computers and was selected to participate in the "LINC Summer of '63." For further information on the LINC, see chap. 4 and Joe November, "LINC: Biology's Revolutionary Little Computer," *Endeavour* 28, no. 3 (2004).

106. Edward A. Feigenbaum interview with author June 20, 2004.

107. Edward A. Feigenbaum, "A Personal View of Expert Systems: Looking Back and Looking Ahead," Knowledge Systems Laboratory Report No. KSL 92-41, 3–4. Simon was referring to his Logic Theory program, the first heuristic program.

108. Pamela McCorduck, *Machines Who Think: A Personal Inquiry into the History and Prospects of Artificial Intelligence* (San Francisco: W. H. Freeman and Co., 1979), 277–78.

109. Ibid., 281.

110. Edward A. Feigenbaum interview with author June 27, 2004.

111. For Feigenbaum's account of his later break with McCarthy, see McCorduck, *Machines Who Think.*

112. Edward A. Feigenbaum interview with author June 20, 2004.

113. Edward A. Feigenbaum interview with author June 27, 2004.

114. Edward Feigenbaum interview with Richard Zemel Jan. 25, 1984, qtd. in Richard Zemel, "Old Ideas and New Viewpoints in Artificial Intelligence: The Birth of Expert Systems," BA thesis, Harvard University, 1984. Zemel wrote this thesis for the Committee on History and Science and particularly Seymour Papert. Zemel conducted extensive interviews of DENDRAL participants. Although I do not draw extensively from Zemel's analysis, which focuses on internal AI debates, his interview data has been invaluable.

115. Ibid.

116. DENDRAL first ran on an IBM 7090, then migrated to a DEC PDP-6, then a DEC PDP-10, and finally resided on the School of Medicine's IBM 360/50. When DENDRAL was tasked to test Meta-DENDRAL's hypotheses, however, the computational immensity of the task overwhelmed even the IBM 360. Edward A. Feigenbaum, "A Personal View of Expert Systems: Looking Back and Looking Ahead," Knowledge Systems Laboratory Report No. KSL 92-41, 9.

117. E. Feigenbaum and J. Lederberg, "Mechanization of Inductive Inference in Organic Chemistry," in *Formal Representation of Human Judgment*, ed. Benjamin Kleinmuntz (New York: John Wiley & Sons, 1968), 216. Regarding time-sharing, they commented, "In retrospect it is quite obvious that the program simply could never have

been written and debugged without the help of the rapid interaction provided by the time-sharing system."

118. "It never occurred to us to worry about funding . . . the president of ARPA was sensitive to the problems of early AI, and let us do what we thought needed to be done" (Edward Feigenbaum interview with Richard Zemel, Jan. 25, 1984, qtd. in Zemel, "Old Ideas and New Viewpoints in Artificial Intelligence").

119. Edward A. Feigenbaum, "A Personal View of Expert Systems: Looking Back and Looking Ahead," Knowledge Systems Laboratory Report No. KSL 92-41, 10.

120. Bruce G. Buchanan, "Towards an Understanding of Information Processes of Scientific Inference in the Context of Organic Chemistry," Stanford Artificial Intelligence Project Memo 99 (1969).

121. The name DENDRAL first appeared in print in Lederberg's proposal to NASA, "DENDRAL-64: A system for computer construction, enumeration, and notation of organic molecules as tree structures and cyclic graphs," NASA CR-57029, STAR No. N65-13158.

122. Edward A. Feigenbaum, "A Personal View of Expert Systems: Looking Back and Looking Ahead," Knowledge Systems Laboratory Report No. KSL 92-41, 10.

123. Edward A. Feigenbaum interview with author June 20, 2004: "We would show him what DENDRAL could do, and he would be so intrigued by what it couldn't do that he couldn't resist the urge to help!" While reviewing this paper on Feb. 23, 2005, Lederberg remarked that Djerassi would take exception to the term "hooked," instead preferring a more suitable term to convey his intellectual motives for spending so much time entering data into DENDRAL's knowledge base.

124. In a draft on a 1965 *Washington Post* article titled, "The Meaning of Mariner IV," Lederberg and Caltech planetary geologist Bruce C. Murray cast the Mariner findings as an "unexpectedly informative 'First Close-Up Look'" at Mars, and dismissed questions such as "Isn't it apparent that Mars is lifeless?" Though Mars appeared barren, they emphasized that these appearances should not deter NASA from pursuing a "large scale and aggressive program of exploration of Mars leading to eventual direct tests for, and analysis of, life forms that may exist there." (Bruce C. Murray and Joshua Lederberg," draft of "The Meaning of Mariner IV," BBBDDC, Joshua Lederberg Papers, National Library of Medicine.)

125. John McCarthy and Joshua Lederberg, "A Proposal for the Study of Computer Control of External Devices and an Automated Biological Laboratory," Oct. 15, 1964, BBGCZC, Joshua Lederberg Papers, National Library of Medicine.

126. It is telling that the correspondence and grant proposals related to Forsythe's attempt to gain NIH support for acquiring a computer for Stanford biomedical researchers are part of the ACME Papers (SC 236) rather than the George and Alexandra Forsythe Papers (SC 098) at the Stanford University Archives. It is likely that Lederberg himself donated Forsythe's papers regarding the NIH-sponsored computer to the archives.

127. Joshua Lederberg, "Advanced Computer for Medical Research," grant application prepared for NIH, Sept. 29, 1965, file 6, box 1, ACME Collection (SC 236), Stanford University Archives, 1.

128. For a thorough discussion of IBM's (and particularly Thomas Watson Jr.'s) motivations for developing the System/360, see Emerson W. Pugh, *Memories That Shaped an Industry: Decisions Leading to IBM System/360* (Cambridge, MA: MIT Press, 1984).

129. Pamela McCorduck, "An Interview with Edward Feigenbaum," Charles Bab-

bage Institute Oral History 14, June 12, 1979, 18. Note the similarity to Warren Weaver's "raise the peaks" rhetoric.

130. Lederberg, "Advanced Computer for Medical Research," 3–4.

131. Ibid., 4. Lederberg made it clear that access to the SCC would not suffice for biomedical research, but he also stressed that "the computer and its supporting staff are intended to complement the services available from the University Computation Center." Once SCC's IBM 360/67 went online in 1967, biomedical researchers were able to use the machines around the clock, every day of the year; when one computer was down, they could simply send their work to the other one.

132. Lederberg and Hundley, "Final Report: LINC Evaluation Program," xiii–9.

133. Lederberg, "Advanced Computer for Medical Research," 4.

134. IBM, "Scientific Marketing Newsletter," Special Issue, no. 16 (1965). IBM played up this aspect of the 360 (and other large, digital computers) in advertisements to biomedical researchers.

135. Lederberg, "Advanced Computer for Medical Research," 4.

136. Ibid., 10.

137. Ibid.

138. Ibid..

139. Research Resources Information Center, National Institutes of Health, *The Seeds of Artificial Intelligence: SUMEX-AIM* (Rockville, MD: NIH, 1980), 18.

140. IBM, "Scientific Marketing Newsletter," Special Issue, no. 16 (1965).

141. Richard S. Zemel, "Old Ideas and New Viewpoints in Artificial Intelligence: The Birth of Expert Systems," 121.

142. Edward A. Feigenbaum interview with author June 21, 2004.

143. DENDRAL Conversation, B. G. Buchanan and R. K. Lindsay, Nov. 20, 1974. Edward Feigenbaum Papers, Stanford University, SC 340, box 2.

144. Robert Lindsay, Edward Feigenbaum untitled interview, 1975. Edward Feigenbaum Papers, box 2—page 9 of transcript erroneously reads "It's baking come alive!"

145. The impetus for Meta-DENDRAL does not entirely derive from Bruce Buchanan, but came originally from Lederberg, who in the late 1950s wanted to be able to determine the structure of alien amino acids—which were presumable distinct from any known amino acids—from afar.

146. Robert K. Lindsay et al., *Applications of Artificial Intelligence for Organic Chemistry* (Stanford: Stanford University Press, 1980), 163. Lindsay's name appears first not because he led the project, but rather because he did the most work in terms of assembling this volume, which was the DENDRAL team's formal attempt to preserve their view of the DENDRAL project for posterity.

147. J. Bronowski, "The logic of the mind," *American Scientist* 54 (1966): 6. Reproduced in Lindsay et al., *Applications of Artificial Intelligence for Organic Chemistry*, 161.

148. Ibid., 166.

149. Ibid., 35.

150. Edward Feigenbaum interview with Richard Zemel Jan. 25, 1984, qtd. in Richard Zemel, "Old Ideas and New Viewpoints in Artificial Intelligence."

151. Joshua Lederberg to Helen Gee (NIH-CRSS), 1965, file 6, box 1, ACME Collection (SC 236), Stanford University Archives.

152. Joshua Lederberg to John Z. Bowers (President, Josiah Macy, Jr. Foundation), 1966, file 6, box 1, ACME Collection (SC 236), Stanford University Archives.

153. Compilers are the software tools that convert instructions encoded in a higher-level language (for example, FORTRAN) into machine code.

154. Gio Wiederhold, CV, http://infolab.stanford.edu/pub/gio/personal/personal .html, accessed Jul. 29, 2011.

155. Gio Wiederhold, "A Summary of the ACME System," presentation given at Office of Naval Research Computer and Psychobiology Conference, 17 May 1996, US Navy Postgraduate School, Monterey, CA. 1, BBGHBT, Joshua Lederberg Papers, National Library of Medicine.

156. Lederberg to Caspersson, Oct. 13, 1965, BBANAV, Joshua Lederberg Papers, National Library of Medicine.

157. Wiederhold, "A Summary of the ACME System," 2.

158. Of course, seeing the "special run" light illuminate on the light box just as one was preparing to settle in for some work on ACME was a frustrating experience. The lack of a queuing system also created congestion at times when there was heavy demand for ACME. Gio Wiederhold interview with author June 23, 2004.

159. ACME/PL was a variant of IBM's PL/1 (Programming Language 1), which had been developed for the 360.

160. David E. Clark, "Computing Requirements of the Hospital and Medical School," (Manchester: Medical Computing Unit, University of Manchester, Jan. 23, 1967), box 1, folder, 9, ACME Collection (SC 236), Stanford University Archives.

161. Ibid., 4.

162. Joshua Lederberg, XDS Sigma-5 Proposal (1970), 1–2, box 1, folder 17, ACME Collection (SC 236), Stanford University Archives.

163. Gio Wiederhold interview with author June 23, 2004. The films run about five minutes each, and feature ACME being used in the context of heart surgery and Lederberg's exobiology work. They also demonstrate Wiederhold's time-sharing system and emphasized that the IBM 360, despite being housed outside the laboratory, could—via terminal access—nonetheless serve as a vital piece of laboratory equipment.

164. R. Jamtgaard, "Quarterly Report for Acme Computing Facility for Stanford University Computer Facilities Committee," 1972, letterbook Jan.–June 1972, box 4, ACME Collection (SC 236), Stanford University Archives.

165. ACME memorandum, file 24, box 1, ACME Collection (SC 236), Stanford University Archives. The ACME Policy Board also regulated hardware purchases, which were supported by the NIH and to a lesser extent the Josiah Macy Jr. Foundation ($160,000). Coincidentally, another Josiah Macy was heavily involved in the LINC project.

166. Staff of the Heuristic Program, "The Stanford Heuristic Programming Project: Goals and Activities," *AI Magazine* 1, no. 1 (1980).

167. Joshua Lederberg, "XDS Sigma 5 Proposal," 1969 box 1, folder 17, ACME Collection (SC 236), Stanford University Archives.

168. Research Resources Information Center, National Institutes of Health, *The Seeds of Artificial Intelligence: SUMEX-AIM* (Rockville, MD: NIH, 1980), 18.

169. Edward A. Feigenbaum, "S U Medical Experimental Computer Resource (SUMEX)," NIH Grant Application, May 27, 1980. This application to renew SUMEX funding was filed following Lederberg's 1978 departure from Stanford to Rockefeller University. After Lederberg left, Feigenbaum became head of the project. Though Led-

erberg had secured five additional years of funding for SUMEX-AIM in 1977, the NIH reduced funding to three years when he left the project.

170. Staff of the Heuristic Program, "The Stanford Heuristic Programming Project: Goals and Activities."

171. Edward Feigenbaum, "Molgen—Applications in Artificial Intelligence to Molecular Biology: Research in Theory Formation, Testing, and Modification." This was Feigenbaum's proposal to the National Science Foundation for funds to support further development of MOLGEN.

172. IntelliGenetics pamphlet, "Computer Aided Design for the Molecular Biologist," 1983.

173. Association for Computing Machinery, ACM Awards, http://awards.acm.org/, accessed Dec. 21, 2010.

Conclusion

Epigraph. Lee Lusted, "The Development of National Biomedical Computing Capability," in Data Acquisition and Processing in Biology and Medicine: Proceedings of the 1961 Rochester Conference vol. 2, ed. Kurt Enslein (New York: Pergamon Press, 1962), 8.

1. E. O. Attinger and A. Anne, "LINC Evaluation Program, Final Report," *Proceedings of the Final LINC Evaluation Program Meeting* (St. Louis: Computer Research Laboratory, Washington University 1965), 9–16.

2. Lee B. Lusted, "Bio-Medical Electronics—2012 A.D," *Proceedings of the IEEE* 50, no. 5 (May 1962): 636–37.

3. Rogers, Lee F. " 'My Word, What Is That?' Hounsfield and the Triumph of Clinical Research," *American Journal of Roentgenology* 180 (2003): 1501.

4. Nathan Ensmenger, "Resistance Is Futile? Reluctant and Selective Users of the Internet," in *The Internet and American Business*, eds. William Aspray and Paul E. Ceruzzi. (Cambridge, MA: MIT Press, 2008), 351–88.

5. Daniel M. Fox, forward to Jeanne Daly, *Evidence-Based Medicine and the Search for a Science of Clinical Care* (Berkeley: University of California Press, 2005), vii.

6. William Rosenberg, Anna Donald, "Evidence-based Medicine: An Approach to Clinical Problem-solving," *British Medical Journal* 310, no. 6987 (Apr. 29, 1995): 1122.

7. Barack Obama, Remarks by the President to a Joint Session of Congress on Health Care, Sept. 9, 2009, US Capitol, Washington, DC.

8. David Leonhardt, "Making Health Care Better," *New York Times Magazine*, Nov. 3, 2009.

9. For discussion of the roots of EBM in the late 1950s and early 1960s computer work of Warner, Ledley, and Lusted, see Joseph A. November, "Early Biomedical Computing and the Roots of Evidence-Based Medicine," *IEEE Annals of the History of Computing* 33, no. 2 (Apr–Jun 2011), 9–23.

10. Simon, *The Sciences of the Artificial* (Cambridge, MA: MIT Press, 1969), 27–28.

11. Strasser, "The Experimenter's Museum: GenBank, Natural History, and the Moral Economies of Biomedicine," *Isis* 102, no. 1 (Mar. 2011): 60–96.

12. David E. Clark, "Computing Requirements of the Hospital and Medical School" (Manchester: Medical Computing Unit, University of Manchester, Jan. 23, 1967), 9, box 1, folder 9, ACME Collection (SC 236), Stanford University Archives.

13. Jochen Moehr transcribed in "Planting the Seeds—A Panel," *A History of Medical Informatics: Proceedings of Association for Computing Machinery Conference on History of Medical Informatics*, eds. Bruce I. Blum and Karen Duncan (New York: ACM Press, 1990), 69.

14. Wesley Clark interview with author June 26, 2004.

15. Freeman Dyson, "When Science & Poetry Were Friends," *New York Review of Books* 56, no. 13 (Aug. 13, 2009). Dyson added: "Candidates for leadership of the modern Romantic Age are the biology wizards Kary Mullis [developer of PCR], Dean Kamen [inventor], and Craig Venter [founder of Celera Genomics], and the computer wizards Larry Page, Sergey Brin [co-founders of Google], and Charles Simonyi [Xerox PARC alumnus and former Microsoft executive]."

ESSAY ON SOURCES

In examining the introduction of digital electronic computers to biology and medicine, this book shows that early computerization of each area was deeply influenced by the priorities of early biomedical computing advocates, the missions and constraints of the institutions that sponsored computer use, and the capabilities and restrictions of the technology itself. As I outline, many crucial tools and resources for biology and medicine have roots in these early efforts. Furthermore, computer technology itself came away from the process profoundly changed, and indeed the particular way most people use computers today owes much to early attempts to make computers more useful to life scientists. To support these claims, this book draws on a wide variety of conventional and unconventional sources. A full bibliography is available online at www.cas.sc.edu/hist/books/november/.

PRIMARY SOURCES

Published Material

The many journals that today are dedicated to the use of computers in biology and medicine did not exist during the period covered by this book, the late 1940s through the mid-1960s, when interest in the subject was forming. Nevertheless, most of the scientists, computer developers, and computing advocates I examine published extensively in peer-reviewed journals and other formal outlets. Besides conveying the methods of computing pioneers, such sources often make explicit their motivations and priorities. For instance, Robert Ledley and Lee Lusted articulated their vision of how physicians should prepare to use computers in "Reasoning Foundations of Medical Diagnosis," *Science* 130 (July 3, 1959): 9–21. Just a few months later in the same journal, Ledley published his plans for the computerization of biology as "Digital Electronic Computers in Biomedical Science," *Science* 130 (Nov. 6, 1959): 1225–34. Both articles were widely read at the time and demonstrably convinced many biologists and physicians, including Joshua Lederberg and Homer Warner (both subjects of this book), to start to use computers. Ledley's 1965 monograph on biomedical computing, *Use of Computers in Biology and Medicine* (New York: McGraw-Hill, 1965), further expanded on his plans, but due to significant changes in computer technology between 1959 and 1965 many of its discussions were outdated by time it was published. In the case of the LINC, Wesley Clark and Charles Molnar made clear their machine's design priorities and capabilities in "A Description of the LINC," in *Computers in Biomedical Research*, Vol. 2, edited by Ralph W. Stacy and Bruce D. Waxman (New York: Academic Press, 1965).

Several conferences, where many of the book's subjects gathered, provide in their published proceedings a wealth of information on their activities and ideas. These include: *Data Acquisition and Processing in Biology and Medicine: Proceedings of the 1961– 1963 Rochester Conferences*, edited by Kurt Enslein (New York: Pergamon Press, 1962– 1964); *Proceedings of the 3rd IBM Medical Symposium* (Endicott, NY: IBM, 1961); and *Proceedings of the Final LINC Evaluation Program Meeting* (St. Louis: Computer Research Laboratory, Washington University, 1965). The last set of proceedings offers a candid look at a wide spectrum of experiences of researchers who began to use computers in their laboratories, and it is unique in that participants were attentive to the changes the new technology brought to their work.

Publicity material provided much insight into the institutional mechanisms of introducing computers to biology and medicine. A brochure circulated by the NIH's Division of Research Facilities and Resources, titled *Special Research Resources for the Biomedical Sciences* (Bethesda: NIH 1965), encouraged NIH grant applicants to consider using computers in their research, and provided explanations of how the NIH could support the use of computers. The National Biomedical Research Foundation's massive promotional book, *NBR Research Accomplishments 1960–1970* (Washington, DC: NBRF, 1973), featured article reprints but also accessible descriptions of the machines and computing resources developed by that organization during its first decade. The effort the foundation put into that book demonstrates the importance of engaging a wide audience in order to obtain support for computing projects. Finally, advertising by computer manufacturers like IBM, DEC, CDC, and Spear Electronics serves to illustrate how these corporations hoped to create a lucrative market for their machines in the life sciences.

Unpublished Material

One of the major challenges in preparing this book was that there are very few well-organized and professionally managed archival collections dedicated to early biomedical computing. The most extensive repository is located at the Stanford University Archives, which in its ACME Collection (SC 236) contains papers related to development of a biomedical computing facility at Stanford, and the Edward Feigenbaum Papers (SC 340), which include the work of Edward Feigenbaum and Joshua Lederberg on DENDRAL and other early expert systems. The Computer History Museum in Mountain View, California, provided me access to the DEC papers it maintains, which contained much discussion of the construction and sale of DEC's LINC variants. The MIT Museum, meanwhile, has a small collection of papers (LINC Collection) related to the development of the LINC and the activities of the ACCR. The National Academy of Sciences, which was involved in late-1950s efforts to stimulate computer use in biomedicine, has preserved, in its Committee on Uses of Electronic Computers in Biological and Medical Sciences Collection, meeting proceedings, memoranda, and material it published in relation to those efforts.

The NIH, despite its deep involvement in biomedical computing, preserved very little material related to its early efforts to introduce computers to biology and medicine. Bureaucratic protocols calling for the destruction of papers more than a few years old have robbed the NIH of large volumes of material that would be useful to historians. Therefore, most of what is known about early NIH biomedical computing activities comes from the National Archives, university archives such as Stanford and MIT, and the private collections of the NBRF and individuals such as Ledley, Clark, and Lederberg. It should be noted that since the 1990s the NIH has been active in preserving externally maintained records of its activities. For instance, the National Library of Medicine is currently in the process of archiving the papers collected by the NBRF. The NLM's Profiles in Science: The Joshua Lederberg Papers, which organizes makes available online the several thousand documents the prolific Lederberg produced or found influential, serves as an example of how information technology can serve historical research.

Due to the limited utility of traditional archives in terms of organizing and preserving material related to early biomedical computing, I made extensive use of personal and private collections in my research. Robert and Terry Ledley provided several boxes of material, which are now being processed by the NLM. Many of the documents describing Ledley's work in OR and his early activities as a promoter of biomedical computing were preserved by the Ledleys. Wesley Clark and his wife, Maxine Rockoff, also collected many important unpublished documents from the early part of Clark's career. Among them is Clark's memorandum "Data Processing Aspects of Biomedical Computing Centers"—Lincoln Laboratory Report C.13.3. (Nov. 22, 1961)—which crucially pinpoints Clark's objections to using conventional general-purpose digital electronic computing centers for life sciences research. Joshua Lederberg, beyond supplying the massive holdings of his NLM Profiles in Science collection, provided material he had kept only at his Rockefeller University office. The smaller collections of Jerome Cox, and Gio Wiederhold all contained otherwise inaccessible documents related to LINC (Cox) and ACME (Wiederhold).

Among the collections of unpublished material I read, several types of documents stood out in terms of providing insight into the early computerization of biology and medicine. Grant applications to the NIH—few of which were preserved by the NIH itself—served as particularly helpful resources because they so clearly conveyed the goals and plans of many important early projects. Heavily cited examples include: Robert S. Ledley, "Biomedical Computer and Biomathematics Research Center," grant application prepared for the National Institutes of Health, Nov. 1, 1959 (Robert S. Ledley Papers, National Biomedical Research Foundation, grant # B-RG-2075, formerly RG 7323); George E. Forsythe and Keith Killam, "Medical Data Processing," grant application prepared for the NIH, June 5, 1962 (Stanford University Archives, ACME Collection); and Joshua Lederberg, "Advanced Computer for Medical Research," grant application prepared for National Institutes of Health, Sept. 29, 1965 (Stanford University Archives, ACME Collection). That two of these three applications were rejected, despite the prominence of the applicants, shows that support for early projects, while generous, was by no means certain, and that sponsors and researchers often misunderstood each other's priorities and constraints.

Office memoranda, at NIH, Stanford, MIT, and Digital Equipment Corporation, convey an intimate narrative of the process of computerization. Frederick Brackett's struggle between 1956 and 1960 to introduce computers to the NIH campus is preserved in the National Archives' NIH Electronic Data Processing Collection (RG 443 G2A 64), which shows clearly Brackett's hopes for using the machines as well as other NIH researchers' reasons for resisting Brackett's call to acquire a general-purpose computer. The day-to-day crises that erupted as Stanford University attempted to introduce computers to its biomedical researchers are captured in gritty detail in the university's collections and the NLM's Lederberg Papers. In many memoranda, especially those held in the

National Academies of Sciences Archive, the fragility of the endeavor of introducing computers to biology and medicine is revealed. As I suggest, institutional support for computing in biomedicine, even when it amounted to millions of dollars, was generally provisional, and it was seldom entirely clear to researchers what criteria had to be satisfied to continue to receive that support.

Technical reports, as well as drafts of research proposals and papers, provided windows to the early phases of projects like LINC and DENDRAL. Clark's "Design Considerations for an Experimental Computer (Lincoln Laboratory Memo 6M-3536; 1955) and "Data Processing Aspects of Biomedical Computing Centers"—(Lincoln Laboratory Report C.13.3. (Nov. 22, 1961)—bring to light the process through which he arrived at his opposition to time-sharing and the design of the LINC. At Stanford, many of the documents preserved by Feigenbaum and Lederberg show how their ambitions converged to create the DENDRAL project. A draft of Lederberg's "An Instrumentation Crisis in Biology" (NIH-1962 Q102 BBGCVS) shows how he thought computers could become useful in his exobiology efforts, while Feigenbaum and Watson's "An initial problem statement for a machine induction research project" (Stanford AI Memo #40, 1965) illustrates Feigenbaum's belief that Lederberg's project would be a fruitful domain for AI.

Interviews and Other Discussions

A great advantage I had in conducting very recent history is that many of the individuals I discuss are not only alive but were active participants in this book's preparation. Besides agreeing to extensive interviews, they furnished—and discussed at length—volumes of valuable unarchived material, provided me access to artifacts, helped me to get in touch with other subjects, and eagerly reviewed manuscript drafts, supplying me with insights that have since become an integral part of this text.

Robert Ledley met me several times during the writing of my doctoral dissertation and then on a near-weekly basis in 2007 and 2008, when I served as a DeWitt Stetten Jr. Memorial Fellow at the NIH. Our dozens of hours of interviews revealed many aspects of his career and of early biomedical computing that simply had never been documented elsewhere. On February 21, 2008, we recapitulated the most interesting aspects of our interviews in a public presentation at the NIH, titled, "A Lifetime of Biomedical Computing: A Conversation with Robert S. Ledley," the captioned video of which is available online at the NIH's website along with supporting visual materials. Ledley commented on early drafts of the manuscript and answered many of my technical questions about his early and more recent work.

I interviewed Wesley Clark on several occasions at various stages of the book's preparation. The interviews ranged from discussions of his early life to in-depth explanations of the technical aspects of computer design. Beyond filling in many of the gaps in the printed record, Clark carefully reviewed many parts of the manuscript, especially those pertaining to his work at the Lincoln Laboratory. In so doing he clarified the origins of his revolutionary approach to designing computers and provided me with a much better understanding of the many forces at work in the world of computing between 1955 and 1965.

A daylong 2004 discussion with John Barlow, Nelson Y. S. Kiang, Ishmael Stefanov-Wagner, and David Steffens at the Massachusetts Eye and Ear Infirmary, in Boston, yielded my initial understanding of LINC's capabilities and the way it interfaced with the rest of a laboratory. To tell the story of LINC, I also draw from a series of interviews I conducted in 2004 with some of the members of the LINC design team, their survivors, and LINC users. These included Severo Ornstein, Donna Molnar (widow of Charles Molnar), and Jerome Cox. My 2008 discussions with James Lynch and William Talbot provided much understanding of what it was like to actually use the LINC in research, and the benefits and costs of using that computer.

My account of the rise of biomedical computing at Stanford draws from interviews I conducted there in 2004. To better understand DENDRAL and biomedical computing on campus, I held several formal, recorded discussions with Edward Feigenbaum. Gio Wiederhold, one of the leaders of the ACME project, showed me artifacts of the IBM 360 that Stanford had used as well as artifacts related to the modifications he made to the system in order to make it more useful the biomedical community. I interviewed Joshua Lederberg twice in 2005 about his activities at Stanford and his reasons for becoming interested in computing.

Artifacts

Intensive collaboration with surviving biomedical computing pioneers has allowed me to treat the computers and programs themselves as historical sources. Computers included the LINC, Ledley's "Metal Brain for Diagnosis," and Stanford's ACME, while DENDRAL was the set of programs most carefully examined. Only by "reading" the computers and programs as artifacts could I determine why they took the forms they did and how they functioned in research and clinical environments. To bring the computers themselves out of the black box I examine them as what Langdon Winner calls "political artifacts." By politics, Winner means "arrangements of power and authority in human associations as well as the activities that take place within those arrangements." As Winner explains, this notion of politics can be brought to bear on artifacts in the course of investigating them: "artifacts can contain political properties . . . instances in which the invention, design, or arrangement of a specific technical device or system becomes a way of settling an issue in the affairs of a particular community"—Langdon Winner, "Do Artifacts Have Politics?" *Daedalus* 109, no. 1 (1980): 121–36. Thus, by investigating how computers embodied their builders' and advocates' particular priorities, be they episte-mological or institutional, I have attempted to illuminate the motivations of those who sought to computerize as well as provide a political context of biologists' use of (and plans to use) computers. Indeed, throughout this book the computer is often cast as a means to an end: in Lee Lusted's case, computers would serve to conglomerate biology into a "big" science; for Robert Ledley, Bruce Waxman, and Joshua Lederberg, computers were a means of "mathematizing" the life sciences; and for the researchers who used Wesley Clark's LINC, the machine's specific design characteristics allowed them to preserve traditional biological experimental practices and institutional norms.

As Winner's numerous critics, most notably Bernward Joerges in "Do Politics Have Artefacts?," have pointed out, examining an artifact's politics presents the danger of attributing qualities to them and motives to their builders (and the societies that used them) that may be unwarranted. But, a close investigation of the forces that brought computers to biology complicate Joerges's claim that "the power represented in built and other technical devices is not to be found in the formal attributes of these things themselves. Only their authorization, their legitimate representation, gives shape to the definitive effects they may have"—Bernward Joerges, "Do Politics Have Artefacts?" *Social Studies of Science* 29 (1999): 411–31. Granted, support for building computers like LINC and software like DENDRAL was authorized by individuals and groups with well-defined priorities, and in several cases it is useful to examine how sponsors' priorities either resonated or conflicted with those of the technology developers. Nevertheless, in the cases of LINC and DENDRAL it is clear that many of the attributes of the artifacts in question were primarily manifestations of their builders' and users' ideals.

SECONDARY SOURCES

Despite its importance, computer use in science and medicine is not an area that has generated much literature by professional historians. Part of the reason is that there is little discussion of the recent history of the life sciences to begin with. To paraphrase Nathaniel Comfort, the roads paved by historians of early twentieth-century biology taper off into rough trails by the time their analyses reach the 1960s and disappear altogether into the trackless "wilderness" of the 1970s and beyond—Nathaniel Comfort, "A History of Molecular Biology (Book Review)," *Quarterly Review of Biology* 75 (2000): 303. Among historians of technology, meanwhile, the interaction of computer technology and the sciences is a newly emerging area of study. The few comprehensive studies of the development of digital electronic computers, such as Martin Campbell-Kelly and William Aspray, *Computer: The History of the Information Machine* (Boulder: Westview Press, 2004) and Paul E. Ceruzzi, *A History of Modern Computing* (Cambridge, MA: MIT Press, 2003), have only touched lightly on the subject of life sciences computing. As with post-1960 biology, the challenge is that the subject is immense—Michael S. Mahoney calls it a "trackless jungle. We pace on the edge, pondering where to cut in"—"The History of Computing in the History of Technology," *Annals of the History of Computing* 10 (1988): 115.

This book, to borrow from Comfort's and Mahoney's metaphors, is an attempt to cut a trail through what is largely trackless subject matter. Due to the paucity of professional work, there are few areas in this book where traditional historiographical techniques, such as reevaluating secondary discussions in light of new primary evidence, can be fruitfully applied. I considered myself fortunate to find more than a handful of professional historians commenting on the material encompassed by a whole chapter. However, several historians who do not directly engage the subject of biomedical computing have still been influential in shaping my narrative, either by providing conceptual tools that I have been able to apply to my discussion or by examining ideas, people, and events that affected biomedical computing.

Chapter 1 draws heavily on Soraya de Chadarevian's account of British crystallographer John Kendrew's OR background and his work with EDSAC in *Designs for Life: Molecular Biology After World War II* (Cambridge, UK: Cambridge University Press, 2002), and it owes much to the connection de Chadarevian makes between OR and Kendrew's very early computer use. Although this chapter does not discuss cybernetics or information theory, it has been strongly influenced by Lily E. Kay's *Who Wrote the Book of Life?: A History of the Genetic Code* (Stanford: Stanford University Press, 2000). Kay's book clarifies the conceptual shifts in biology in the mid-twentieth century, many of which created in their wake an environment conducive to applying information technology to biological problems. My analytic framework of early computer use in molecular biology was, due to the work of several historians, able to avoid the pitfalls of the pervasive Informational School/Structural School narrative introduced by members of Delbrück's circle in 1967, as manifest in John Cairns, Gunther S. Stent, James D. Watson (eds.) *Phage and the Origins of Molecular Biology* (Cold Spring Harbor: CSH Press, 1967) and widely transmitted via Kendrew's contrary cheerleading in "How Molecular Biology Started," *Scientific American* 216 (1967): 141–44, and Stent's response to Kendrew in "That Was the Molecular Biology That Was," *Science* 160 (1968): 390–95. Works that have been particularly helpful in avoiding the seductive dichotomy set up by Kendrew and Stent are: Pnina G. Abir-Am, "'New' Trends in the History of Molecular Biology," *Historical Studies in the Physical Sciences* 26 (1995): 167–96; David N. Berol, "Living Materials and the Structural Ideal: The Development of the Protein Crystallography Community in the 20th Century" (Ph.D. diss., Princeton University, 2001); and Angela N. H. Creager, "The Paradox of the Phage Group," *Journal of the History of Biology* 43, no. 1 (Feb. 2010): 183–93.

Chapter 2 incorporates elements of Nicholas Rasmussen's discussion of the AEC's promotion the "physics of life" in "The Midcentury Biophysics Bubble: Hiroshima and the Biological Revolution in America, Revisited," *History of Science* 35 (1997): 245–99 in order to help explain the military's somewhat counterintuitive investment in civilian biomedical computing starting in the mid-1950s. My examination of skepticism toward computing among leading NIH researchers in the mid- and late 1950s is indebted to Thomas Haigh's discussion of the corporate world's hesitancy to adopt computers in "The Chromium-Plated Tabulator: Institutionalizing an Electronic Revolution: 1954–1958," *IEEE Annals of the History of Computing* 23,no. 4 (2001): 75–104. I caught an initial glimpse of the radical and far-reaching nature of the NIH-ACCR's plans to transform biology and medicine in Timothy Lenoir's "Shaping Biomedicine as an Information Science," *Proceedings of the 1998 Conference on the History and Heritage of Science Information Systems*, ed. Bowden et al. (Medford, NJ: Information Today, Inc., 1999).

While I was unable to engage much work of professional historians in chapters 3 and 4 because of the sheer lack of coverage of the development of the LINC or early computer use among biologists and physicians, I was able to draw from science writer M. Mitchell Waldrop's *The Dream Machine: J. C. R. Licklider and the Revolution That Made Computing Personal* (New York: Viking, 2001) to situate Clark's work in the broader context of the development of timesharing of real-time interactive computers. I also employed Bruno Strasser's analyses of Margaret Dayhoff's ironic marginalization in the sequencing community that used her *Atlas* as a central clearinghouse. Bruno J. Strasser, "Collecting, Comparing, and Computing Sequences: The Making of Margaret O. Dayhoff's *Atlas of Protein Sequence and Structure*, 1954–1965," *Journal of the History of Biology* 43, no. 4 (Dec. 2010): 623–60, and Bruno J. Strasser, "The Experimenter's Museum: GenBank, Natural History, and the Moral Economies of Biomedicine," *Isis* 102, no. 1 (Mar. 2011): 60–96.

My discussion of biomedical computing at Stanford in chapter 5 is centered around several professional studies that provided analyses of the university's postwar war development. C. Stewart Gillmor's *Fred Terman at Stanford: Building a Discipline, a University, and Silicon Valley* (Stanford: Stanford University Press, 2004) and Robert Kargon and Stuart Leslie, "Imagined Geographies: Princeton, Stanford and the Boundaries of Useful Knowledge in Postwar America," *Minerva* 32 (Summer 1994): 121, shed much light on administrators' aspirations for the school, without which the growth of computing projects there would not have occurred. The influence of the school's priorities on the study of life is elucidated by Lenoir in several unpublished or informally published essays on science at Stanford—for example, "Visions of Theory: Fashioning Molecular Biology as an Information Science" (unpublished) and "Biochemistry at Stanford: A Case Study in the Formation of an Entrepreneurial Culture" (*Lenoir Second Quarter Progress Report*, Apr. 21, 2002)—and by Eric J. Vettel, "The Protean Nature of Stanford University's Biological Sciences 1946–1972," *Historical Studies in the Physical and Biological Sciences* 35, no.1 (2004) : 95–113.

Published memoirs and recollections of early participants in biomedical computing are an integral part of my account. Cited heavily throughout the book are many of the firsthand accounts published in Bruce I. Blum and Karen Duncan (eds.), *A History of Medical Informatics: Proceedings of Association for Computing Machinery Conference on History of Medical Informatics* (New York: ACM Press, 1990). That volume gives a voice to many of the book's subjects who otherwise would be accessible only through primary sources, most importantly Lee Lusted, Charles Molnar, and Bruce Waxman. Similarly, commemorative essays in DeWitt Stetten (ed.), *NIH: An Account of Research in Its Laboratories and Clinics* (New York: Academic Press, 1984) provided a window into life at the NIH during the years in which the agency began to adopt computer technology. Severo M. Ornstein's colorful memoir, *Computing in the Middle Ages: A View from the Trenches 1955–1983* (Bloomington, IN: 1st books Library, 2002), offered a broad view of LINC's development as well as a sense of what it was like to become captivated by what the little machine stood for. Finally, Morris Collen's encyclopedic *A History of Medical Informatics in the United States* (Bethesda: American Medical Informatics Association, 1995) was by far the most comprehensive repository of information about early medical computing projects.

INDEX